Series Editor

Prof. Dr. Michael J. Parnham
PLIVA
Research Institute
Prilaz baruna Filipovica 25
10000 Zagreb
Croatia

Immunomodulatory Agents from Plants

Hildebert Wagner

Editor

Springer Basel AG

Editors

Prof. Dr. Dr. h.c. H. Wagner
Institut für pharmazeutische Biologie
Ludwig-Maximilians-Universität München
Karlstrasse 29
D-80333 München

A CIP catalogue record for this book is available from the Library of Congress, Washington D.C., USA

Deutsche Bibliothek Cataloging-in-Publication Data
Immunomodulatory agents from plants / ed. by H. Wagner - Basel ; Boston ;
Berlin : Birkhäuser, 1999
(Progress in inflammation research)
ISBN 978-3-7643-5848-8 ISBN 978-3-0348-8763-2 (eBook)
DOI 10.1007/978-3-0348-8763-2

Printed on acid-free paper produced from chlorine-free pulp. TCF ∞
Cover design: Markus Etterich, Basel
Cover illustration: With the friendly permission of Mayer & Partner GmbH, Frankf. Str. 119, D-63303 Dreieich

ISBN 978-3-7643-5848-8

9 8 7 6 5 4 3 2 1

Contents

List of contributors

Rudolf Bauer, Institute of Pharmaceutical Biology, Heinrich-Heine-Universität, Universitätsstr. 1, D-40225 Düsseldorf, Germany;
e-mail: Rudolf.Bauer@uni-duesseldorf.de

Goro Chihara, Ajinomoto Co. Ltd, 49-15 Tanacho, Aoba-ku, Yokohama 227-0064, Japan

Sharadini A. Dahanukar, Ayurveda Research Centre, Department of Pharmacology and Therapeutics, Seth GS Medical College, Parel, Mumbai 400 012, India;
e-mail: kemarc@bom3.vsnl.net.in

Tess E. De Bruyne, Department of Pharmaceutical Sciences, University of Antwerp, Universiteitsplein 1, B-2610 Antwerp, Belgium

Andreas C. Emmendörffer, Department of Immunobiology, Fraunhofer Institute for Toxicology and Aerosal Research, Hannover, Germany

Tibor Hajto, Department of Internal Medicine, University Hospital Zürich, P.O. Box 77, CH-4132 Muttenz, Switzerland

Katarina Hostanska, Department of Internal Medicine, University Hospital Zürich, P.O. Box 77, CH-4132 Muttenz, Switzerland

Yoichi Itakkura, Pharmacology and Safety Assessment Laboratory of Institute for OTC Research, Wakunaga Pharmaceutical Co., Ltd., 1624 Shimokotachi, Koda-cho, Takata-gun, Hiroshima 739-11, Japan

Ksenija Jurcic, Institute of Pharmaceutical Biology, Ludwig-Maximilians-University Munich, Karlstrasse 29, D-80333 Munich, Germany

Shigeo Kasuga, Pharmacology and Safety Assessment Laboratory of Institute for OTC Research, Wakunaga Pharmaceutical Co., Ltd., 1624 Shimokotachi, Koda-cho, Takata-gun, Hiroshima 739-11, Japan

Hiroaki Kiyohara, Oriental Medicine Research Center, The Kitasato Institute, Minato-ku, Tokyo 108-8642, Japan

Stefan Kraus, Institute of Pharmaceutical Biology, Ludwig-Maximilians-University Munich, Karlstrasse 29, D-80333 Munich, Germany

Eikai Kyo, Pharmacology and Safety Assessment Laboratory of Institute for OTC Research, Wakunaga Pharmaceutical Co., Ltd., 1624 Shimokotachi, Koda-cho, Takata-gun, Hiroshima 739-11, Japan

Marie-Aleth Lacaille-Dubois, Laboratoire de Pharmacognosie, Faculté de Pharmacie, Université de Bourgogne, 7, Bd Jeanne d'Arc, F-21033 Dijon Cedex, France

Klaus Linde, Münchener Modell – Centre for Complementary Medicine Research, Technical University/Ludwig-Maximilians-University, Kaiserstr. 9, D-80801 Munich, Germany; e-mail: Muenchener.Modell@lrz.uni-muenchen.de

Chang-Xiao Liu, Tianjin Institute of Pharmaceutical Research, State Pharmaceutical Administration of China, 308 An-Shan West Road, Tianjin, 300193, P.R. China; Fax: 86-22-27381305; e-mail: Lcx@publicitpt.tj.cn

Marie-Luise Lohmann-Matthes, Department of Immunobiology, Fraunhofer Institute for Toxicology and Aerosal Research, Hannover, Germany

Yukiko Y. Maeda, Department of Laboratory Animal Science, The Tokyo Metropolitan Institute of Medical Science, 3-18-22 Honkomagome, Bunkyo-ku, Tokyo 113-8613, Japan; e-mail: maeda@rinshoken.or.jp

Dieter Melchart, Münchener Modell – Centre for Complementary Medicine Research, Technical University/Ludwig-Maximilians-University, Kaiserstr. 9, D-80801 Munich, Germany; e-mail: Muenchener.Modell@lrz.uni-muenchen.de

Michael J. Parnham, Institute of Pharmacology for the Natural Sciences, Goethe University Frankfurt, D-60439 Frankfurt am Main, Germany
Present address: PLIVA d.d., Research Institute, Prilaz baruna Filipovića 25, HR-10000 Zagreb, Croatia; e-mail: plivaii@zg.tel.hr

Luc A.C. Pieters, Department of Pharmaceutical Sciences, University of Antwerp, Universiteitsplein 1, B-2610 Antwerp, Belgium

Nirmala N. Rege, Ayurveda Research Centre, Department of Pharmacology and Therapeutics, Seth GS Medical College, Parel, Mumbai 400 012, India

Rainer Samtleben, Institute of Pharmaceutical Biology, Ludwig-Maximilians-Universität Munich, Karlstr. 29, D-80333 Munich, Germany

Hiromichi Sumiyoshi, OTC Development Department, Wakunaga Pharmaceutical Co., Ltd., 1624 Shimokotachi, Koda-cho, Takata-gun, Hiroshima 739-11, Japan

Urmila M. Thatte, Ayurveda Research Centre, Department of Pharmacology and Therapeutics, Seth GS Medical College, Parel, Mumbai 400 012, India

Naoto Uda, Pharmacology and Safety Assessment Laboratory of Institute for OTC Research, Wakunaga Pharmaceutical Co., Ltd., 1624 Shimokotachi, Koda-cho, Takata-gun, Hiroshima 739-11, Japan

Arnold J. Vlietinck, Department of Pharmaceutical Sciences, University of Antwerp, Universiteitsplein 1, B-2610 Antwerp, Belgium; e-mail: vlietinck@uia.ua.ac.be

Hildebert Wagner, Institute of Pharmaceutical Biology, Ludwig-Maximilians-University Munich, Karlstrasse 29, D-80333 Munich Germany;
e-mail: H.Wagner@lrz.uni-muenchen.de

Pei-Gen Xiao, Institute of Medicinal Plant Development, Chinese Academy of Medical Sciences, Beijing, 100094, P. R. China; e-mail: xiaopg@public.bta.net.cn

Haruki Yamada, Oriental Medicine Research Center, The Kitasato Institute, Minato-ku, Tokyo 108-8642, Japan; e-mail: yamada-h@kitasato.or.jp

Preface

The human immune system, despite having its own sophisticated defence mechanisms, is inferior to bacteria and viruses with respect to adaptability. Furthermore, our immune system is increasingly exposed to detrimental effects, that is immunosuppressive environmental consequences, unhealthy living, and chronic illnesses. Excessive chemotherapy threatens our immune system even further. This situation demands compensatory prophylactic therapeutic regimes. One of these – specific immunostimulation – is more difficult to achieve than the immunosuppression currently used in transplantation surgery and the medical treatment of autoimmune diseases.

The earliest attempts to develop suitable medication for immunostimulation were based on traditional remedies which embodied the accumulated experience of several centuries. Medicinal plants are already being used prophylactically as standardized and efficacy-optimized preparations for the treatment of various recurrent infections, or in combination with chemotherapeutics in standard medical practice.

In order to rationally apply immunostimulants of plant origin, however, it is necessary to search for the active principles of these substances and to produce them in a pure form. Because suitable screening methods have become available only recently, research in this field is in its very beginning. Further progress can be expected from systematic basic research on the mechanisms underlying immunomodulation. This also applies to verification of clinical efficacy, which is a prerequisite for the acceptance of medications with purported immunostimulatory properties.

This book attempts to provide a synopsis of the most important research results to date in the field of immunomodulators of plant origin. It is also intended to offer suggestions and to provide a scientific basis for further research, which has become ever more urgent since recombinant cytokines have yet to fulfill their promise as effective immunotherapeutic agents.

München (Germany), July 1998 H. Wagner

Search for potent immunostimulating agents from plants and other natural sources

Hildebert Wagner, Stefan Kraus and Ksenija Jurcic

Institute of Pharmaceutical Biology, University of Munich, Karlstrasse 29, D-80333 Munich, Germany

What are immunostimulants?

Immunostimulants [1, 2] or immunopotentiators are drugs leading predominantly to a non-specific stimulation of immunological defence mechanisms. Most of them are not real antigens but antigenomimetics or so-called mitogens. Non-specific and non-antigen dependent stimulants do not affect immunological memory cells and, since their pharmacological efficacy fades comparatively quickly, they have to be administered either in intervals or continuously. Some immunostimulants may also stimulate T-suppressor cells and thereby reduce immune resistance, hence the term immunomodulation or immunoregulation, denoting any effect on, or change of, immune responsiveness is also very often used.

Immunostimulants can be applied either orally or intravenously. The effects generated depend on the dosage, time and mode of administration as well as on the immune status of the patient. In this book only drugs which activate the unspecific immune system are described.

Different from immunostimulants are the immunoadjuvants (i.e. complete or incomplete Freund's adjuvants) which are added to antigenes (vaccines) and hereby increase the production of antibodies without acting as antigens themselves (see Lacaille-Dubois, this volume).

Why do we need immunostimulants?

The human body is continuously exposed to a series of stress factors [1, 2], which more or less weaken the function of the immune system and hereby generate immunosuppression. Immunosuppression can be generated by severe bacterial and viral infections, cancer, environmental agents such as pesticides or allergens, excessive long term chemo- or radiotherapy, malnutrition, psychic stress, or endogenic autoimmune reactions. There exists a dramatic increase in microorganisms resistant to antibiotics and chemotherapeutic agents, new plagues (e.g. AIDS) have emerged, and many old ones such as tuberculosis have returned. The application of recombi-

Immunomodulatory Agents from Plants, edited by H. Wagner

nant cytokines is limited and has not fulfilled the expected hopes of the nineties. We have no effective vaccines against some severe infections or parasitic diseases, and many chronic diseases are the consequence of an unbalanced or impaired immune system. Among them, the recurrent opportunistic infections, skin and intestine inflammations are the most important ones, and we should realize that the incidence of some severe infections such as AIDS might be positively influenced by a restoration of the chronically suppressed immune system.

What do we expect from immunostimulants?

Non-specific immunostimulation [1, 2] might be useful and very effective when the immune system of the host is impaired. Therefore, it can be indicated to counteract immunosuppressions or an ineffectively working immune system, which might be the consequence of excessively applied chemotherapy or long term treatment with immunosuppressive drugs. In these cases immunostimulants can be applied adjuvant to a conventional chemotherapy. According to Drews [3], immunostimulants are an attractive alternative to conventional chemotherapy when mixed infections, infectious hospitalism, chronic infectious diseases, persistent infections and their immunopathogenic sequels, or chemotherapy resistent bacterial and viral infections have to be treated.

Another field of application is the prophylaxis of opportunistic infections in patients. Here, due to a lack of suitable medication, the prophylaxis of viral infections in particular plays a significant role.

In the treatment of cancer, immunostimulants might be effective for the prophylaxis of metastases after removal of the primary tumor.

Whereas herbal medicines with immunostimulatory potential are only appropriate for the prophylaxis and therapy of moderate infections of the respiratory organs, such as the infectious bronchitis or recurrent infections of the urogenital system, for the treatment of severe bacterial and viral infections only chemically-defined constituents have a rationale.

Whereas for oral application plant extracts are the appropriate form, for parenteral use only isolated, pure compounds are the adequate drugs.

Since immunostimulants are often administered over a longer period of time, it must be guaranteed that they are safe and do not generate any severe adverse effects (i.e. allergies, anaphylactic shock).

Immunostimulatory drugs available today

Of the old shock therapies [1, 2, 4] ("Reizkörpertherapie") or the injection of the body's own blood or milk proteins (autologous or heterologous proteins) and s.c. terpentine- or crotonoil-injection, only the "Baunscheidt's method" has been retained. This old method aims at the restoration of an impaired immune system in cases of chronic inflammations. All other preparations have been abandoned due to uncertain, unforeseeable, often also severe side effects. Suspensions of attenuated microorganisms such as *Escherichia coli*, *Myobacterium tuberculosis*, *Corynebacterium parvum* or *Plasmodium malariae* have been used primarily for the treatment of cancer. Today, the BCG vaccine from *Bacillus Calmette Guérin* is the only bacterial preparation that is still on the market being used in the therapy of prostate bladder cancer. As adjuvants, complete or incomplete Freund's adjuvant with certain minerals and plant oils with or without added mycobacteria have been applied [5]. At present, aluminium hydroxide and a saponin from *Quillaja saponaria* (QS 21) [6] (see Lacaille-Dubois, this volume) are the only compounds added to vaccine preparations. In Germany and other countries of Europe a great variety of plant extracts such as those from *Echinacea purpurea*, *Thuja occidentalis* and *Baptisia tinctoria* have been registered as extracts mainly for oral prophylaxis and therapy of bacterial and viral infections of the respiratory organs and the urogenital system. Since only some of these preparations are chemically or biologically standardized, they are not appropriate for rational medication. Among the pure constituents isolated from plants or other sources, for which an immunostimulatory activity has been claimed, the glucan Lentinan from *Lentinus edodes* is used in Japan in combination with mitomycin and 5-fluoruracil for i.v. therapy of various cancer species (see Maeda and Chihara, this volume). An arabinogalactan produced from a tissue culture of *Echinacea purpurea* is also undergoing clinical trials (see Emmendörffer et al., this volume). Recently, one major immune stimulatory compound of mistletoe, the recombinant galactose-specific ML-lectin I, was made available as the first plant constituent produced using gene technology to be applied for clinical studies in cancer therapy (see Samtleben et al., this volume).

In this context the recombinant human cytokines and colony stimulating factors such as interferones, interleukines 1 and 2 and granulocyte-colony stimulating factor (G-CSF) and granulocyte-monocyte-colony stimulating factor (GM-CSF) have to be mentioned. The application of these substances, which are used mainly for the restoration of the immune system as well as for its activation, will not be discussed here, since they do not fit into the scope and aim of this book. Apart from that, it has to be stated that the success obtained with the body`s own immune regulators are not yet very convincing and one must underline the necessity to search for new immunostimulants from other sources.

Screening methods for the detection of immunostimulating compounds

The results of more than 15 years of screening experience in the author's laboratory has shown that the best short cut to finding *in vivo* effective immunostimulants are investigations using experimental animals and infectious stress or immunosup-

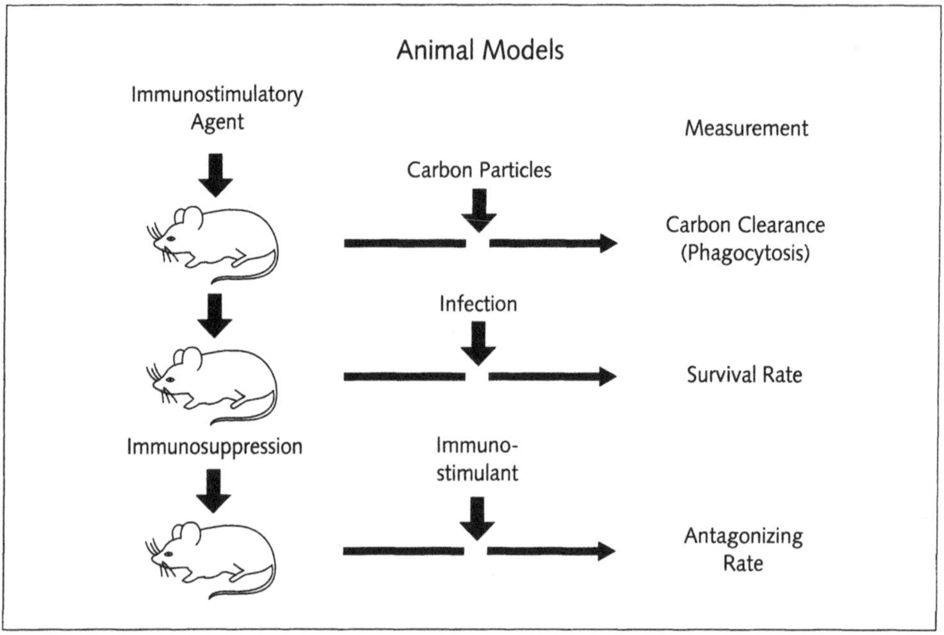

Figure 1
Animal models for screening immunostimulants.

pression models. They indicate whether or not, and to what extent, an agent is able to antagonize a severe or lethal infection and through this prove the protective or therapeutic potential of a drug. The immunosuppression models reveal to what extent a drug under test can restore the partly impaired immune system (Fig. 1).

For mass screening, however, the various *in vitro* bioassays are the most adequate methods, since they provide at the same time hints on the possible mechanism of action of a drug. Since the results obtained *in vitro* must not necessarily have a correlation *in vivo*, it is necessary to confirm them by *in vivo* experiments. *Vice versa* it is possible that positive *in vivo* results cannot be substantiated in any *in vitro* assay. This can happen when several cooperating cells or mediator systems not present in an *in vitro* cell system are responsible for the *in vivo* effect.

In general, it is necessary to carry out several *in vitro* assays since there is no immunological master or key cell system which regulates and governs all various immune pathways.

Immunological *in vitro* and *in vivo* assays

The most important *in vitro* test systems among the immunological assays available at present (see [7, 8] and also Emmendörffer et al., Pieters et al. and Yamada and

Kiyohara, this volume) are those that allow us to determine the functional state and efficiency of the mononuclear phagocyte system (Figs. 2 and 3). Ranked second are tests that measure the influence of compounds on the complement and on T-lymphocyte populations.

Phagocytosis is the uptake and programmed elimination of microorganisms or other particles by phagocytes. Phagocytes are derived from white cells in the blood stream and are called polymorphonuclear granulocytes (leukocytes) (PMNL ≅ 70% of the white blood cells) and mononuclear cells (≅ 30% of the white blood cells). The latter are composed of 25% lymphocytes and 5% monocytes/macrophages. In addition, there are bone marrow macrophages, peritoneal macrophages, Langerhanns cells (skin macrophages) and Kupfer cells in the liver. PMN can only phagocytize particles that are opsonized by antibodies plus complement, whereas macrophages can endocytize without opsonins or with complement as the only opsonin (alternative pathway). The main product involved in the killing of microorganisms by PMNL or macrophages are reactive oxygen species which can be estimated by the chemiluminescence assay. For the *in vitro* phagocytosis and chemiluminescence assays, human granulocyte fractions are isolated by Ficoll density centrifugation from heparinized blood. Bone marrow macrophages can be obtained from seven day old C57 BL/6 bone marrow-cell cultures (mice femurs), and peritoneal macrophages from mice pretreated i.p. with thioglycolate or starch injections.

Microscopy smear test according to Brandt ([9], modified in [7])

The granulocyte fraction is separated, purified, and adjusted to a certain cell density (3×10^6 cells/ml), and incubated for 30 min with 9.25×10^6 baker's yeast cells, the substance to be analyzed and pool serum for opsonization. The phagocytosis is terminated with 0.2 M EDTA and the suspension distributed on microscope slides and dried. The smear is stained according to Pappenheim, and the phagocytosis index (PI) (mean number of ingested yeast cells in 100 granulocytes) determined by counting under the microscope. Cell viability is measured by trypan blue dye exclusion. This test can also be performed with macrophages or monocytes.

Stimulation is calculated, using the following equation:

$$\text{stimulation}^{1}\ (\%) = \frac{(PI_{test} - PI_{control}) \times 100}{PI_{control}}$$

1 or suppression

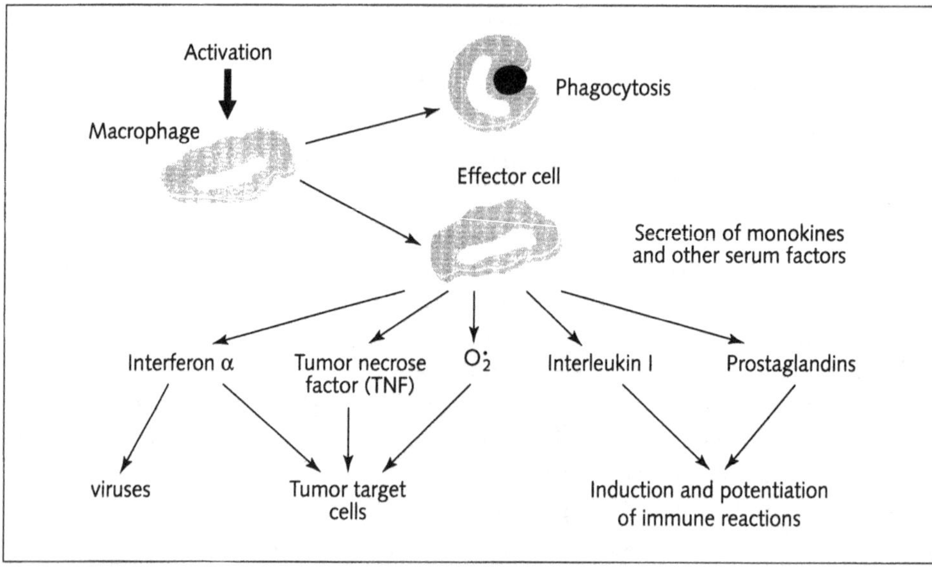

Figure 2
Mechanism of non-specific stimulation of monocytes (macrophages).

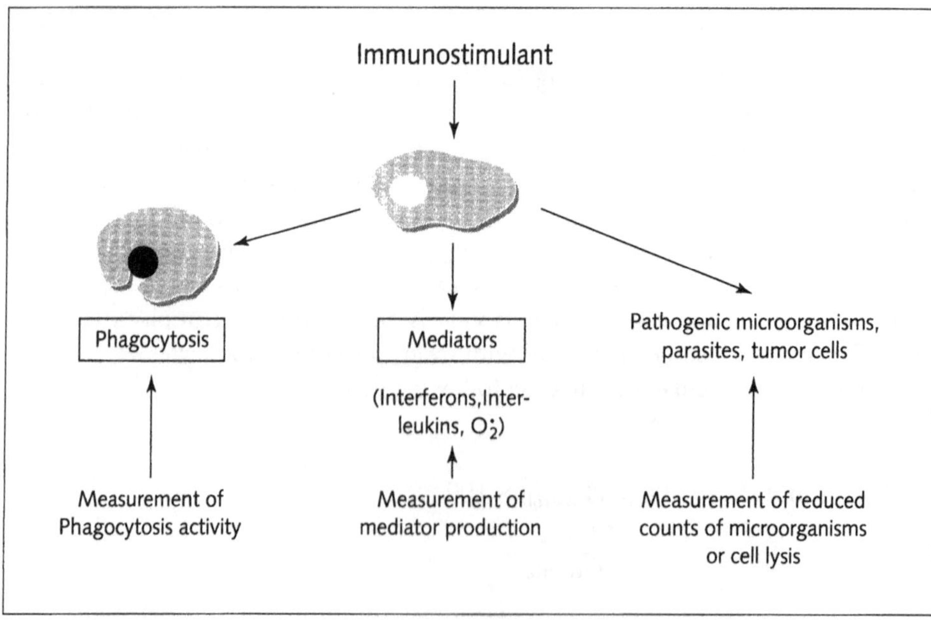

Figure 3
In vitro *test models for screening immunostimulants.*

Flow cytometric assay according to Wagner and Jurcic [10]
The test is a whole blood assay and uses fluorescence-labelled latex particles which are added to the heparinized whole blood sample. The PMN phagocytize the opsonised latex particles and the PMNL, having ingested fluorescent beads, are separated in a cell sorter and the size and fluorescence of the PMNL are determined. The mean fluorescence is equal to the number of latex particles ingested per cell. The phagocytosis index and percentage are calculated from the proportion of cells which underwent phagocytosis and that of the control.

Chemiluminescence assay [11,12]
Here the quantity of oxygen radicals produced during granulocyte or macrophage phagocytosis is measured using luminol or lucigenin which are excited to chemiluminescence by the oxygen radicals $O_2^{\cdot}$, $O^{\cdot}H$ and $^1O_2$. Zymosan, a mixture of polysaccharides obtained from yeast by cell wall disruption, PAF (platelet aggregation factor), TPA (tripalmitoylphorbol acetate), or calcium ionophore can be used as challengers. The oxygen production of a granulocyte macrophage suspension of known cell density is measured in a 6-channel Biolumat over a period of 1–2 h, by measuring photons with a photomultiplier (cpm).

Note:
- although the measured formation of oxygen radicals may correlate with the degree of increased phagocytosis, the two processes are different and not necessarily interdependent.
- The chemiluminescence test can also be performed routinely with monocytes or liver Kupffer cells.

In vivo *phagocytosis assay (carbon clearance test [13])*
The test substance is administered i.p. or p.o. to mice. After 24 h, each mouse receives an intravenous injection of Indian Ink (colloidal carbon particle, Schwarz Nr. 591017, Rotringwerke, Riepe KG, Hamburg) in 0.3 ml dispersion per 30 g body weight. Blood samples are taken from the retro-orbital venous plexus at intervals of 3, 6, 9 , 12 and 15 min after the i.v. injection. The "carbon clearance", i.e. the rate of elimination of carbon from the blood, is determined by turbidimetric spectrophotometry at 650 nm. Density reading, plotted against time on a logarithmic scale, give the regression lines. The stimulation rate is obtained as the ratio of the mean regression coefficient of the substance (Rc_{tr}) to the regression coefficient of the control (Rc_c). In the presence of immunostimulants, the coefficients vary between 0 and 3.0. Values of 0–1.2 are devoid of activity, values of 1.3–1.5 are registered as moderately active, and those > 1.5 as highly active. The highest clearance values observed in our screening program were around 3.0.

In vitro *complement assay [14, 15]*

The complement system belongs to the non-specific humoral defence system. It plays an important part in antigen processing and is involved in the defence against viruses and tumors. Activation of complement leads to increased destruction and lysis of cells that possess a lipoprotein membrane, i.e. bacteria, viruses, and tumor cells. Conversely, complement is partly responsible for some inflammatory processes that occur in a state of hyper-reactivity and is able to eliminate immune aggregates. The complement system can be subdivided into the classical and alternative activation pathway. The classical pathway is dependent on antibodies (IgM and IgG), whereas the alternative pathway can be activated by microorganisms on their own or in combination with IgA antibodies.

Interference of drugs with the complement system can be studied *in vitro* where the lysis of foreign erythrocytes and the released hemoglobin, estimated photometrically, is taken as the parameter. Measurement of hemolytic complement activity can be used for the classical (CP) as well as for the alternative (AP) complement pathways.

The classical pathway hemolysis (CPH_{50}) test is performed with rabbit antibodies, sensitized sheep erythrocytes, and guinea pig complement, in a buffer system containing Ca^{2+} and Mg^{2+}. The alternative pathway hemolysis (APH_{50}) test uses rabbit erythrocytes with human pool serum as the source of complement and Mg^{2+}-EGTA buffer. After incubation at 37° C, the degree of hemolysis in the supernatant is determined spectrophotometrically at 412 nm.

Comment:

- A decrease in lysis may result from either activation or inhibition of the complement system. Activated components are consumed and therefore removed so that the effect on the total system resembles that of inhibition. The exact mechanism of action can only be elucidated by specific reactions with the individual complement components.
- In plant extracts high amounts of chlorophyll or tannins can interfere with the assay and lead to false positive reactions.

Lymphocyte-assays

Lymphocytes (B and T lymphocytes with their subpopulations C-4, C-8) belong to the cellular immune system. They play an important role in practically all defence mechanisms and can be activated directly by antigens and mitogens, or indirectly by cytokines or substances released from macrophages.

Method I

Lymphocyte proliferation assay according to a modified method of Wagner and Jurcic [7]

This test can be performed with the total peripheral blood lymphocyte population or with individual lymphocyte subpopulations (B lymphocytes, T_4 and T_8 lymphocytes) isolated from the total human lymphocyte fraction by monoclonal antibody separation. The rate of lymphocyte proliferation under influence of mitogens is measured through determination of the rate of incorporation of ^{3}H-thymidine into the DNA of the lymphocytes.

The lymphocyte fraction is separated from heparinized blood by Ficoll gradient centrifugation and the lymphocytes adjusted to a cell density of 10^5 cells/ml. For prestimulation of the lymphocytes, phytohemagglutinin (PHA-M) or concanavalin A are used as mitogens. The prestimulated lymphocytes together with the substance to be tested are transferred to microtitre plates and incubated for 70 or 80 h. ^{3}H-thymidine is added and the incubation continued for a further 18 h. The quantity of ^{3}H-thymidine incorporated is determined by scintillation counting (cpm). Percent stimulation is taken as the difference between the incorporated ^{3}H-thymidine of the test and control incubations, multiplied by 100, and divided by the control value.

As reference compounds, certain lectins, phorbol esters or endoxins can be used. Note that prestimulation is not always necessary, some compounds can stimulate lymphocytes directly, without presensitization.

Method II

CD69 antigen expression-test [16]

The CD69 antigen is one of the earliest cell markers expressed on all activated T-, B-, and NK-lymphocytes, which can be stimulated by a variety of mitogenic agents. The stimulus used can influence the distribution of CD69 expression on lymphocyte subsets. These properties suggest that CD69 represents a generic marker for lymphocyte activation and is well suited for rapid analysis of discrete subsets of responding cells. The assay utilizes fluorescence triggering on CD3-positive lymphocytes in the F13 channel and subsequent two-color analysis of the activation marker CD69 PE versus the subpopulation markers such as CD4 FITC or CD8 FITC. T-cell activation is measured as a function of the percentage of T-cell subsets (F11) that express CD69 (F12).

Immune-induced cytotoxicity assay [17, 18]

Macrophages can be transformed into effector cells by induction, and thus stimulated to release cytotoxic effector substances. One of the most important effector is the membrane-bound tumor necrosis factor (TNFα) which necrotizes or lyses tumor cells. There are several modifications of these tests. In principle, they vary according to whether the tumor cells (i.e. WEHI 164 fibrosarcoma tumor cells) are labeled with ^{51}Cr or ^{3}H-thymidine.

Adherent, thioglycolate-induced, starch-induced peritoneal mouse or bone marrow macrophages are incubated for 24 h with the substance to be investigated. The supernatant of the culture is then discarded, the macrophages washed, and coincubated with the ^{51}Cr labeled tumor cells for 24 h.

The supernatants and the sediments are separated and the radioactivity of both fractions measured in a γ-counter. The specific ^{51}Cr release is taken as the difference of the ^{51}Cr release between target cells cultured in the presence and absence of control or activated macrophages.

Cytokine (e.g. IL-1, IL-2, IFN-β_2, TNFα) induction assays [18, 19]

Cytokines, released by various immunocompetent cells after activation, play a great role in the regulation and potentiation of non-specific and specific immune reactions. The cytokine induction tests can be performed with macrophages or thymocytes, measuring the concentration of released cytokines in the supernatant by specific antibodies or by ^3H-thymidine incorporation in replicating cells.

Infectious stress assays with mice [20]

These experiments aim at evaluating any claimed immunostimulating agent for its protective potential and therapeutic effect against a systemic lethal infection (see also Fig. 1).

The immunostimulants are injected i.v. in mice (day 1) followed by i.v. injection of the pathogenic microorganism (i.e. *Candida albicans* or *Listeria monocytogenes*) after 24 h (day 0). A second injection of the same dose of immunostimulant is administered on day 1. The protective effect can be measured as follows:

(1) registration of the survival or death rate after a certain time,
(2) current estimation of blood parameters (counts of leukocytes, T- and B-lymphocytes etc.) in infected and pretreated mice,
(3) 24 or 48 h after infection the spleen, liver or kidneys of mice are removed, homogenized, aliquoted amounts transferred to agar plates, and the number of CFU (colony forming units) measured.

Note:

- *Listeria monocytogenes* infections are mainly macrophage dependent, whereas, in a *Candida albicans* infection, granulocytes play the major role.
- The experiments can be carried out with immunocompromized mice, which are pretreated with cyclosporin A, cyclophosphamide or radiation i.e. which have a suppressed T-lymphocyte system. In these cases it might be necessary to reduce the number of pathogenic microorganisms to be injected by a factor of 50 or 100.

Selection of plants and isolated compounds for screening

In old literature on traditional medicine or ethnopharmacology the term immunostimulant cannot be found. Hence, other criteria have to be used for selection.

It can be assumed, however, that plants of traditional medicine, which have been, and still are, used as teas and were recommended for their antibacterial, antiviral, antifungal or antitumoral activities, might be suitable candidates for screening. Moreover, it can be suggested that the beneficial effects of cancer drugs or anti-infection agents, because of the relatively low quantities of pharmacologically active principles applied of those plants, might be caused by an immune-induced activity rather than by a direct antitumoral activity. This observation is underlined by recently performed immunological *in vitro* studies which showed that numerous classical cytotoxic drugs such as vincristine, methotrexate, taxol, or podophyllotoxin can be converted into immunostimulants when applied in very low concentrations [21]. This finding is consistent with the observation that substances, which in former times were used for so called "shock therapy", and are characterized as irritants or inflammatory agents such as phorbol esters (croton oil), pungent agents, saponins, mustard oils or sesquiterpenlactones, can exert a marked immunostimulatory activity. In our last screening studies besides some bitter-tasting substances, diacylglycerol derivatives and protein- or tyrosine kinase C-inhibitors have also been found to be potent immunostimulants [22].

Screening results

Raw drugs or drug extracts

From a databank obtained from NAPRALERT[2] and Phytodoc[3] in 1997 we obtained over 200 citations on plant extracts or fractions and more than 30 citations on isolated natural products, which describe immunostimulatory potential. In the following paragraph the most intensively studied plants and plant constituents are listed and their immunological potential described.

Of around 130 plant crude drugs investigated, ca. 90% belong to the higher plants and ca. 10% to the class of mushrooms, fungi, algae and lichens. From more

2 NAPRALERT database copyrighted from 1975 to date by the Board of Trustees. The University of Illinois, maintained by the Program of Collaborative Research in the Pharmaceutical Sciences, within the Department of Medicinal Chemistry and Pharmacognosy in the College of Pharmacy of the University of Illinois at Chicago, 833 South Wood Street (m/c 877), Chicago, IL 60612. N.R. Farnsworth, Director and Editor in Chief. Information: http://pcog8.pmmp.uic.edu/mcp/or: http://info.cas.org/ONLINE/DBSS/napralertss.html. Fax: 001-312-413-5968.

3 Phytodoc, Dr. H. Schmidt, Geigenbergerstr. 11, D-81477 München (Solln), Germany.

Table 1 - Plant extracts and fractions which have been immunologically studied

Acanthopanax senticosus	*Cnidium officinale*
(Eleutherococcus senticosus)	*Coffea arabica*
Achyranthes bidentata	*Combretum micranthum*
Achyrocline satureoides	*Cordyceps sinensis*
Aconitum carmichaelli, A. napellus	*Coriolus versicolor*
Actinidia arguta	*Croton tiglium*
Aeginetia indica	*Curcuma longa*
Albizzia julibrissin	*Daucus carota*
Aloe vera	*Echinacea angustifolia,*
Alsophila spinulosa	*E. pallida, E. purpurea*
Angelica acutiloba, A. sinensis	*Echinosphora koreensis*
Anthurium wagnerianum	*Epimedium alpinum*
Aralia mandshurica	*Eupatorium cannabinum*
Aristolochia clematitis	*Euphorbia hirta*
Arnica montana	*Fagopyrum cymosum*
Artemisia capillaris, A. iwayomogi	*Forsythia koreana*
Asarum europaeum	*Galax aphylla*
Astragalus membranaceus	*Ganoderma lucidum*
Astragalus onobrychis	*Geranium macrorrhizum*
Atractylodes japonica, A. lancea	*G. sanguineum*
A. macrocephala	*Glycine maxima*
Avena sativa	*Glycyrrhiza glabra*
Azadirachta indica	*Grifola frondosa*
Baptisia tinctoria	*Guatteria spruceana*
Benincasa cerifera	*Gymnema sylvestre,*
Bryonia dioica	*G. pentaphyllum*
Bupleurum chinense	*Hedysarum polybotrys*
Caesalpinia sappan	*Herpestis monniera*
Calendula officinalis	*Houstonia purpurea*
Camellia sinensis	*Jacaranda rhombifolia*
Carthamus tinctorius	*Janaica arayalpathra*
Caulophyllum thalictroides	*Laetipurus sulphureus*
Cetraria islandica	*Morus alba*
Chelidonium majus	*Nectandra globosa,*
Chlorella prenoidosa	*N. trucillensis*
Choerospondias acillaris	*Nicotiana tabacum*
Cimicifuga simplex	*Nocardia rubra*
Cinnamomium cassia	*Nyctanthes arbor-tristis*
Cistanche salsa	*Ocimum sanctum*

Table 1 (continued)

Ophiopogon japonicus	*Rynchosia phaseoloides*
Paeonia albiflora	*Rudbeckia bicolor*
Panax Ginseng	*Saccharum officinale*
Petivera alliacea	*Sapium sebiferum*
Phellinus linteus	*Schisandra chinensis*
Phellodendron amurense	*Serenoa repens*
Picrorhiza kurroa	*Selenostemma argel*
Pinellia ternata	*Sophora subprostata*
Pinus armandii,	*Spirulina platensis*
Pinus caribaea	*Tabebuia barbata*
P. sylvestris, P. taeda,	*Taraxacum platycarpum*
P. strobilius	*Tinospora cordifolia*
Polygala tenuifolia	*Tremellia fuciformis*
Polyporus umbellata	*Trichosanthes kirilowii*
Polystictus versicolor	*Tripterygium wilfordii*
Poria cocos	*Ulva lactuca*
Porphyra tenora	*Viscum album*
Potentilla tormentilla	*Uncaria tomentosa*
Pseudostellaria heterophylla	*Zea mays*
Quillaja saponaria	*Zingiber officinale*
Rehmannia glutinosa	*Ziziphus jujuba*

than 70% of the plants the ethanol and water extracts (decoction) or the powdered drugs were investigated. From the remaining ca. 30%, more or less chemically-defined fractions, i.e. polysaccharides, glycoproteins, saponins, lignans, flavonoids or alcaloid enriched fractions were administered to animals. The dosages applied and the parameters measured vary so widely that no conclusion can be drawn or comparison can be made between the immunological potential of the various plants. In Table 1 the immunologically investigated plants are listed.

The intragastrically or orally administered crude drug powder (decoction or extract) ranges from 100 mg to some grams with a dominance of 100 to 200 mg/kg mouse, rat or guinea pig. The i.p. or s.c. dosages applied were dependent on the manner of the extraction procedure or the enriched state of a fraction respectively. The most used dosages for this form of administration were in the range of 10–11 mg/kg. As far as the experimental animal models are concerned, the phagocytosis clearance model, with carbon particles or bacteria as challenges, was one of the most used models. In second place were the infectious stress or immunosuppression models. All experiments resulted in an increase in the number of immunocompetent cells such as polymorphonuclear leukocytes, macrophages, NK cells, T and B cells and/or an enhancement of cytokine liberation (interferons, interleukines) as well as the liberation of antibodies. In a few experimental animal infection models, some plant preparations were found to protect animals to some extent against bacterial and viral infections (i.e. *Listeria*, *Candida* or *Herpes*). Some clinical studies were also carried out with humans (cancer patients, debilitated children with hypoimmunity, adults with chronic, recurrent infections of the air ways, influenza, *Candida* mycosis etc.), however, with the exception of phytopreparations from *Echinacea* spec., *Viscum album* (mistletoe), and some Chinese drug preparations, no double blind studies or placebo-controlled studies have been carried out in accordance with good clinical practice (GCP) requirements.

Results obtained with the many drug prescriptions of traditional Chinese medicine are also lacking therapeutic relevance (see also Xiao and Liu, this volume).

From the following plant drugs, detailed results on the *in vitro* and *in vivo* immunological effects can be found in other chapters of this book: *Echinacea* spec. (see Emmendörffer et al.), *Viscum album* (see Samtleben et al.), *Lentinus edodes* (see Maeda and Chihara), *Tinospora cordifolia* (see Dahanukar et al.), *Eleutherococcus sent.*, *Ganoderma lucidum*, *Panax Ginseng* and *Glyzyrrhiza glabra* and other Chinese drugs (see Xiao and Liu).

Isolated compounds of low molecular weight

The low molecular weight compounds claimed to act as immunostimulants (see Tab. 2) and reported in the literature up to 1985 have been investigated only for their general enhancing effects on the unspecific and specific immune parameters. Due to lack of available specific immunological assays, the value of the immunological results is questionable and has to be confirmed by novel detailed investigations. The corresponding references can be found in review articles written by Wagner and Probst [1] and Lindquist and Teuscher [3].

Although no clear structure activity relationships in the class of naturally occurring immunostimulants can be seen so far, in the following classes of compounds a relatively high percentage of effective immunostimulants have been found. It is remarkable that among the high molecular weight compounds, polysaccharides of various structures are predominant (Tab. 3).

One of the first compounds found to exert immunostimulating activity was the N-containing aristolochic acid (**1**). The compound exhibited a pronounced enhancement of phagocytosis of leukocytes and peritoneal macrophages [24, 25]. Exploiting the immunocytoadherence phenomenon, Sieving and Müller [26] demonstrated that aristolochic acid was capable of preventing a reduction of rosette numbers induced by prednisolone (5 mg/kg) in rats. Prednisolone appeared to be equally

Table 2 - Low molecular weight compounds with claimed immunomodulatory activity

Aristolochic acid (3,4-methylendioxy-8-methoxy-10-nitrophenanthren carboxylic acid)	*Aristolochia clematitis*
Cepharanthine (biscoclaurin alcaloid)	*Stephania cepharantha* and *S. susaka*
Emetine	*Uragoga ipecacuanha*
Colchicine, Demecolcine*	*Colchicum autumnale*
Helenalin, tenulin, eupaphyssopin (sesquiterpenlactones)	*Arnica/Eupatorium* spp.
Zexbrevins A + B (sesquiterpenlactones)	*Zexmenia brevifolia*
Diketocoriolin B (sesquiterpenoid)	*Coriolus consors*
Alantolactone* (sesquiterpenlactone)	*Inula helenium*
Withanolide* (Steroidlactone)	*Withania somniferum, Solanum dulcamara, S. nigrum*
Cleistanthin (lignan derivative)	*Cleistanthus collinus*
Curculigoside (alkylglucoside)	*Curculigo orchioides*
Urushiol (alkylcatecholes)	*Toxicodendron* spp.
Gossypol	*Gossypium marsupium*
Ubiquinones Q_7 + Q_8	Various sources of plant and animal origin
Furanocumarins	*Psoralea*-spp.
Tetrahydrocannabinol*) (THC)	*Cannabis sativa*
Lysolecithin	Various sources of plant and animal origin and synthetic analogs
Trichothecium-mycotoxins*	*Fusarium*- and *Trichothecium* spp.

* *According to the reported protocols only immunosuppressive activities could be registered. This does not exclude, however, that the same compounds also exert immunostimulating activities when applied in much lower concentrations [21].*

Table 3 - Classes of compounds in which immunostimulants have been found

Low molecular weight compounds	**High molecular weight compounds**
alkylamides	proteins (lectins)
phenolic compounds	peptides
alcaloids	polysaccharides
quinones	glycolipids (lectins)
saponins	
sesquiterpenes, di- and triterpenoids	

effective as aristolochic acid at 0.005 mg/kg body weight. The biological activity was interpreted as being the result of competitive inhibition of lymphocyte surface receptors. Lemperle [27] could show that the reduction of phagocytosis induced by chloramphenicol and tetracycline could be compensated by simultaneous administration of aristolochic acid. In a double blind study, 0.9 mg/day administered orally over 21 days, showed a significant enhancement of phagocytosis with a maximum on the 6th/8th day [28]. Aristolochic acid has been suspected of being carcinogenic, in experiments performed with mice. It could be shown that mice treated with 0.1–10 mg/kg/day for three months developed gastric tumors (Fig. 4).

Another alcaloid, the biscoclaurine alkaloid cepharanthine (**2**) from *Stephania cepharantha* and *S. susaki* was reported to stimulate the production of antibodies in animal experiments and to exert a protective effect on the suppression of hematopoesis induced by cytostatic agents [29]. Emetine and some oxindol alcaloids from the Peruvian plant *Uncaria tomentosa* (e.g. isopteropodine) increased *in vitro* granulocyte-phagocytosis at a concentration of 1–10 ng/ml [30]. Vincristine was found to increase antibody production in mice after prestimulation with antigens in a dosis of 5–30 µg/100g body weight [31]. Camptothecine induced interferon at a concentration of 100 µg [32]. The observation that classical cytostatic compounds can also exert immunostimulating activity has prompted us to investigate other cytostatic compounds more closely for their immunostimulating potential [21]. Vincristine (**3**), Podophyllotoxin, Taxol and Staurosporine, exerted immunosuppressive or cytotoxic effects when used at high doses and exhibited immunostimulatory properties at very low doses as measured by *in vitro* granulocyte/macrophage phagocytosis and lymphocyte proliferation assays [21–33] (Fig. 5).

The same or similar dose-dependent reversal effects on human granulocytes and T lymphocytes were also observed with naturally occurring naphthoquinones (e.g. plumbagin, lapachone, chimaphilin, alkannin and shikonin) [21]. The stimulating *in vitro* effects of plumbagin (**4**) were found in a concentration range of 2.5 pg–2.5 g/ml, whereas the dehydro-iso-α-lapachone from *Tabebuia ochracea*, a furanoquinone, and β-lapachone exerted a phagocytosis enhancing effect only at a concentration of 10 µg/ml (Fig. 6). This immunostimulating effect could also be confirmed in plumbagin-treated BALB/C mice, which were infected with *Staphylococcus aureus*. The immunoinduced antiinfectious effect resulted in an enhanced killing of bacteria [34].

In the course of our *Echinacea* research, the compound cichoric acid, isolated from the water soluble fraction of *E. purpurea* roots, was found to activate phagocytosis *in vitro* and *in vivo* [35].

Since it has been reported that cells whose activities are suppressed are more sensitive to stimulating agents than cells under homoeostatic conditions, lymphocytes were exposed to a cold shock (4° C for 1 h) before incubation with vincristine using the same concentration ranges as in non-cold treated cells. As shown in Figure 5, cold shocked cells were found to be more sensitive to stimulation than non-

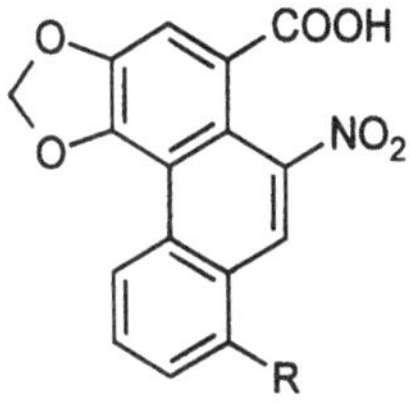

(**1**) Aristolochic acid

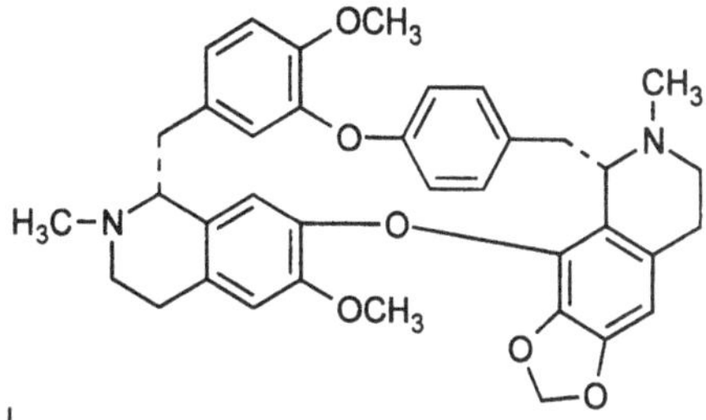

(**2**) Cepharanthine

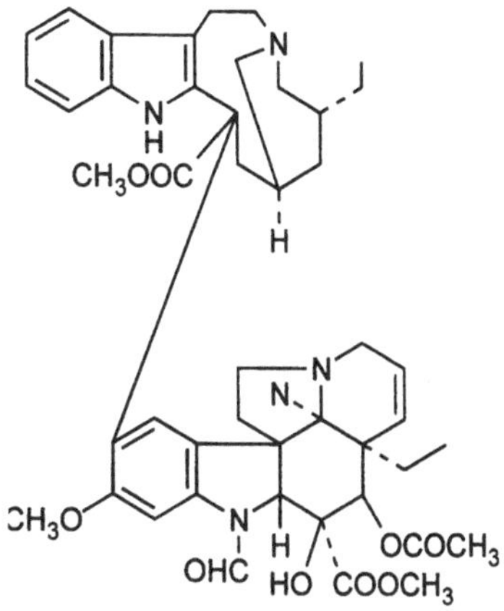

(**3**) Vincristine

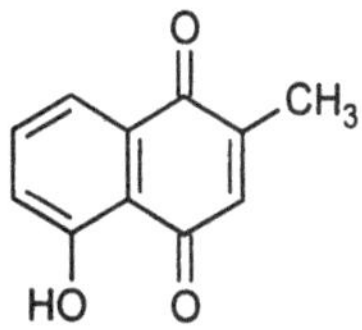

(**4**) Plumbagin

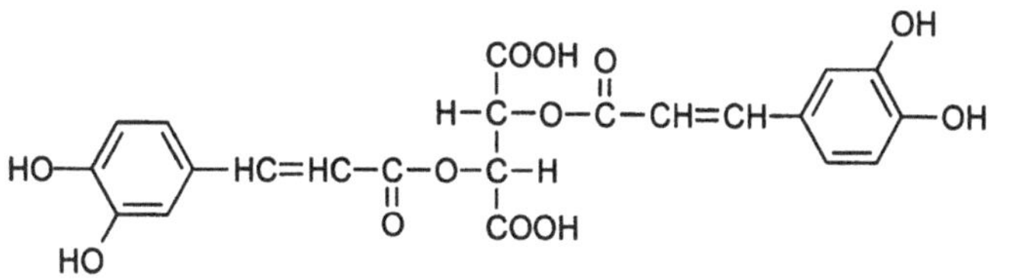

(**5**) Cichoric acid

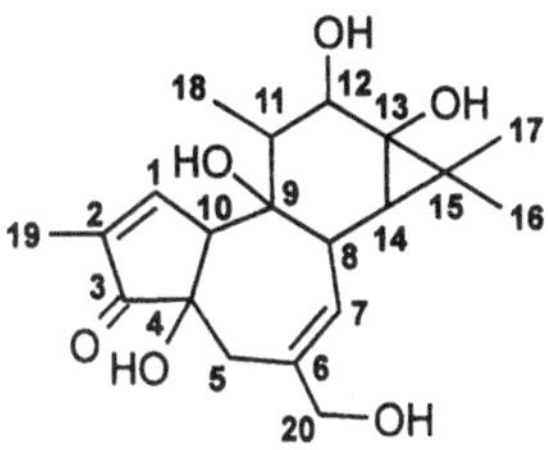

(**6**) Phorbolester

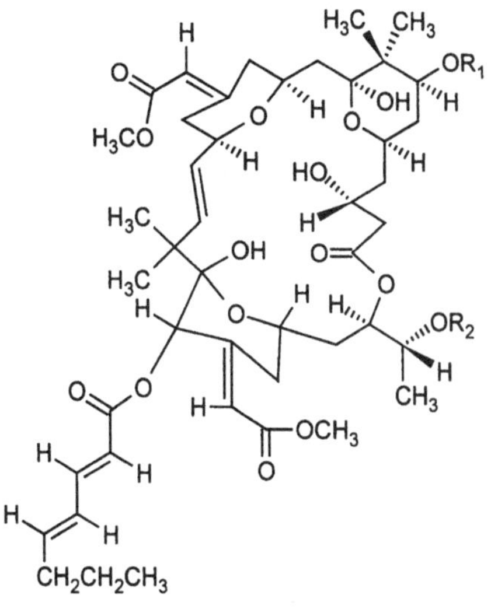

(**7**) Bryostatin 1

Figure 4
Structures of some plant immunostimulants.

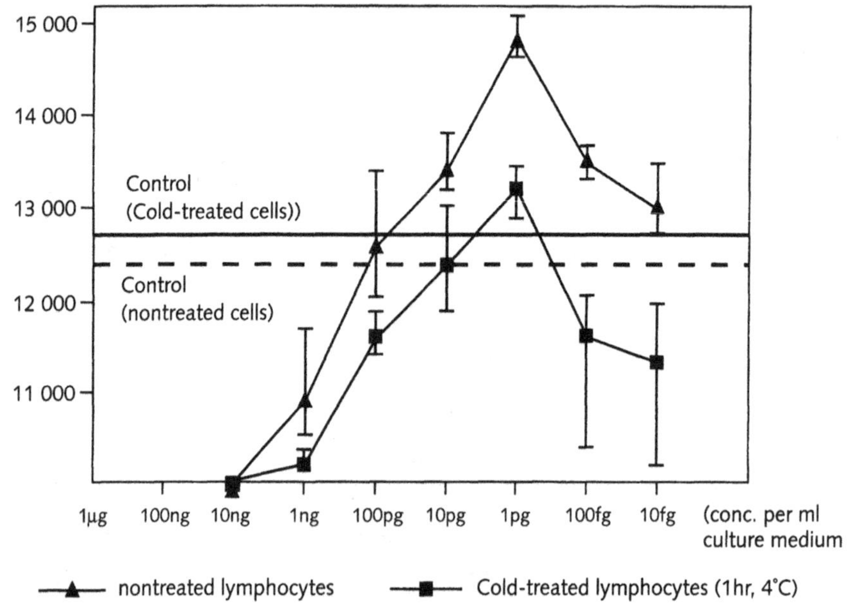

Figure 5
Dose-dependent influence of Vincristine on the ^{3}H-thymidine incorporation rate of human T lymphocytes.

pretreated cells [21]. The same effect was observed when the lymphocytes were exposed to a heat shock (40° C for 30 min.). The immunostimulating potential of very low doses of classical antitumor compounds has also been demonstrated with phorbolesters (e.g. TPA) (**5**) and the recently isolated antitumoral bryostatins (**6**) from the marine organism *Budula neritina*. The macrocyclic lactones (bryostatins) are known to show antitumoral activity in many *in vitro* and *in vivo* models [36, 37]. In low doses, however, bryostatins also show maximal stimulating effects on lymphocytes and granulocytes in the concentration range of 100 pg and 10*f*g/ml [38] (Fig. 7). Bryostatins 1, 2 and 5 stimulated the phagocytosis of human granulocytes *in vitro* up to 233% in a conentration range of 1 µM to 10 nM. This high phagocytic potential could be confirmed for bryostatin 1 in the *in vivo* carbon clearance model (conc. 100 µg/kg, 350% stimulation). Strong immunostimulating effects were also measured in the *in vitro* chemiluminescence test [38]. The finding of May et al. [39] that bryostatins, in addition to their known antineoplastic activities, show a multipotential stimulating effect on human hematopoetic progenitor cells, indicates that bryostatins can mimic many effects of the multipotential recombinant human granulocyte-macrophage colony stimulating factor (HGM-CSF). In

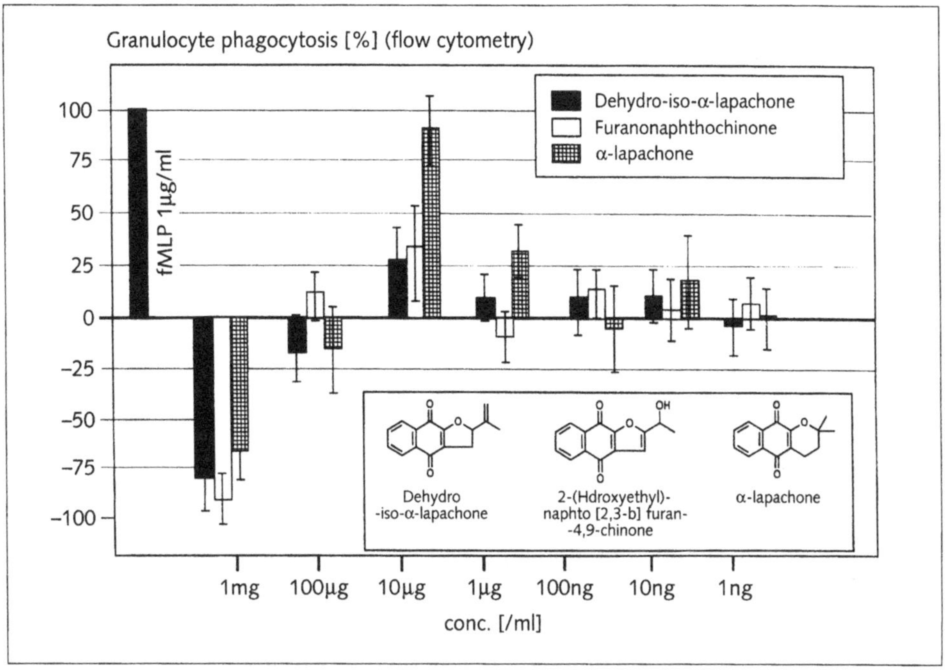

Figure 6
Dose-dependent modulation of the phagocytosis of human granulocytes by Tabebuia quinones.

contrast to TPA, bryostatins completely lack tumor-promoting ability [40]. The same cytostatic agents might result at low doses in another interesting effect on tumor growth. According to Sachs [41] various synthetic and microbial cytostatic agents (e.g. cytosin arabinoside, methotrexate or adriamycin) are able to achieve, at doses of 3–7 ng/ml, a differentiation of myeolotic leukemia cells *in vitro* and thereby a reversion of malignancy. Induction of differentiation was explained by the production of colony stimulating inducer proteins (MG T-2) acting as modulators or inhibitors of oncogene expression, respectively. If this triggering effect on cell differentiating processes by low doses of immunostimulatory agents could be veryfied *in vivo*, a new and promising concept of tumor therapy would be available [42].

In the light of all these findings, it is plausible to assume that some cancer drugs of plant origin such as mistletoe (*Viscum album*) or the South American lapacho (*Tabebuia avellanedae*), which are applied in very low concentrations with regard to the active constituents present in the preparations of traditional medicine, exert their antitumor activities by a total or partial immune or apoptosis inducing mechanism of action.

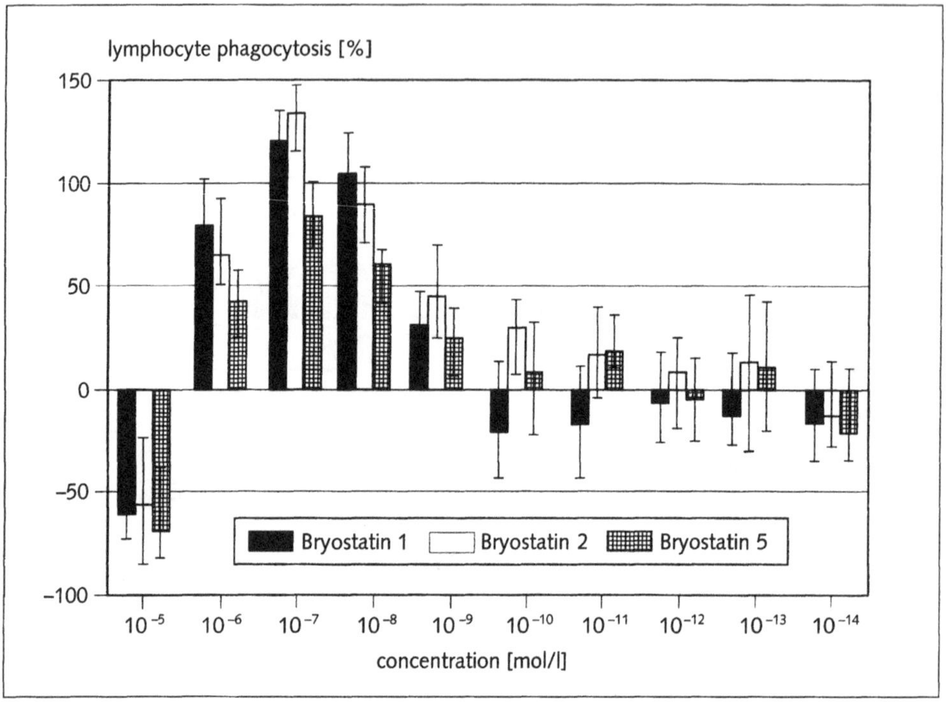

Figure 7
Dose-dependent influence of Bryostatins on the proliferation rate of human T lymphocytes.

Of several compounds isolated from marine organisms, only the oligopeptide dolastatin 10 and the macrolactone halistatin 1 showed stimulating effects in the *in vitro* chemiluminescence and phagocytosis tests [22].

Following the immunological results generated in the previously mentioned shock therapy we investigated several irritants and bitter substances for their immunomodulating potentials. Whereas the bitter substances amarogentin, chinine and quassiin exerted no *in vitro* effects, in the *in vivo* carbon clearance model, however, all showed after oral administration of 10 μg, 1 mg and 10 mg/kg clearance rates with index-values[4] ranging between 1.4 and 1.6 [22]. Similarly, the pungent capsaicin and safrol increased the clearance after i.v. administration of 10 μg/kg, by index values of 1.7 and 1.8 respectively, and after oral administration at 100 μg/kg by an index up to 1.4. The lack of *in vitro* effects of irritants and bitter substances shows that the *in vivo* activation of the non-specific immune system might be caused by an increased release of irritating mediators such as histamin, bradykinin and

4 Index values < 1.3–1.5, moderate activity; Index values > 1.5, high activity.

prostaglandins and a direct or indirect inducing effect on the intestine-associated immune system.

This mediated activation of the immune system might be explained also by the so-called 'counter irritant effect' [43].

Isolated compounds of high molecular weight

In this class of compounds, the number of possible polyclonal ligands that may react with surface structures of immunocompetent cells appears, at first glance, to be unlimited. However, the relatively small number of compounds that have reached the drug market until now demonstrates that the ability of a compound to effectively stimulate the immune system is dependent on several factors, such as secondary and tertiary structure, conformation, molecular weight, solubility, etc. Proteins, polysaccharides and glycopeptides are among the most preferred natural products with immunostimulatory activity.

Lectins

The first polymers attracting the interest of immunologists were some plant lectins that were first discovered in plants and called phytohemagglutinins due to their ability to agglutinate cells and glycoconjugates. Lectins are sugar-binding carbohydrate-specific proteins or glycoproteins, which, apart from their hemagglutinating properties and diagnostic value for blood group typing, are of additional interest because some of them bind predominantly to lymphocytes and induce mitosis. Other lectins inhibit protein synthesis in eucaryotic cells and some lectins agglutinate malignant cells better than normal cells [44]. In addition to these types of lectins, e.g. those of *Phaseolus vulgaris* (PHA), *Canavalia ensiformis*, *Lens culinaris*, *Rizinus communis* and *Phytolacca americana*, a galactose specific lectin from *Viscum album* (mistletoe lectin I) (see Samtleben et al., this volume) and an N-Acetylglucosamin specific lectin from *Urtica dioica* (UDA) [45] were found of interest in recent years due to their multiple immunostimulating (e.g. Interferon inducing) potential. The advanced immunological test systems available today may lead to a renaissance of the lectin research in the coming years with particular focus on immunological activities.

Proteins

Kojima et al. [46] have isolated a protein from the leaves of *Artemisia princeps* by means of ultrafiltration and Sephadex chromatography. This protein has a molecular weight of 500,000–1000,000 Da and induces interferon when administered orally and parenterally. In recent years the ribosome inactivating proteins (RIPs) have gained particular interest due to their multiple effects on HIV-infections. Whereas the type II RIPs, such as ricin or abrin from *Ricinus communis* and *Abrus precatorius*, are extremely toxic, the type I RIPs are practically non-toxic to cell systems since they cannot penetrate through cell membranes. Type I RIPs show antiviral activity by inhibiting the protein synthesis through RNA N-glycosidase activity. Trichosanthin from *Trichosanthes kirilowii* is able to reduce the retroviral protein and RNA levels in acutely infected T lymphoblast cultures and cultures of chronically infected monocytes/macrophages. In a clinical phase I/II study on HIV patients, a significant reduction of the p24 level (24kDa protein of the nucleocapsids) and an enhancement of the $CD4^+$ cell number could be shown [47, 48]. Three other RIPs, the bryodin from *Bryonia cretica* ssp. *dioica*, peponin from *Cucurbita pepo* and ecballin from *Ecballium elaterum* also inhibited at a concentration of 2–3 µg/ml culture medium the growth of chronically infected T lymphoma cells (TCID50). At this concentration the RIPs exerted only little influence on the growth of non-infected T lymphocytes. Since the anti HIV-effect of peponin and ecballin is due to inhibition of recombinant HIV-1 reverse transcriptase, it is likely that HIV-infected cells possess an increased membrane permeability, which elevates the uptake of the proteins into the cells [49, 50]. From these results it can be concluded that the proteins are not only able to inhibit the spreading of the infection through inhibition of the proliferation of chronically infected cells, but also to reduce the acute infection of non-infected T lymphocytes. It is well-known that infected cells which have expressed HIV-antigens on the cell surface, are able to destroy non-infected T cells by binding to them through CD4 receptors and forming lethal syncytical cells. The immunomodulating role of RIPs has been described in detail by Ng et al. [51], but needs further investigation.

Antitumoral and antiinfectious polysaccharides (except anti HIV polysaccharides)

The first polysaccharides found to stimulate the "reticuloendothelial system" were isolated from fungi, algae and lichens and have been described in several review articles [1, 52–54]. As shown in Table 4, the glucans with β-1,3-linkages in the back bone and further β-1,6-branching points are the dominating types.

As far as the fungal polysaccharides are concerned, most of them have been reported to be active against a series of allogenic and syngenic tumors and at the moment three of them (lentinan, schizophyllan and krestin) are in clinical use as single preparations in combination with chemotherapy (see also Maeda and Chihara, this volume). Meanwhile, a great number of polysaccharides with immunostimulating activity have also been isolated from higher plants [1, 2] (see also Emmendörffer et al., this volume).

The immunostimulating potential of these polysaccharides is described as enhancing phagocytosis of granulocytes and macrophages, inducing the interferon-, interleukine- and tumor necrosis factor-production, and as complement-activating or

Table 4 - Immunostimulating polysaccharides from fungi, lichens and algae

	Polysaccharides	type	linkage	M.W. (Da)
Fungi	Zymosan	glucan	β1→3	50–120,000
	Mannozym	mannan	β1→3	5–20,000
			β1→3	50–65,000
			β1→4	
	Lentinan	glucans	β1→3	ca. 500,000
	Pachyman		(β1→2	– 1 Mill
	Pachymaran		β1→6)	
	Schizophyllan	glucan	β1→3 ↓	ca. 400,000
			β1→6	
	Krestin (PSK)	glucan	β1→4 ↓	50–100,00
			β1→6	
			+ coval. proteins	
Lichens, algae			glucans	
	Pustulan		β1→6	
	Lichenan		β1→3	
			β1→4	
	Isolichenan		α1→3	100–500,00
			α1→4	
	Laminaran		β1→3	
			β1→6	

antitumoral. The term "antitumoral", first defined for several polysaccharides from fungi and algae, includes several kinds of interactions in which macrophages as well as T lymphocytes, NK cells, and their mediators can be involved. The expression "complement activating" can be interpreted either as an antigen processing mechanism or as an antiinflammatory activity since most of the complement tests measure the complement comsumption only (see also Yamada and Kiyohara, this volume).

Since it is obvious that the various polysaccharides do not have the same sites of interaction with the immune system it is, at present, hardly possible to suggest a clear structure activity relationship or to indicate what structural features are essential for an optimal immunostimulating activity. As far as phagocytosis and macrophage stimulation is concerned, it is remarkable that neutral xyloglucans and glycuronic acid containing arabinogalactans or 4-0-methyl-glucuronoxylans are predominating. Most of the active polysaccharides are highly branched with anionic structural units and m.w. in the range of 20 kDa to 50 kDa or more. They are derived from primary cell walls, have pectic or protopectic properties and some are viscous, belonging to the class of gums and mucilages. In the class of potent complement-activating polysaccharides, acidic polygalakturonan structures with arabinogalaktan side chains are frequently found (see also Emmendörffer et al., this volume).

As prototypes for both classes the acidic arabinorhamnogalaktan from *Echinacea purpurea* tissue cultures [55] (see Emmendörffer et al., this volume) and the heteroglycanes of *Achyrocline satureioides* [56] and *Urtica dioica* [57] can be considered. The first one, with a m.w. of 75 kDa, was effective in activating macrophages to cytotoxicity against tumor cells and against pathogenic microorganisms both *in vivo* as well as *in vitro* (i.e. *Leishmania enrietii*, *Listeria cytogenes*, *Candida albicans*) (see Emmendörffer et al., this volume).

The great advantage of the polysaccharide of *Echinacea purpurea* is that it acts selectively on macrophages and that it is non-toxic over a wide concentration range (acute toxicity > 4 g/kg i.p. or i.v.). This polysaccharide, which is now produced biotechnologically on an industrial scale, is considered a promising candidate for clinical trials. The *Achyrocline* polysaccharides (AS3 and AS4), two glycanogalakturonans, strongly enhanced granulocyte and macrophage phagocytosis, they also showed a moderate effect on the TNF-α-induction but exerted a strong anticomplement activity in both the classical and the alternative pathway. It is likely that these anticomplement properties are responsible for the antiinflammatory activities of both polysaccharides as measured in the rat paw edema model (25–30% inhibition at 3 mg/kg i.v.). The *Urtica* polysaccharides consist of neutral and acidic polysaccharides with molecular weights ranging between 20 and 200 kDa [57].

The observation that several polysaccharides exert significant antiinflammatory activities also after parenteral administration, has stimulated investigations on the putative mechanism of action. From the results available so far, one can conclude that the polysaccharides interfere with the complement system and/or the cytokine release, whereas a significant influence on the arachidonic acid pathway can be excluded.

Anti-HIV polysaccharides

Gerber et al. [58] were the first to report antiviral activity of agar polysaccharides and carrageenan of seaweed. This report was followed by others on the inhibition of replication of *Herpes simplex*, Coxackie Δ9, yellow fever, or poly-viruses by various sulfated glucosamine glycans from *Dumontiacea*. Meanwhile, an anti-HIV-activity could also be demonstrated for these polysaccharides [59, 60]. In a series of investigations carried out by Yoshia et al. [61], arabinosyl curdlan, galactosyl or glucosyl curdlan were sulfated and tested for anti-HIV-1 activity. The survival rate, the expression of viral antigens in HIV-1 infected cells and the inhibition of syncytia formation were measured.

Lentinansulfate, arabinosyl curdlan sulfate and galactosyl curdlan sulfate were observed to possess a prominent inhibitory activity on HIV-1 replication at a concentration of 10 µg/ml. The relation between anti-HIV-1 activity, degree of sulfation and molecular weight was investigated for curdlan sulfate resulting in an anti-HIV-1-activity at a concentration of 3.3 µg/ml. The m.w. of curdlan sulfate was > 5.0×10^4 Da and the sulfur content > 13.5%. In contrast to this finding lentinan did not show a direct inhibition on HIV-1 replication in Mat-4, Skw-3, U-937 and CEM cell lines [62]. However, when 100 µl/ml were combined with 5 µl/ml 3'-azido-2',3'-dideoxythymidine (AZT) in a cell culture, lentinan enhanced the inhibitory activity of AZT against HIV-1. The same tendency was also observed by using other cell lines. In a second experiment it was investigated if infectivity of the virus would appear again in a curdlan sulfate-depleted cell culture following co-cultivation of the same compound with infected cells and target cells. The antigen expression of HIV-1 on the cell surface in curdlan sulfate-depleted cell cultures disappeared entirely after co-cultivation of infected cells with curdlan sulfate (5 µg/ml) for 168 h and normal cell proliferation was observed [63]. This result might be explained by a binding of the sulfated polysaccharides to the viral surface resulting in a complete inhibition of viral binding to, and entry into, the cell surface. It is noteworthy that the neutral polysaccharides exerted a host-mediated antitumoral, but not antiviral effect, whereas the sulfated polysaccharides showed a direct inhibitory activity on the HIV-1 replication but were inactive against tumor growth.

In Germany, Bayer and Hoechst investigated a polysulfated polyxylan (Hoe/Bay 946)[5] with the m.w. 6 kDa for its *in vitro* anti-HIV-activity [64]. The polyanion polysaccharide was able, at a concentration of 25 µg/ml, to totally inhibit the HIV-reverse transcriptase and the HIV-induced syncytia formation of T lymphocytes. The *in vitro* and experimental animal studies were followed by an open, clinical trial with HIV-infected patients (phase I, III and IV, cluster of differentiation classification (CDC)). Hoe/Bay 946 was applied orally in a concentration of 3×150 mg and 3×450 mg/day for 12 months. The therapy was well tolerated by all patients. In patients in phase II + III, the peripheral lymphocytes increased from 2500 to 2785/µl, the T_4 lymphocytes from 460 to 560/µl whereas the T_4/T_8 ratio decreased from 0.50 to 0.475.

In the 12 months period of investigation, one patient out of 14 died. In phase IV a similar tendency of improved immune parameters could be observed. From 20 patients five patients died in a 12 months period. All others developed severe opportunistic infections (i.e. *Candidiasis*, pneumonia e.o.). It was reported that Hoe/Bay 946 was three to four times more effective than dextransulfate in laboratory experiments. These results clearly show that the direct interaction of the polymers with

5 xylanpoly (hydrogensulfate)-dipotassium salt

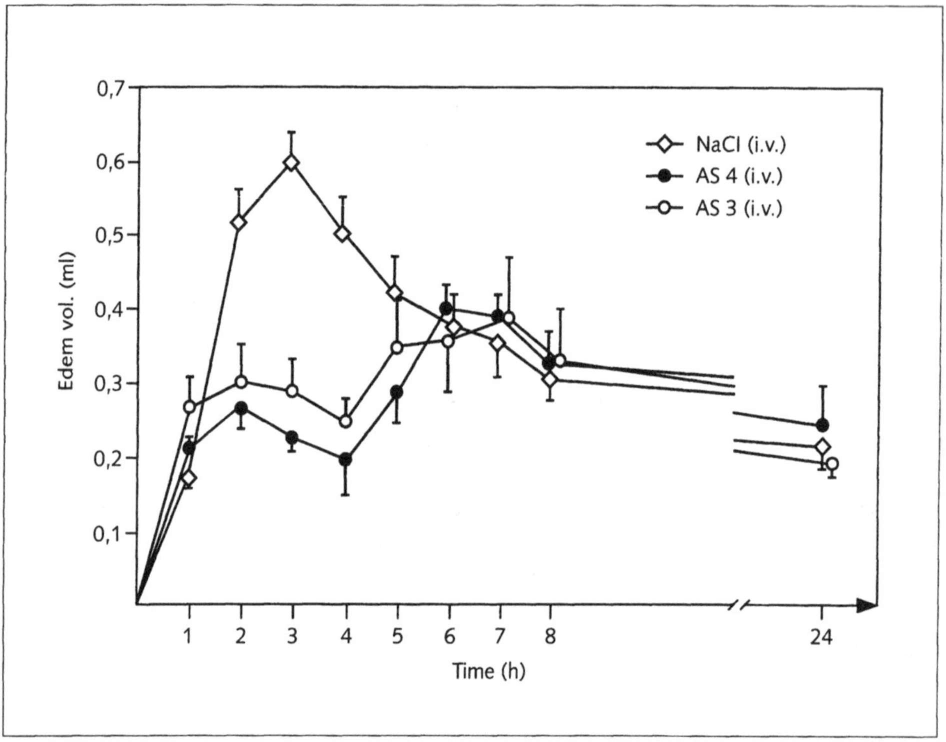

Figure 8
Antiphlogistic activity of polysaccharides AS3 and AS4 of Achyrocline satureioides *in the rat paw carragenan induced edema model. 1 h after s.c. injection of 0.05 ml 1% carragenan sol. 3 mg each of AS3 and AS4/ml were i.v. injected. The volumes were recorded by plethysmometry. Ref. compound: indometacin (10 mg/kg).*

the virus must be accompanied by an immunoenhancing effect. Another polyanion, chondroitinsulfate (m.w. 3000–30,000 Da) has been tested in the MT-4 cell assay and was found to be more active than dextransulfate, heparin, pentosanpolysulfate, dermatan-sulfate, AZT and suramin.

Antiinflammatory polysaccharides

The observation that several polysaccharides, e.g. polysaccharides of *Achyrocline satureoides*, at parenteral administration exert significant *in vivo* antiinflammatory activities, as measured in the rat paw edema model (Fig. 8), raises the question on their mechanisms of action. The great structural diversity of polysaccharides, ranging from linear glucans to highly branched acidic polygalacturonans, which were found to exert antiinflammatory activities, favours multiple mechanisms of action. From a pathophysiological point of view many mediators liberated from immunocompetent cells and plasma enzymatic systems can be involved in the inflammatory process.

One target for the antiinflammatory polysaccharides could be the complement system, which is part of the non-specific humoral immune system and known to be involved in inflammatory processes. This suggestion would be consistent with the anticomplement effect found for many neutral glucans, mannans, galactans and arabinogalactans as well as acidic galacturonans and rhamnogalacturonans in Yamada's as well as our own laboratory (see also Yamada and Kiyohara, this volume) (Tab. 5). However, since it has been shown that a reduced serum complement level caused by cobra venom factor or by the polysulfonated urea derivative Suramin (a known complement inhibitor) did not result in an inhibition of carrageenan-induced rat paw edema [65, 66], it is likely that the polysaccharides exert their antiinflammatory activity indirectly through other immunological or non-immunological mechanisms of action.

In this context, the role of adhesion molecules and complement receptors found on macrophages, neutrophils and NK-cells and the role of leukocyte chemotaxis might be of importance and should therefore be investigated. Furthermore, the influence of polysaccharides on endocrine functions (counter irritant effect), on prostaglandin metabolism, or on the NO-mediators have to be taken into consideration.

Chemotaxis

An activation of the complement cascade results in generation of the chemotactic cleavage product C5a. Through this activation, polysaccharides are able to increase leukocyte migration in an *in vitro* chemotaxis assay when incubated in the presence of serum [67, 68].

In contrast to this increased chemotaxis mediated by the complement cascade we could show that UPS I, an α-glucan from the rhizome of *Urtica dioica* L., is able to stimulate leukocyte migration by itself. At a concentration of 12.5 mg/ml the chemotactic answer was eight times higher when compared to a negative control [69]. Since Silva et al. [70] could demonstrate that even 4h after an intraperitoneal administration of a β-glucan from *Paracoccidioides brasiliensis*, the polymorphonuclear cell recruitment into the peritoneal cavity of rats was strongly increased, it is plausible that, as a result of this influx of leukocytes, the amount of inflammatory cells in the blood vessels is reduced and an antiinflammatory effect generated. This would be in agreement with the findings of Damas et al. [71], who could show that the carrageenan edema in rats can be inhibited by leukopenia. On this basis, the antiinflammatory effect of UPS I, a 60% reduction of the rat paw edema volume at an i.p. administration of 10 mg/kg, can be explained at least in part.

Table 5 - Antiinflammatory polysaccharides

Name	Type	MW (Da)	Biological activity	Plant source	Reference
AS3	Glykanogalacturonan	7,600	- antiinflammatory (rat paw edema) - anticomplementary - immunostimulating (Carbon Clearance)	*Achyrocline satureioides*	[87]
AS4	Glykanogalacturonan	15,000	- antiinflammatory (rat paw edema) - anticomplementary - immunostimulating (Carbon Clearance)	*Achyrocline satureioides*	[87]
U-3-A	Glucuronoxylomannan	2,4 Mio	- antiinflammatory (rat paw edema) - antihyperalgesic	*Auricularia* species	[88]
Carrageenan	(1-3)-β-galp-2-sulfat-(1-4)-α-D-galp-2,6-disulfat (λ-Carrageenan)	2 Mio	- antiinflammatory (rat paw edema)	*Chondrus crispus* *Gigartina stellata*	[78, 79, 89]
T-5-N	β-Glucan		- antiinflammatory (rat paw edema) - antihyperalgesic	*Dictyophora indusiata*	[90, 91]
GIIa	Arabinoglucan	8,400	- antiinflammatory (mouse paw edema)	*Melia azadirachta*	[92]
GIIIa	Arabinofucoglucan	8,000	- antiinflammatory (mouse paw edema)	*Melia azadirachta*	[92]
OL-2	β-Glucan	610,000	- anticomplementary - antitumoral - release of IL-1, IL-6, TNFα	*Omphalia lapidescens*	[93–95]
S-4001	β-Glucan		- antiinflammatory (croton oil mice ear edema, yeast induced ankle swelling)	Omphalia *lapidescens*	[73]
	Glycogen		- antiinflammatory (rat paw edema)	*Perna canaliculus* (mussel)	[96, 97]

Pinellian G	Glucan	15,000	- anticomplementary - immunostimulating (enhanced phagocytosis)	*Pinellia ternata*	[98]
Pinellian PA	Galactan	118,000	- anticomplementary - immunostimulating (enhanced phagocytosis)	*Pinellia ternata*	[99]
BX-W	Amylose	4,100	- antiinflammatory (mouse paw edema)	*Pinellia ternata*	[100]
NAS2	Polygalacturonan	13,000	- antiinflammatory (rat paw edema)	*Sedum telephium*	[101]
TIIc	α-1,6-Glucan	24,000	- antiinflammatory (mouse paw edema, adjuvant arthritis)	*Tetragonia tetragonoides*	[102]
RP 2	Amylopectin	50,000	- anticomplementary - immunostimulating (enhanced proliferation of lymphocytes	*Urtica dioica*	[57, 103, 104]
UPS I	α-1-4-Glucan	10,000	- anticomplementary - chemotactic activity - antiinflammatory (rat paw edema)	*Urtica dioica*	[69]

Adhesion molecules and complement receptors

As well as chemotactic factors generated by the activated complement cascade, complement receptors can also be involved in the regulation of the inflammatory process. These complement receptors play a key role in the removal of immune complexes and in the engulfing of opsonized particles. The complement receptor 3 (CR3 = Mac1, Integrin CD11b/CD18) possesses adhesion molecule functions and mediates the sticking of leukocytes to activated endothelium, an important step in the extravasation of inflammatory cells. Since Thornton et al. [72] demonstrated that β-glucans bind specifically to CR3, thus blocking the binding of antibodies directed against CR3, β-glucans should be able to decrease the extravasation of leukocytes by blocking cell interactions between the endothelium and leukocytes. S-4001, a β-glucan, which exactly matches the structural requirements for binding to CR3, has been isolated from *Omphalia lapidescens*. This polysaccharide was found to have significant antiinflammatory activity in various experimental animal models including croton oil-induced ear edema [73]. The fact that inhibitory action on leukocyte migration was observed, indicates that the blocking of cell adhesion molecules could be another mechanism of action for the antiinflammatory activity of this β-glucan.

Futher evidence for the importance of adhesion molecules as targets for antiinflammatory polysaccharides was provided by Dong and Murphy [74, 75]. They showed, using an *in vivo* mouse model that a glucuronoxylomannan from *Cryptococcus neoformans* inhibits leukocyte extravasation into sites of acute inflammation. They propose that binding to CD18 (part of the cell adhesion molecule Mac1) on human neutrophils is responsible for the observed inhibition of leukocyte migration.

Counter irritant effects

Since Rocha e Silva et al. [76] have reported that a number of sulphated polymers show antiinflammatory potential, counter irritation has been discussed as one possible mechanism. Beside turpentine [71] and sulphated polysaccharides, a neutral glucan was also found to possess irritating and inflammation-inducing activity [77]. Most likely this class of polysaccharides also exhibits antiinflammatory effects in the carrageenan rat paw edema through counter irritation. This could be of great importance in acute animal inflammation models, since Ferreira et al. [78] demonstrated that counter irritant effects were able to reduce edema formation as early as 2 h after administration of the irritating substance.

Inhibitors of the adrenocorticoid synthesis [79] neutralize counter irritation effects suggesting participation of the symphato-adrenal system. The first evidence for the involvement of neutral glucans in the induction of adrenocorticoid release was reported by Wang and Zhu [73]. A β-glucan from *Omphalia lapidescens*, which has shown antiinflammatory activity in animal models, was able to increase the plasma content of corticosterone in rats. In addition to this β-glucan, other glucans like UPS I from *Urtica dioica*, can be expected to exhibit an antiinflammatory effect through corticoid release. The time course of corticoid release, having a maximum 7 h after the injection of carrageenan as stressor [80] could explain why the maximum of the antiinflammatory activity of UPS I was found after 24 h.

Prostaglandin pathway

For polysulfated pentosan an inhibition of the leukocyte 5-lipoxygenase has been found [81]. According to our knowledge, an involvement of non-sulphated polysaccharides in the arachidonic acid cascade and a resulting decrease of pro-inflammatory prostanoids has so far not been reported. Panossian [82] tested different polysaccharides (including carrageenan and *Echinacea* polysaccharide) for their effect on the release of arachidonic acid metabolites from stimulated and non-stimulated human PMNL. None of the tested polysaccharides was able to activate or inhibit this pathway. In their search for the mechanism of action of the antiinflammatory polysaccharide T-2-HN (a partially O-acetylated α-D-mannan from *Dictophora indusiata*) Ukai et al. [83] found only a slight influence on the arachidonic acid metabolism. An inhibition of the generation of vasoactiv kinine, which is postulated by many authors to be a key mediator in the carrageenan-induced rat paw edema model [84], has so far not been seen.

NO-mediators

The function of nitric oxide in the carrageenan inflammation model has been investigated by several research groups. Salvemini et al. [85] propagate nitric oxide as a key mediator in the early and late phases of carrageenan-induced rat paw inflammation. Meller et al. [86] reported the participation of nitric oxide in the development and maintenance of the hyperalgesia produced by intraplantar injection of carrageenan in the rat.

In conclusion, a lot of evidence points to the fact that immunological cells and humoral factors play a great role in the antiinflammatory activity of polysaccharides, but it is likely that other mechanisms of action discussed here are also involved.

Studies on the immunological mechanism of action of polysaccharides in general

The immunological screening of hundreds of polysaccharides from natural sources in a variety of *in vitro* and *in vivo* assays has revealed that all of them exert a more or less stimulating activity on various parts of the immune system, but no clear information could be obtained on how a polysaccharide has to be structurally designed in order to have an optimal inducing effect on certain immune cells. If one calculates the number of possible permutations for four sugar monomers one comes up with over 35,000 different ways of linking the monomers, whereas for example four amino acids yield only 24 permutations [105]. This enormous potential variability provides the kind of flexibility needed for the precise control of cell-cell interactions in a living system like the immune system. Since it can be suggested that the polysaccharides analogous to lipopolysaccharides have to be bound to certain receptor domains of the cell membrane surface in order to induce a signal chain, several attempts have been made to optimize the immune-induced antitumoral and immunomodulating activity of polysaccharides by modifying their structures by enzymatic, oxidative or acidic degradation, introducing alkyl and acid groups into the molecule through esterification, or simply by treating them with solubilizers (i.e. urea) [106].

These results confirm the hypothesis that the immunological activity of a polysaccharide is dependent on a specific conformational feature and the presence of a certain number of anionic domains. In our opinion, the approach to a rational drug design has to include the production of radio-, fluorescence- or gold-labeled polysaccharides and antibodies. These tools will help to explain the requirements for an optimal polysaccharide-immune cell interaction. This technique could also be useful for localizing the site of binding on the surface of the immune cell thus giving information on the pharmacokinetic and bioavailability of polysaccharides after oral and parenteral application.

References

1 Wagner H, Proksch A (1985) Immunostimulatory drugs of fungi and higher plants. In: N Farnsworth, H Wagner (eds): *Economic and medicinal plant research*, Vol 1. Academic Press, London, 113–153

2 Wagner H (1990) Search for plant derived natural compounds with immunostimulatory activity (recent advances). *Pure & Appl Chem* 62: 1217–1222

3 Drews J (1980) Möglichkeiten der Immunstimulierung. *Swiss Pharma* 2:9 (49)

4 Seiler FR, Hofstaetter T, Kolar C, Kraemer HP, Schorlemmer HU, Sedlacek HH (1985) Immunmodulation: Immunstimulation and Immunsuppression In: Ruschig H (ed): *Arzneimittel Fortschritte 1972–1985*. VCH-Verlag, Weinheim, 1367–1433

5 Freund J (1956) The mode of action of immunologic adjuvants Adv Tuberc Res 7: 130

6 Gupta RK, Siber GR (1995) Adjuvants for human vaccines – current status, problems and future prospects. *Vaccine* 13: 1263–1276

7 Wagner H, Jurcic K (1991) In: Dey PM, Harborne JB, Hostettmann K (eds): *Methods in plant biochemistry*, Vol 6. Academic Press, London, New York, 195–217

8 Weir DM (1978) *Application of immunological methods. Handbook of experimental immunology*, 3rd ed. Blackwell Scientific Publications, Oxford

9 Brandt I (1967) Studies on the phagocytic activity of neutrophilic leukocytes. *Scand J Haematol* (Suppl 2)

10 Wagner H, Jurcic K (1996) A new flowcytometric assay for measuring the leukocyte phagocytosis activity of immunostimulating plant extracts, polysaccharides and various low molecular weight compounds. *Phytomedicine* 3 (Suppl 1): 31

11 Allen RC (1981) In: DeLuca MD, Mc Elroy WD (eds): *Bioluminescence and chemoluminescence*, Vol 3. Academic Press, New York, London, 63

12 D'Onofrio C, Lohmann-Matthes ML (1984) Chemoluminescence of macrophages depends upon their differentiation stage: Dissociation between phagocytosis and oxygen radical release. *Immunbiology* 167: 414–430

13 Biozzi G, Benacerraf B, Halpern BN (1953) Quantitative study of the granulopectic activity of R.E.S. II. A study of the kinetics of the granulopectic activity of the R.E.S. in relation to the dose of carbon injected. Relationship between the weight of the organs and their activity. *Brit J Expo Pathol* 34: 441

14 Kabat EA, Mayer MM (1961) In: Thomas CC (ed): *Kabat and Mayer's experimental immunochemistry*, 2nd ed., chapter 4, Springfield, 133–239

15 Platts-Mills TAE, Ishizaka KJ (1974) Activation of the alternate pathway of human complements by rabbit cells. *J Immunol* 113: 348–357

16 Nakamura S, Sung SSJ, Bjorndal JM, Fu SM (1989) Human T-cell activation. IV T-cell activation and proliferation via early activation antigen EA-1. *J Exp Mod* 169: 677– 689

17 Meerpohl HG, Lohmann-Matthes ML, Fischer H (1976) Studies on the activation of mouse bone-marrow derived macrophages by the macrophage cytotoxicity factor (MCF). *Eur J Immunol* 6: 213–217

18 Luettig B, Steinmüller C, Gifford GE, Wagner H, Lohmann-Matthes ML (1989) Macrophage activation by the polysaccharide arabinogalactan isolated from plant cell cultures of *Echinacea purpurea. J Nat Canc Institute* 81: 669–675

19 Stimpel M, Proksch A, Wagner H, Lohmann-Matthes ML (1984) Macrophage activation and induction of macrophage cytotoxicity by purified polysaccharide fractions from the plant *Echinacea purpurea. Infections and Immunity* 46: 845–849

20 Roesler I, Steinmüller Ch, Kiderlen A, Emmendörffer AC, Wagner H, Lohmann-Matthes ML (1991) Application of purified polysacharides from cell cultures of the plant *Echinacea purpurea* to mice mediates protection against systemic infection with *Listeria* monocytogenes and *Candida albicans. Int J Immunopharmac* 13: 27–37

21 Wagner H, Kreher B, Jurcic K (1988) *In vitro* stimulation of human granulocytes and lymphocytes by pico- and femtogram quantities of cytostatic agents. *Arzneim-Forsch/Drug Res* 38: 237–275

22 Eisemann K (1996) *Methodenentwicklung und Screening von Pflanzenextrakten und isolierten Naturstoffen auf immunmodulierende Wirkung*. PhD-Thesis, University of Munich, Germany

23 Lindequist U, Teuscher E (1985) Pflanzliche und mikrobielle Wirkstoffe als Immunmodulatoren. *Pharmazie* 40: 10–16

24 Möse JR (1963) Versuche über die Wirksamkeit von Artistolochiasäure. *Planta Med* 11: 72–91

25 Möse JR (1966) Weitere Untersuchungen über die Wirkung der Aristolochia-Säure. *Arzneimittel-Forsch* 16: 118–122

26 Sieving H, Müller HJ (1981) Gegensätzliche Wirkung von Glukokortikoiden und Aristolochiasäure auf das Immunozytoadhärenzphänomen. *Arzneimittel-Forsch* 31: 1260–1262, 31(II)

27 Lemperle G (1972) *Funktion des retikuloendothelialen Systems bei chirurgischen Erkrankungen.* Habil-Schrift der Med Fakultät, Universität Freiburg, Germany

28 Kluthe R, Vogt A, Batsford S (1982) Doppelblindstudie zur Beeinflussung der Phagozytosefähigkeit von Granulozyten durch Aristolochiasäure. *Arzneim-Forsch* 32: 443–445

29 Mori M, Nakamoto S, Arashima Y, Seno S (1979) Protective effect of Cepharanthine on suppression of hemopoesis by antitumor agents. *Gato Kagaku Ryoho* 6: 175

30 Wagner H, Kreuzkamp B, Jurcic K (1985) Die Alkaloide von *Uncaria tomentosa* und ihre Phagozytosesteigernde Wirkung. *Planta Med* 419–423

31 Schwarz JA, König P, Scheuden PG (1974) Beeinflussung der humoralen Immunantwort durch Vincristinsulfat und Vincristin/Cyclophosphanoid. *Verh Dtsch Ges Inn Med* 80: 1597

32 Atherton AC, Burke DC (1978) The effects of some different metabolic inhibitors on interferon superinduction. *J Gen Virol* 41: 229–237

33 Zheng QY, Kiranowska M, Sadlik JR, Hadden JW (1987) Purified podophyllotoxins (CPH-86) inhibits lymphocyte proliferation but augments macrophage proliferation. *J Immunopharmac* 9: 539

34 Abdul KM, Ramchender RP (1995) Potentiation of macrophage bactericidal activity. *Immunopharmacology* 30: 231

35 Bauer R, Remiger P, Jurcic K, Wagner H (1989) Beeinflussung der Phagozytose-Aktivität durch *Echinacea*-Extrakte. *Z Phytother* 10: 43–48

36 Pettit GR, Herald CL, Doubek DL, Herald DL (1982) Isolation and Structure of Bryostatin 1. *J Am Chem Soc* 104: 6846–6848

37 Schuchter LM, Esa AH, May S, Laulis MK, Pettit GR, Hess AD (1991) Successful treatment of murine melanoma with Bryostatin 1. *Cancer Res* 51 (2): 682–687

38 Eisemann K, Totola A, Jurcic K, Pettit GR, Wagner H (1995) Bryostatins 1, 2 and 5 activate human granulocytes and lymphocytes: *in vitro* and *in vivo* studies. *Pharm Pharmacol Lett* 1: 45–48

39 May WS, Sharkis SJ, Esa AH, Gebbia V, Kraft AS, Pettit GR, Sensenbrenner LL (1987) Antineoplastic bryostatins are multipotential stimulators of human hemotopoietic progenitor cells. *Proc Natl Acad Sci USA* 84: 8483

40 Kraft AS, Reeves JA, Ashendel CL (1988) Differing modulation of proteinkinase C by bryostatin 1 and phorbolesters in IB6 mouse epidermal cells. *J Biol Chem* 263: 8437

41 Sachs L (1982) Normal development programms in myeloid leukemia: Regulatory proteins in the control of growth and differentiation. *Cancer Surveys* 1: 321–342

42 The chemotherapy of malignant diseases (1989) In: Eckhart S, Holzner JH, Nagel GA (eds): *Contribution to Oncology*. Karger, Basel

43 Atkinson DC, Hicks R (1975) The antiinflammatory activity of irritants. *Agents and Actions* 5: 239–249

44 Lis H, Sharon N (1973) The biochemistry of plant lectins (Phytohemagglutinins). *Ann Rev Biochem* 42: 541

45 Wagner H, Willer F, Samtleben R (1994) Lektine und Polysaccharide – die Wirkprinzipien der *Urtica*-Wurzel? In: G Boos (ed): *Benigne Prostatahyperplasie*. pmi-Verlag, Frankfurt, 115–122

46 Kojima Y (1980) Antineoplastic effect of TGDS synthetic acid polysaccharides on human cervical cancer Experimental therapy of HeLa-S3 cell cancer transplanted to nude mice. *Nippon Monaikei Gakhai haishi* 19 (4): 261

47 McGrath MS, Santulli S, Gaston I (1999) Effects of GLQ 233 TM on HIV-replication in human monocyte/macrophages chronically infected *in vitro* with HIV. *AIDS Res Human Retroviruses* 6: 1039–1043

48 Byers VS, Levin AS, Waites LA, Starrett BA, Mayer RA, Clogg JA, Price MR, Robins RA, Delaney M, Baldwin RW (1990) A phase I/II study of trichosanthin treatment of HIV disease. *AIDS* 4: 1189–1196

49 Gerhäuser C, Samtleben R, Tau GT, Pezzuto JM, Lottspeich F, Wagner H (1993) Peponin, a new ribosome-inactivating protein isolated from the seeds of *Cucurbita pepo* L inhibits human immunodeficiency virus type I reverse transcriptase. *Pharm Pharmacological Lett* 3: 71–75

50 Wachinger M, Samtleben R, Gerhäuser C, Wagner H, Erfle V (1993) Bryodin, a single ribosome-inactivating protein selectively inhibits the growth of HIV-1 infected cells and reduces HIV-1 production. *Res Exp Med* 193: 1–12

51 NG TB, Chan WY, Yeung HW (1992) Proteins with abortifacient ribosome inactivating, immunmodulatory, antitumor and anti-AIDS activities from *Cucurbitaceae* plants. *Gen Pharmac* 23: 575–590

52 Whistler RL, Bushway AA, Singh PP, Nakahara W, Tokuzen R (1976) Noncytotoxic antitumor polysaccharides. *Adv Carbohydr Chem Biochem* 32: 235–275

53 Chihara L, Hamuro J, Maeda YY, Shiio T, Surija T (1987) In: Niebugs NE (ed): *Immunbiology of cancer and AIDS*. AR Liss Inc, New York, 423–438

54 Franz G (1989) Polysaccharides in Pharmacy: Current Applications and Future Concepts. *Planta Med* 55: 493–497

[55 Wagner H, Stuppner H, Schäfer W, Zenk M (1988) Immunological active polysaccharides of *Echinacea purpurea* cell cultures. *Phytochemistry* 27: 119–126

56 Puhlmann J, Knaus U, Tubaro L, Schäfer W, Wagner H (1992) Immunologically active metallic ion-containing polysaccharides of *Achyrocline satureoides*. *Phytochemistry* 31: 2617–2621

57 Wagner H, Willer F, Samtleben R and Boos G (1994) Search for the antiprostatic principle of stinging nettle (*Urtica dioica*) roots. *Phytomedicine* 1: 213–224

58 Gerber P, Dutcher JD, Adams EV, Sherman JH (1958) Protective effect of seaweed

extracts for chicken embryos infected with influenza B or mumps virus. *Proc Soc Exp Biol Med* 99: 590–593

59 Nakashima H, Kido Y, Kobayashi N, Motoki Y, Neushul M, Yamamoto N (1987) Purifications and characterization of an avian myoblastosis and human immunodeficiency virus reverse transcriptase inhibitor sulfated polysaccharides extracted from sea algae. *Antimicrob Agents Chemoth* 31: 1524–1528

60 Ito M, Baba M, Sato A, Pauwels R, de Clercq E, Shigeta S (1987) Inhibitory effect of dextran sulfate and heparin on the replication of human immunodeficiency virus (HIV) *in vitro. Antiviral Res* 7: 361–367

61 Yoshida O, Nakashima H, Yoshida T, Kaneko Y, Yamamoto I, Matsuzaki K, Uryu T, Yamamoto N (1988) Sulfation of the immunomodulating polysaccharide lentinan: a novel strategy for antivirals to human immunodeficiency virus (HIV). *Biochem Pharmacol* 37: 2887–2891

62 Tochikura St, Nakashima H, Kaneko Y, Kobayashi N, Yamamoto N (1987) Suppression of human immunodeficiency virus replication by 3'-azido-3'-deoxythymidine in various human hematopoietic cell lines *in vitro*: Augmentation of the effect by lentinan. *Jpn J Cancer Res* (Gann) 78: 583–589

63 Kaneko Y, Yoshida O, Nakagawa R, Yoshida T, Dato M, Ogihara S, Shioya S, Matsuzawa Y, Nagashima N et al (1990) Inhibition of HIV-1 infectivity with curdlan sulfate *in vitro. Biochem Pharmacol* 39: 793–797

64 Biesert L, Suhartono H, Winkler I, Meichsner C, Helsberg M, Hewlett G, Klimetzek V, Molling K, Schlumberger HD, Schrinner E et al (1988) Inhibition of HIV and virus replication by polysulphated polyxylan: Hoe/Bay 946, a new antiviral compound. *AIDS* 2: 449–457

65 Vinegar R, Truax JF, Selph JL (1976) Quantitative studies of the pathway to acute carrageenan inflammation. *Fed Proc* 35 (13): 2447–2456

66 Calhoun W, J Chang, RP Carlson (1987) Effect of selected antiinflammatory agents and other drugs on zymosan arachidonic acid, PAF and carrageenan induced paw edema in the mouse. *Agents Actions* 21 (3–4): 306–309

67 Torisu M, Hayashi Y, Ishimitu T, Fujimura T, Iwasaki K, Katano M, Yamamoto H, Kimura Y, Takesue M, Kondo M, Nomoto K (1990) Significant prolongation of disease-free period gained by oral polysaccharide K (PSK) administration after curative surgical operation of colorectal cancer. *Cancer Immunol Imunother* 31: 261–268

68 Pereira Crott LS, Lucisano YM, Siila CL, Barbossa JE (1993) The role of complement system in the neutrophil functions stimulated *in vitro* by an alkali-insoluble cell wall fraction of *Paracoccidioides brasisliensis. Journal of Medical and Veterinary Mycology* 31: 17–27

69 Kraus S, Wagner H (1998) UPS I, a chemotactic polysaccharide isolated from *Urtica dioica. Phytomedicine; in press*

70 Silva CL, Alves LMC, Figueiredo F (1994) Involvement of cell wall glucans in the genesis and persistence of the inflammatory reaction caused by the fungus *Paracoccidioides brasiliensis. Microbiology* 140: 1189–1194

71 Damas J, Remacle-Volon G, Deflandre E (1986) Further studies of the mechanism of counter irritation by turpentine. *Naunyn-Schmiedeberg's Arch Pharmacol* 332 (2): 196–200
72 Thornton BP, Vetvicka V, Pitman M, Goldman RC, Ross GD (1996) Analysis of the sugar specificity and molecular location of the beta-glucan-binding lectin site of complement receptor type 3 (CD11b/CD18). *J Immunol* 156(3): 1235–1246
73 Wang WJ, Zhu XY (1989) The antiinflammatory and immunostimulation activities of S-4001, a polysaccharide isolated from *Lei Wan Polyporus-Mylittae. Acta Pharm Sin* 24(2): 151–154
74 Dong ZM, Murphy JW (1995) Intravascular cryptococcal culture filtrate (CneF) and its major component, glucuronoxylomannan, are potent inhibitors of leukocyte accumulation. *Infect Immun* 63(3): 770–778
75 Dong ZM, Murphy JW (1997) Cryptococcal polysaccharides bind to CD18 on human neutrophils. *Infect Immun* 65(2): 557–563
76 Rocha e Silva M, Cavalcanti RQ, Reis ML (1969) Anti-inflammatory action of sulfated polysaccharides. *Biochem Pharmacol* 18(6): 1285–1295
77 Abe S, Takahashi K, Tsubouchi J, Aida K, Yamazaki M, Mizuno D (1984) Different local therapeutic effects of various polysaccharides on MH-134 hepatoma in mice and its relation to inflammation induced by the polysaccharides. *Gann* 75(5): 459–465
78 Ferreira SH, Lorenzetti BB, Correa FMA (1978) Central and peripheral antialgesic action of aspirin-like drugs. *Eur J Pharm* 53: 39–48
79 Bhattacharya SK, Das N, Rao PJ (1987) Effect of pre-existing inflammation on carrageenan-induced paw oedema in rats. *J Pharm Pharmacol* 39(10): 854–856
80 Stenberg VI, Bouley MG, Katz BM, Lee KJ, Parmar SS (1990) Negative endocrine control system for inflammation in rats. *Agents Actions* 29(3–4): 189–195
81 Freyburger G, Larrue F, Manciet G, Lorient-Roudaut MF, Larrue J, Boisseau MR (1987) Hemorheological changes in elderly subjects-effect of pentosan polysulfate and possible role of leukocyte arachidonic acid metabolism. *Thromb Haemost* 57(3): 322–325
82 Panossian AG (1996) Personal communication
83 Ukai S, Hara C, Kiho T (1982) Polysaccharides in fungi IX, a beta-D-glucan from alkaline extract of *Dictyophora indusiata*, Fisch. *Chem Pharm Bull* 30(6): 2147–2154
84 Damas J, Remacle-Volon G (1982) Kinins and edema induced by different carrageenans (author's transl). *Pharmacol* 13(2): 225–239
85 Salvemini D, Wang Z-Q, Wyatt PS, Bourdon DM, Marino MH, Manning PT, Currie MG (1996) Nitric oxide: a key mediator in the early and late phase of carrageenan-induced rat paw inflammation. *Br J Pharm* 118: 829–838
86 Meller ST, Cummings CP, Traub RJ, Gebhart GF (1994) The role of nitric oxide in the development and maintenance of the hyperalgesia produced by intraplantar injection of carrageenan in the rat. *Neuroscience* 60(2): 367–374
87 Puhlman J (1989) *Immunologisch aktive Polysaccharide aus den Herbadrogen von* Achyrocline satureioides *(Lam) DC und* Arnica montana *L sowie aus* Arnica montana *L Zellkulturen.* PhD Thesis, University of Munich, Germany

88 Kiho T, Sakai M, Ukai S, Hara C, Tanaka Y (1985) Anti-inflammatory effect of the polysaccharide from the fruit bodies of *Auricularia* species. *Carbohydr Res* 142(2): 344–351

89 Damas J, Volon G (1979) Sur l'inhibition de l'oedème à la carragénine par la carragénine elle-même [Inhibition of carrageenan edema by carrageenan itself]. *CR Soc Biol* 173(3): 637–643

90 Hara C, Kiho T, Tanaka Y, Ukai S (1982) Anti-inflammatory activity and conformational behavior of a branched (1-3)-beta-D-glucan from an alkaline extract of *Dictyophora indusiata* Fisch. *Carbohydr Res* 110(1): 77–88

91 Hara C, Ukai S (1995) Kinugasatake, *Dictyophora indusiata* Fisch: Biological activities. *Food Reviews International* 11(1): 225–230

92 Fujiwara T, Takeda T, Ogihara Y, Shimizu M, Nomura T, Tomita Y (1984) Further studies on the structure of polysaccharides from the bark of *Melia azadirachta. Chem Pharm Bull* 32(4): 1385–1391

93 Saito K, Nishijima M, Ohno N, Nagi N, Yadomae T, Miyazaki T (1992) Activation of complement and *Limulus* coagulation systems by an alkali-soluble glucan isolated from *Omphalia lapidescens* and its less-branched derivatives (Studies on fungal polysaccharide XXXIX). *Chem Pharm Bull* 40(5): 1227–1230

94 Suzuki, T, Ohno N, Saito K, Yadomae T (1992) Activation of the complement system by (1-3)-beta-D-glucans having different degrees of branching and different ultrastructures. *J Pharmacobio-Dyn* 15(6): 277–285

95 Ohno N, Saito K, Nemoto J, Kaneko S, Adachi Y, Nishijima M, Miyazaki T, Yadomae T (1993) Immunopharmacological characterization of a highly branched fungal (1-3)-beta-D-glucan OL-2 isolated from *Omphalia lapidescens. Biol Pharm Bull* 16(4): 414–419

96 Knaus U (1989) *Komplementaktive Verbindungen aus der grünlippigen Muschel Perna canaliculus (Gmelin) sowie niederen und höheren Pflanzen.* PhD Thesis, Ludwig-Maximilians-Universität, München, Germany

97 Miller TE, Dodd J, Ormrod DJ, Geddes R (1993) Anti-inflammatory activity of glycogen extracted from *Perna canaliculus* (NZ green-lipped mussel). *Agents Actions* 38(SPEC CONF ISSUE): C139–C142

98 Tomoda M, Gonda R, Ohara N, Shimizu N, Shishido C, Fujiki Y (1994) A glucan having reticuloendothelial system-potentiating and anti-complementary activities from the tuber of *Pinellia ternata. Biol Pharm Bull* 17(6): 859–861

99 Gonda R, Tomoda M, Shimizu N, Ohara N, Takagi H, Hoshino S (1994) Characterization of an acidic polysaccharide with immunological activities from the tuber of *Pinellia ternata. Biol Pharm Bull* 17(12): 1549–1553

100 Zhang DY, Mori M, Hall IH, Lee KH (1991) Anti-inflammatory agents V. Amylose from *Pinellia ternata. Int J Pharmacognosy* 29(1): 29–32

101 Sendl A (1992) *Chemisch-Analytische und Pharmakologische Untersuchungen von Allium ursinum L und Sedum telephium L.* PhD Thesis, Ludwig-Maximilians-Universität, München, Germany

[102 Kato M, Takeda T, Ogihara Y, Shimizu M, Nomura T, Tomita Y (1985) Studies on the structure of polysaccharide from Tetragonia tetragonoides I. *Chem Pharm Bull* 33(9): 3675–3680

103 Wagner H, Willer F, Kreher B (1989) Biologisch aktive Verbindungen aus dem Wasserextrakt von *Urtica dioica. Planta Med* 55(5): 452–454

104 Willer F (1992) *Chemie und Pharmakologie der Polysaccharide und Lektine von Urtica dioica (Lin)*. PhD Thesis, Ludwig-Maximilians-Universität, München, Germany

105 Hodgson I (1991) Carbohydrate-based therapeutics. *Biotechnology* 9: 609–613

106 Kraus J (1990) Biopolymere mit antitumoraler und immunmodulierender Wirkung. *Pharmazie in unserer Zeit* 19(4): 157–164

Chemistry, analysis and immunological investigations of *Echinacea* phytopharmaceuticals

Rudolf Bauer

Institut für Pharmazeutische Biologie, Heinrich-Heine-Universität, Universitätsstr. 1, D-40225 Düsseldorf, Germany

Introduction

Echinacea phytopharmaceuticals represent the most popular group of herbal immunostimulants in Europe and in the USA [1, 2]. According to a recent report, *Echinacea* products have been the best selling herbal products in natural food stores in the USA in 1997 with 11.93% (1996: 9.6%) of herbal supplement sales [3]. Including homeopathic preparations, more than 800 *Echinacea*-containing drugs are currently on the market in Germany. Most of the preparations contain the expressed sap of *Echinacea purpurea* aerial parts, or hydroalcoholic tinctures of *E.* pallida or *E. purpurea* roots. They are mainly used for the treatment of colds and infections [4]. Clinical effects have been demonstrated for the expressed sap of the aerial parts of *Echinacea purpurea* in the adjuvant therapy of relapsing infections of the respiratory and urinary tracts, as well as for alcoholic tinctures of *E. pallida* and *E. purpurea* roots as adjuvants in the therapy of the common cold and flu [5, 6]. In the USA, it is mostly encapsulated powders from roots and aerial parts, but also tinctures from the roots and aerial parts that are used. Many investigations of the constituents of *Echinacea* have been undertaken. So far, compounds from the classes of caffeic acid derivatives, flavonoids, polyacetylenes, alkamides, pyrrolizidine alkaloids, polysaccharides and glycoproteins have been isolated [7]. For the main interest of finding the active component, but also for standardization purposes, the question on the chemical composition of *Echinacea* herbs and preparations is essential. Therefore, the present knowledge on the chemical constituents, analysis, and immunomodulatory effects of *Echinacea* preparations shall be reviewed.

Botanical variation of *Echinacea* phytopharmaceuticals

The genus *Echinacea* is endemic in North America and comprises nine species and two varieties [8]. Three species are used medicinally: *Echinacea purpurea* (L.)

Moench, *E. angustifolia* DC. and *E. pallida* (Nutt.) Nutt. Preparations are either prepared from the roots (mainly from *E. angustifolia* and *E. pallida*, but also from *E. purpurea*), from the aerial parts (*E. purpurea*), or from the whole plant (homeopathic tinctures of *E. angustifolia* and *E. pallida*).

Echinacea angustifolia was the plant originally used by H.C.F. Meyer and by Lloyd-Brothers Inc. in the USA in the last century [9]. Also the Native Americans preferred that species [10]. However, *E. pallida* is much more abundant and much taller with bigger roots than *E. angustifolia*. When the monograph in the National Formulary of the US was published in 1916, the roots of both *E. angustifolia* and *E. pallida* were made official, with the result that differentiation between these two species was further neglected. It ended in the very confusing situation, that most of "*Echinacea angustifolia*" available in the market and in botanical gardens in Europe was in fact *E. pallida* [11, 12]. *E. purpurea* was introduced as a medicinal plant in Europe in the middle of this century by G. Madaus [13]. The roots and the aerial parts are used for medicinal purposes in a similar way as the other *Echinacea* species.

When dealing with the pharmaceutical quality and pharmacological activity of *Echinacea* preparations, it is important to distinguish between the different species, parts of the plants, and the various extraction modes. Since aerial parts and roots of *Echinacea purpurea*, and the roots of *Echinacea angustifolia* and *Echinacea pallida* are the most important raw materials of *Echinacea* phytopharmaceuticals, the constituents and immunological effects of these parts shall be especially reviewed.

Preparations from *Echinacea angustifolia* roots

Chemical constituents and analysis

Essential oil

The roots of *Echinacea angustifolia* usually contain only ca. 0.1% essential oil [5, 14, 15]. Bischoff [16], who reported an essential oil content of 1.25–1.5%, must have used the roots of *E. pallida* for his studies. The main components of the essential oil of *E. angustifolia* are compounds such as dodeca-2,4-diene-1-yl-isovalerate, as well as palmitic and linoleic acids [14]. One other major constituent (44% of the oil) has been identified as pentadeca-1,8Z-diene, a minor one as 1-pentadecene [17]. A further volatile compound, (*E*)-10-hydroxy-4,10-dimethyl-4,11-dodecadiene-2-one ("Echinolon"), published as a constituent of "*Echinacea angustifolia* roots" [18], is probably from the adulterant *E. pallida*. Pentadeca-8Z-en-2-one, already reported by Schulte et al. [19] as a major constituent of "*Echinacea angustifolia*", is presumably derived from *E. pallida*, since Heinzer et al. [14] found it as one of the main components only in the root oil of *E. pallida*. It is also very probable that this compound is identical with the substance reported by Verelis [20] as geranyl-isobutyrate, because Heinzer et al. [14] failed to detect geranyl-isobutyrate in *E. angustifolia* and *E. pallida*, but found the former compound at a concentration of about 0.4%.

Neugebauer [21] was the first to suggest determination of the essential oil content for the quality control of *Echinacea* preparations. Since the content in *Echinacea angustifolia* is so low, this seems not to be a suitable method for this species. Gas chromatography (GC) analysis of the essential oil, however, can be used for the discrimination and identification of the roots of the three major *Echinacea* species (Fig. 1) [14].

Polyacetylenes

According to our present knowledge, the polyacetylenes published as constituents of "*Echinacea angustifolia* roots" [19, 22] are presumably derived from *E. pallida*. It was shown by Heinzer et al. [14] that authentic *Echinacea angustifolia* contains only traces of pentadeca-8Z,11Z-dien-2-one, pentadeca-8Z,13Z-dien-11-yn-2-one and tetradeca-8Z-en-11,13-diyn-2-one which can be detected by GC (Fig. 1).

Alkamides

In total, 15 alkamides have been identified in *E. angustifolia* roots as major lipophilic constituents [23–25]. They are mainly derived from undeca- and dodecanoic acid, and differ in the degree of unsaturation and the configuration of the double bonds (Fig. 2). The predominant structural type is a 2-monoene-8,10-diynoic acid isobutylamide, but also some 2'-methyl-butylamides have been found. The main constituents are the isomeric dodeca-2*E*,4*E*,8*Z*,10*E*/*Z*-tetraenoic acid isobutylamides. In addition, the isobutylamides of undeca-2Z-en-8,10-diynoic acid, dodeca-2*E*-en-8,10-diynoic acid, dodeca-2*E*,4*Z*-dienoic acid and hexadeca-2*E*, 9Z-dien-12,14-diynoic acid, as well as the 2'-methyl-butylamides of undeca-2Z-en-8,10-diynoic acid and dodeca-2*E*-en-8,10-diynoic acid were found in lipophilic extracts of *E. angustifolia* roots. Another constituent, undeca-2*E*-en-8,10-diynoic acid isobutylamide, has already been isolated from *Acmella ciliata* [26]. The isobutylamides of undeca-2*E*,4*E*-dien-8,10-diynoic acid, undeca-2*Z*, 4*E*-dien-8,10-diynoic acid and dodeca-2*E*,4*Z*-dien-8,10-diynoic acid are present only in very low concentrations in *E. angustifolia* roots, but were found as major constituents in the roots of *E. purpurea* (Fig. 9) [25, 27].

According to the literature [28, 23], the roots of *E. angustifolia* contain 0.01% of a polyunsaturated alkamide "echinacein" (dodeca-2*E*,6*Z*,8*E*,10*E*-tetraenoic acid isobutylamide), which has never been detected since. Greger [29] also doubts that a compound with the structure quoted (= neoherculin) occurs in *Echinacea*. Verelis [20] found the isobutylamides of dodeca-2*E*,4*E*-dienoic acid and deca-2*E*,4*E*,6*E*-trienoic acid in "*E. angustifolia* roots", but it can be suspected that he has examined *E. pallida*.

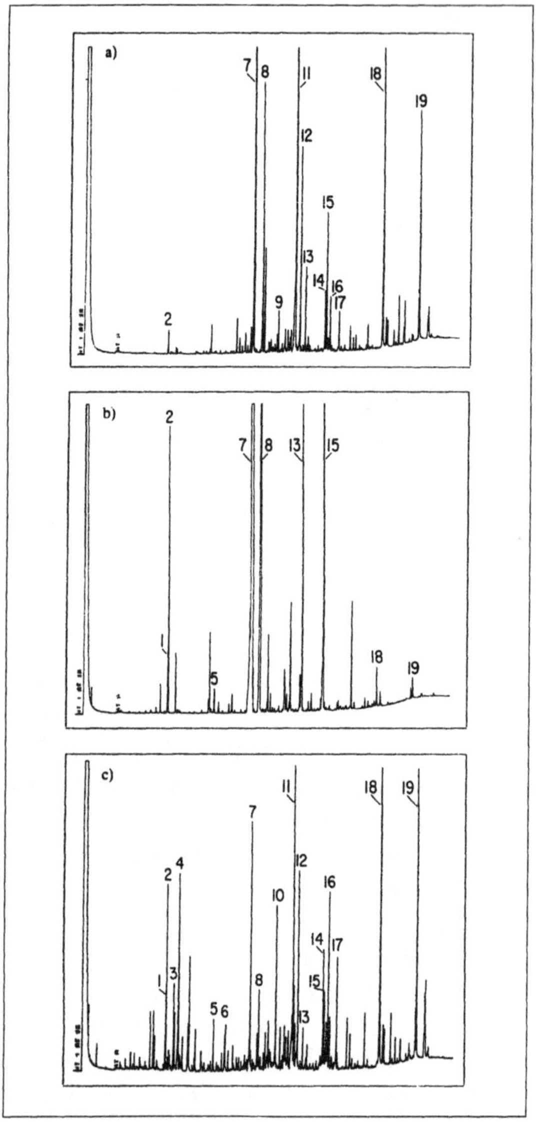

Figure 1

Gas chromatograms of the essential oils from the roots of Echinacea angustifolia *(a), E. pallida (b) and* E. purpurea *(c). From [14].*

1 = 1-Pentadecene; 2 = 1,8-pentadecadiene; 3 = 1,8,11-pentadecatriene; 4 = germacrene D; 5 = a tridecen-2-one; 6 = epishyobunol; 7 = 8Z-pentadecen-2-one; 8 = pentadeca-8Z,11Z-dien-2-one; 9 = dodeca-2,4-dien-1-ol; 10 = α-cadinol (?); 11 = dodeca-2E,4E-dien-1-yl-isovalerate; 12 = a dodecatrienyl-isovalerate (?); 13 = pentadeca-8,13-dien-11-yn-2-one; 14 = tetradeca-8-en-11,13-diyn-2-one; 15, 16, 17 = n.n. alkenyl-isovalerates; 18 = palmitic acid; 19 = linoleic acid.

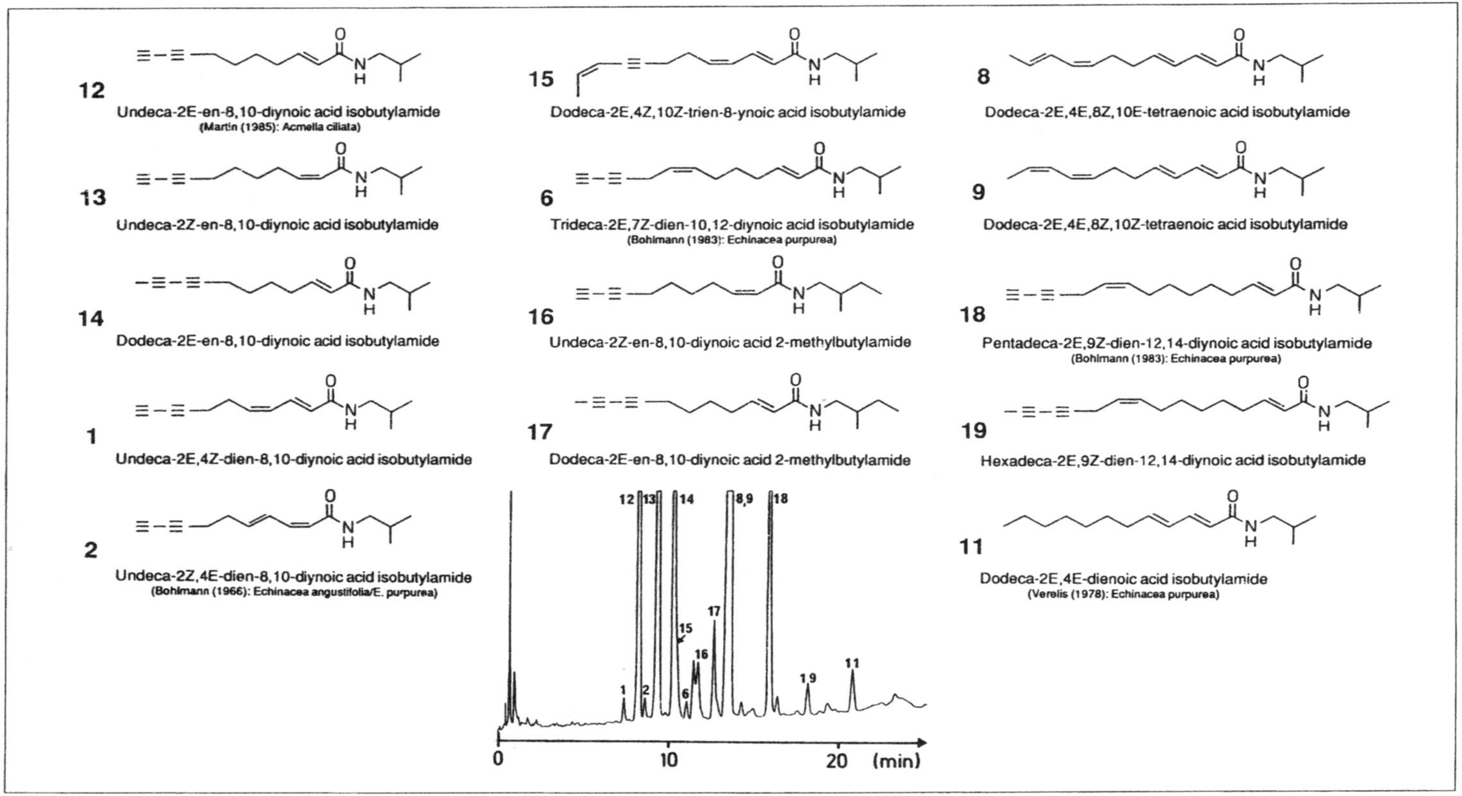

Figure 2
HPLC separation of an alcoholic extract from Echinacea angustifolia *roots with alkamides. From [4].*
Separation parameters: column: Hibar 125-4 with LiChrospher 100 CH-18 (2), 5 μm (Merck); solvents: A = water, B = acetonitrile; gradient: 40–80% B linearly in 30 min; flow rate: 1.0 ml/min; detection: 210 nm.

By HPLC analysis (RP 18; solvent gradient: 40–80% acetonitrile/water; flow: 1.0 ml/min) and photodiode array detection, the different types of alkamides can easily be identified by their retention times and UV-spectra [30]. HPLC analysis is therefore especially suitable for the identification of *E. angustifolia* roots in phytopreparations (see Fig. 2). It is also the most reliable way for the discrimination of extracts from *E. angustifolia* and *E. pallida* roots (see Fig. 7) [31] and for the detection of adulterations with roots of *Parthenium integrifolium* (Fig. 10) [32]. Also TLC can be used (silica gel; solvent: *n*-hexane-ethylacetate (2:1); detection: anisaldehyde/sulfuric acid), but with less significance [30].

HPLC can also be used for the quantitative determination of the alkamides using external standard calibration [30, 31]. Roots of *E. angustifolia* were shown to contain 0.01–0.15% alkamides and therefore a higher amount than *E. purpurea* roots [30]. Consequently, the alkamides are well suited for the standardization of corresponding phytopharmaceuticals.

Alkaloids

The occurrence of a "colourless alkaloid" in *Echinacea angustifolia* was first reported by Lloyd [33]. Heyl and Staley [34] doubted the occurrence of classical alkaloids in *E. angustifolia* roots, and Heyl and Hart [35] finally isolated betaine hydrochloride as the only N-containing compound. Röder et al. [36] and Britz-Kirstgen [37] detected the pyrrolizidine alkaloids tussilagin and isotussilagin in *E. angustifolia* roots and reported a content of 0.006% tussilagin for the dried drug. According to the structure-toxicity relationships elucidated by Mattocks [38], a 1,2-unsaturated necine ring system is necessary for the hepatotoxicity of pyrrolizidine alkaloids. Since neither tussilagin nor isotussilagin contain this structure, they are unlikely to cause liver damage.

Caffeic acid derivatives

Stoll et al. [39] isolated echinacoside from the roots of *Echinacea angustifolia*. It is the major polar constituent and is present at a concentration of 0.3–1.7% [15, 31, 39–41]. It occurs in *E. pallida* at a similar concentration and is therefore not suitable for the discrimination of these two species [42]. However, they can be distinguished by the occurrence of 1,3- and 1,5-O-dicaffeoyl-quinic acids (Fig. 3), which are only present in the roots of *E. angustifolia* [31].

For quality control, extracts can be analyzed either by TLC (silica gel; ethylacetate/formic acid/acetic acid/water 100:11:11:27; detection: natural product reagent/UV 360 nm) or by HPLC (RP 18 solvent gradient: 5–25% acetonitrile/phosphoric acid; flow: 1.0 ml/min; detection: 280 nm) as shown in Fig. 4 [31]. Echinacoside is used as an analytical marker compound to test batch-to-batch consistency and for the standardization of preparations from *E. angustifolia* roots. However,

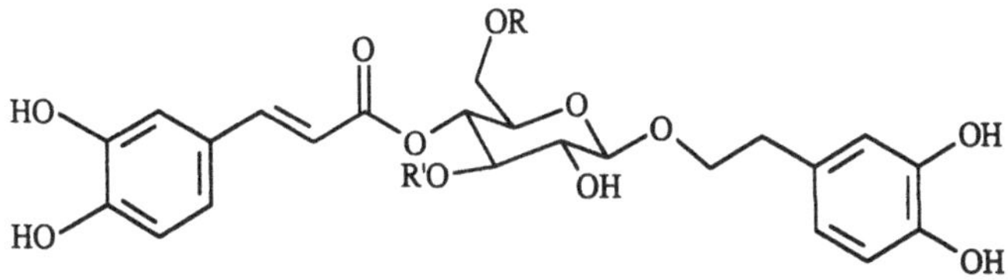

	R	R'
Echinacoside	Glucose (1,6-)	Rhamnose (1,3-)
6-O-Caffeoyl-echinacoside	6-O-Caffeoyl-glucose (1,6-)	Rhamnose (1,3-)
Verbascoside	H	Rhamnose (1,3-)
Desrhamnosyl-verbascoside	H	H

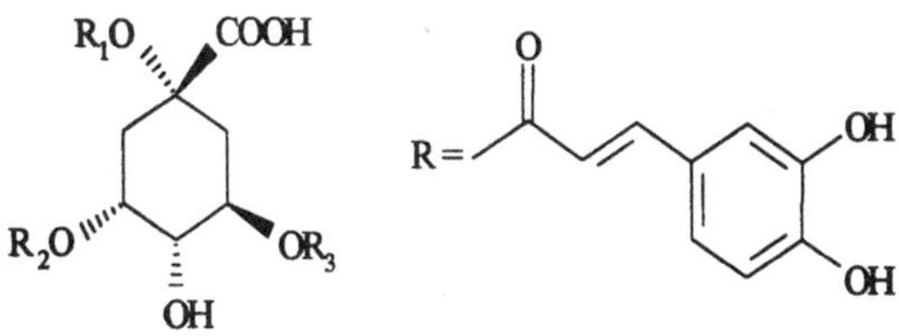

	R_1	R_2	R_3
Quinic acid	H	H	H
Chlorogenic acid	H	R	H
1,3-Dicaffeoyl-quinic acid (Cynarin)	R	R	H
1,5-Dicaffeoyl-quinic acid	R	H	R

Figure 3
Phenylpropanoid glycosides and quinic acid derivatives found in Echinacea *species.*

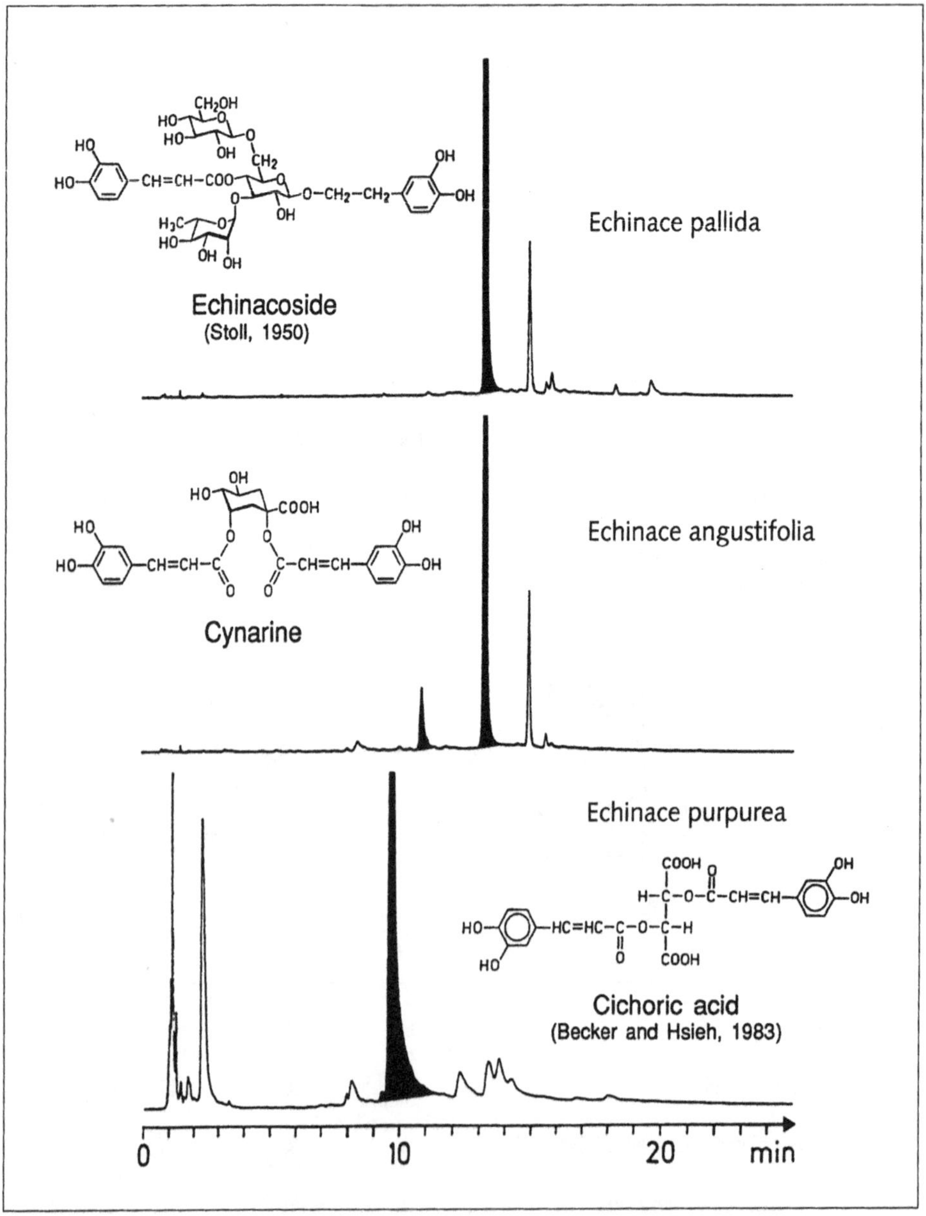

Figure 4
HPLC profiles of alcoholic extracts from Echinacea roots with caffeic acid derivatives. From [4].
Separation parameters: column: Hibar 125-4 with LiChrospher 100 CH-18 (2), 5 µm (Merck); solvents: A = water + 1% 0.1 N-phosphoric acid, B = acetonitrile + 1% 0.1 N-phosphoric acid; gradient: 5–25% B linearly in 20 min; flow rate: 1.0 ml/min; detection: 330 nm.

methods using cynarine as an internal standard [43] should not be used since cynarine is a genuine constituent of *E. angustifolia.*

Capillary electrophoresis (micellar electrokinetic chromatography MEKC) has also proven to be an effective method for the analysis of caffeic acid derivatives [44]. The method provides an excellent resolution and a very high sensitivity and enables the discrimination of the species (see Fig. 5).

Recently, automated multiple development (AMD) thin layer chromatography has been applied for the analyis of caffeic acid derivatives in *E. angustifolia* root extracts [45, 46]. The separation was performed on silica plates (Sil G-50 UV 254) and AMD was achieved in 25 steps using methanol, ethylacetate, toluene, 1,2-dichloroethane, 25% ammonia solution, and anhydrous formic acid as modifiers. For the screening of echinacoside in crude plant extracts, a fast-atom-bombardment tandem mass spectrometry method has been developed [47, 48].

Polysaccharides and glycoproteins

Heyl and Staley [34] reported an inulin content of 5.9% for the roots of *Echinacea angustifolia.* Bonadeo et al. [49] isolated a pseudocrystalline substance ("echinacina B") from *E. angustifolia* with weak anti-hyaluronidase activity. It was characterized as a polysaccharide mixture, consisting mainly of an acidic mucopolysaccharide. A raw polysaccharide fraction from *E. angustifolia* roots was also isolated by Wagner et al. [50]. However, this has not yet been characterized in detail.

Giger et al. [51] investigated the fructan content of *E. angustifolia* and found that the content of total fructose in the roots was lowest in May, increasing during the summer and autumn.

Three glycoproteins, MW 17,000, 21,000 and 30,000 Da, containing ca. 3% protein, have been isolated from *E. angustifolia* and *E. purpurea* roots. The dominant sugars were found to be arabinose (64 - 84%), galactose (1.9–5.3%) and glucosamines (6%). The protein moiety contained high amounts of aspartate, glycine, glutamate and alanine [52]. An ELISA method has been developed for the detection and determination of these glycoproteins in *Echinacea* preparations [53]. It seems that *E. angustifolia* and *E. purpurea* roots contain similar amounts of glycoproteins, while *E. pallida* contains less [57].

Immunological effects

Since *E. angustifolia* and *E. pallida* have been mixed up frequently in the past, it is hard to say in older studies (before 1985) which species has been used.

An ethanolic extract obtained from the roots of *E. angustifolia* (1:10) in a concentration of 10^{-3}% enhanced phagocytosis of yeast particles by human polymorphonuclear neutrophils (PMN) *in vitro* by 17%. There was no activity observed

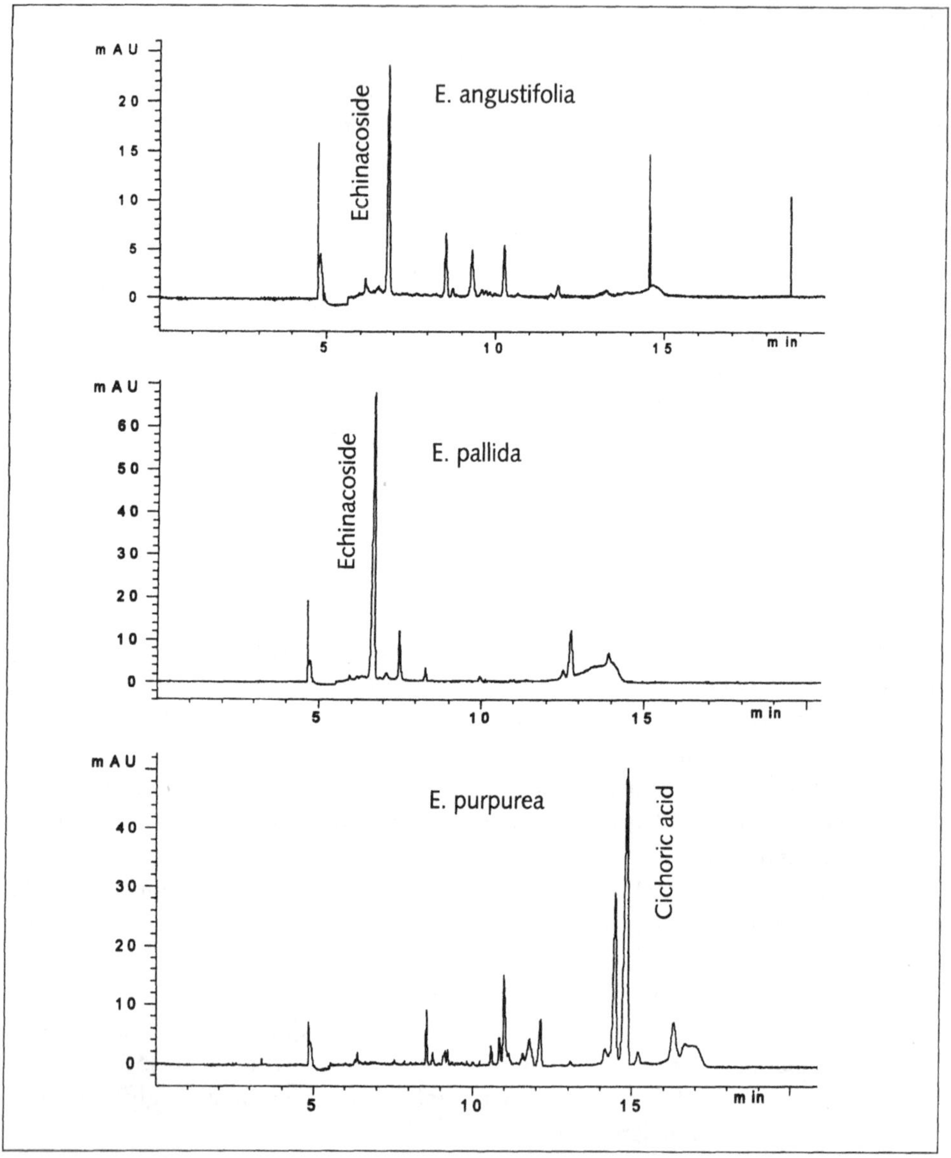

Figure 5

Electropherograms of a mixture of phenolic constituents in Echinacea root extracts separated by MEKC analysis. From [44].

Separation parameters: 3DCE system with diode array detector (Hewlett-Packard, Waldbronn, Germany); uncoated fused-silica capillary 58 cm (50 cm to the detector) ×50 μm i.d.; 3D extended light path (bubble cell) from Hewlett-Packard; running buffer: 25 mM tetraborate, pH 8.6, containing 30 mM SDS; injections by positive pressure (50–200 mbar × sec corresponding to about 1–4 nl); voltage: +20 kV; temperature: 30° C; detection: 320 nm.

below a concentration of 10^{-5}%. The chloroform soluble part of the extract, which contained the alkamides, stimulated phagocytosis by 34% at a concentration of 10^{-4}% (Fig. 6) [54, 55]. Also *in vivo*, in mice, *per os* administration of 10 ml/kg b.w./day of a solution of 0.5 ml of the ethanolic extract in 30 ml normal saline solution enhanced phagocytosis of carbon particles by a factor of 1.7 [54]. The lipophilic alkamide fraction at a dose of 0.33 mg/kg b.w./day enhanced phagocytosis in the carbon-clearance assay by a factor of 1.5 [55]. The main constituent, dodeca-2*E*,4*E*,8*Z*,10*E*/*Z*-tetraenoic acid isobutylamide, only exhibited weak activity. Therefore, the most effective constituent remains to be found.

Alkamides also displayed marked inhibitory activity *in vitro* in the 5-lipoxygenase (porcine leukocytes) and cyclooxygenase (microsomes from ram seminal vesicles) assays. Dodeca-2*E*,4*E*,8*Z*,10*E*/*Z*-tetraenoic acid isobutylamides inhibited cyclooxygenase-1 at a concentration of 50 µg/ml by 54.7% and 5-lipoxygenase at a concentration of 50 µM by 62.2% [56].

A raw polysaccharide fraction of *Echinacea angustifolia* (*E. pallida*?) roots stimulated phagocytosis in mice, determined in the carbon-clearance assay, at a dosis of 10 mg/kg b.w. and also enhanced phagocytosis of human PMN *in vitro* by 32% at a concentration of 0.01 mg/ml [50]. Purified extracts containing a glycoprotein-polysaccharide complex exhibited B-cell stimulating activity and induced the release of interleukin 1, TNFα und IFNα,β both *in vitro* and *in vivo* [57–59].

Echinacoside protected dose-dependently the free radical-induced degradation of Type III collagen by a reactive oxygen scavenging effect [60]. The authors conclude a protective activity of *Echinacea* polyphenols against photodamage of the skin. Echinacoside and other phenylpropanoid glycosides from *Pedicularis* were able to protect against oxidative hemolysis *in vitro* [61].

A stimulatory effect was observed on the lysosomal and peroxidal activity of peritoneal macrophages and splenic cells after five days *in vivo* treatment of C57BL6 inbred mice with the ethanolic extract of the roots of *E. angustifolia* [62, 63].

By flow cytometric analysis, phagocytosis of flourescent labelled latex particles by human PMNs was measured *in vitro* after 30 min preincubation with different concentrations of a *E. angustifolia* (*E. pallida*?) mother tincture. At a concentration of 10^{-4}% a maximal stimulation of 29.5% was observed [64].

In an *in vivo* study with mice, which received *per os* or i.p. a lyophilisate of *E. angustifolia* (*E. pallida*?) mother tincture (2.5, 25 or 250 mg/kg b.w.), no influence on carbon clearance was observed [65]. However, the identity of the mother tincture is not clear and the preparation seems to have been void of active lipophilic constituents. Therefore, the results need also to be reconfirmed.

When 0.1 ml/kg b.w. *E. angustifolia* (*Echinacea pallida*?) mother tincture was applied per os to normal leghorn (HNL) chicken, 5–9 days after application 32% elevated IgG (day 7) and IgA (day 9) levels were found. The IgM value was increased by only 8% (day 7). A dose of 0.4 ml/kg b.w. only enhanced the IgA level

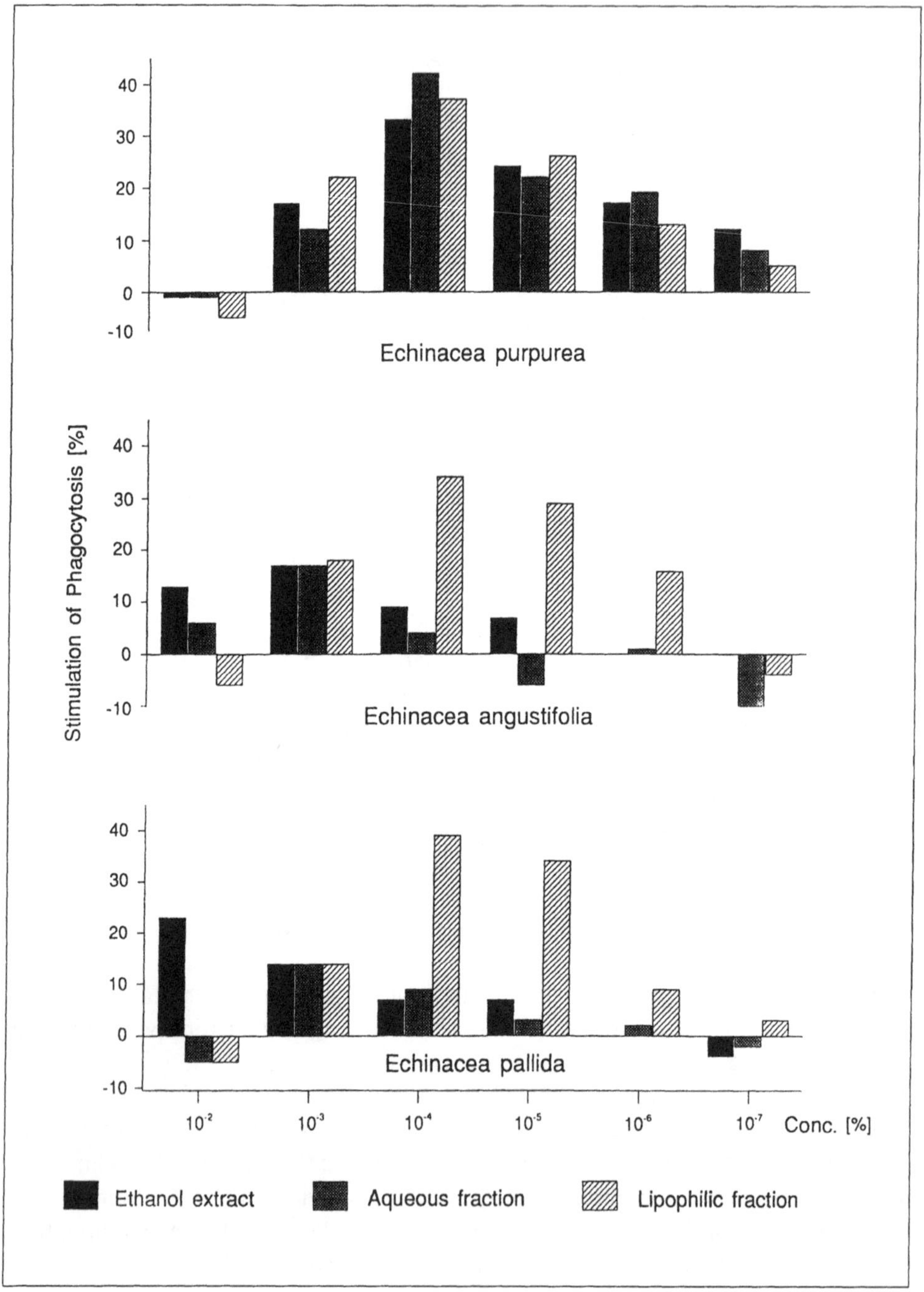

Figure 6

Effects of ethanolic extracts (DEV 6:1) of Echinacea *roots and fractions prepared thereof on phagocytosis of human granulocytes* in vitro. *From [54].*

by 28% [66]. Since the identity and the quality of the mother tincture is not clear, the results need also to be reconfirmed.

The essential oil of *E. angustifolia* reduced tumour weight in rats with Walker Carcinosarcoma 256 (WA) by 69% at a dosis of 400 mg/kg b.w. and increased survival time of mice with P-388 lymphatic leukemia (PS) by 100%. (*Z*)-1,8-Pentadecadiene, which was isolated from the oil, increased survival time by 27% at 100 mg/kg b.w. and reduced tumour weight by 86% [17].

4 Preparations from *Echinacea pallida* roots

Chemical constituents and analysis

Essential oil and polyacetylenes

Echinacea pallida roots contain a high amount (0.2–2.0%) of essential oil [5, 14, 15, 21, 67–69]. Main constituents are pentadeca-8*Z*-en-2-one [19], pentadeca-1, 8*Z*-diene (44% of the oil) and 1-pentadecene (Fig. 1) [17, 70]. In addition, pentadeca-8*Z*,11*Z*-dien-2-one, pentadeca-8*Z*, 13*Z*-dien-11-yn-2-one and tetradeca-8*Z*-en-11,13-diyn-2-one are occurring [14] and probably also (*E*)-10-hydroxy-4,10-dimethyl-4,11-dodecadien-2-one ("echinolon") [18]. These ketoalkenes and ketoalkynes are also the major lipophilic constituents of *E. pallida* roots. Other constituents of this type are pentadeca-8*Z*-ene-11,13-diyn-2-one, pentadeca-8*Z*,11*Z*, 13*E*-triene-2-one, and pentadeca-8*Z*,11*E*,13*Z*-triene-2-one (Fig. 7) [12, 19, 71]. According to Schulte et al. [19], who probably examined *E. pallida* instead of *E. angustifolia*, only 2 mg% polyacetylenes (calculated on airdried material) with trideca-1-en-3,5,7,9,11-pentayne and ponticaepoxide as main compounds are present.

It has been observed that these compounds were oxidized by atmospheric oxygen, especially when the roots are stored in powdered form [71]. When this occurrs, hydroxylated artifacts, 8-hydroxy-tetradeca-9*E*-ene-11,13-diyn-2-one, 8-hydroxy-pentadeca-9*E*-ene-11,13-diyn-2-one, and 8-hydroxypentadeca-9*E*,13*Z*-diene-11-yn-2-one can be detected in the roots (see Fig. 8), often with only small residual quantities of the native compounds [72]. The artifacts are presumably produced by autoxidation (allyl oxidation) of the native constituents, as already described by Bohlmann et al. [22] for similar compounds. Therefore, the roots should be stored in whole form.

The ketoalkenyns cannot be detected in *E. angustifolia* and *E. purpurea* roots. So they are suitable markers for the identification of preparations from *E. pallida* roots. They can be analysed by TLC (silica gel; toluene-ethylacetate 7:3; detection: anisaldehyde/sulfuric acid) or (better) by HPLC (RP 18; solvent gradient: 40–80% acetonitrile/water; flow: 1.0 ml/min; detection: 210 nm) (Figs. 7 and 8) [31]. Since they are not stable, they are not suitable for standardization purposes.

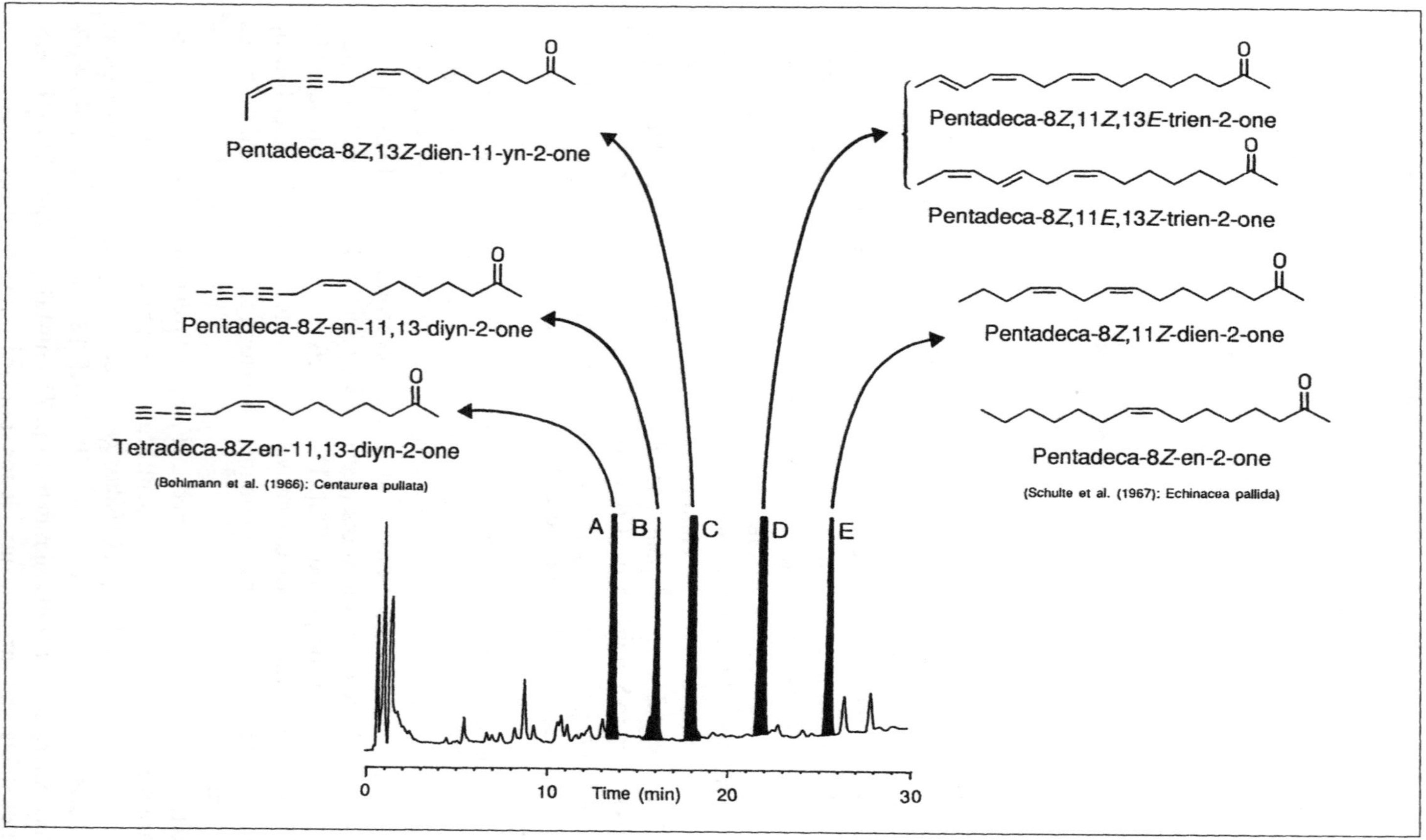

Figure 7
HPLC separation of a methanolic extract of Echinacea pallida *roots with the genuine pattern of ketoalkenes and ketoalkenyns. Separation parameters: see Fig. 2.*

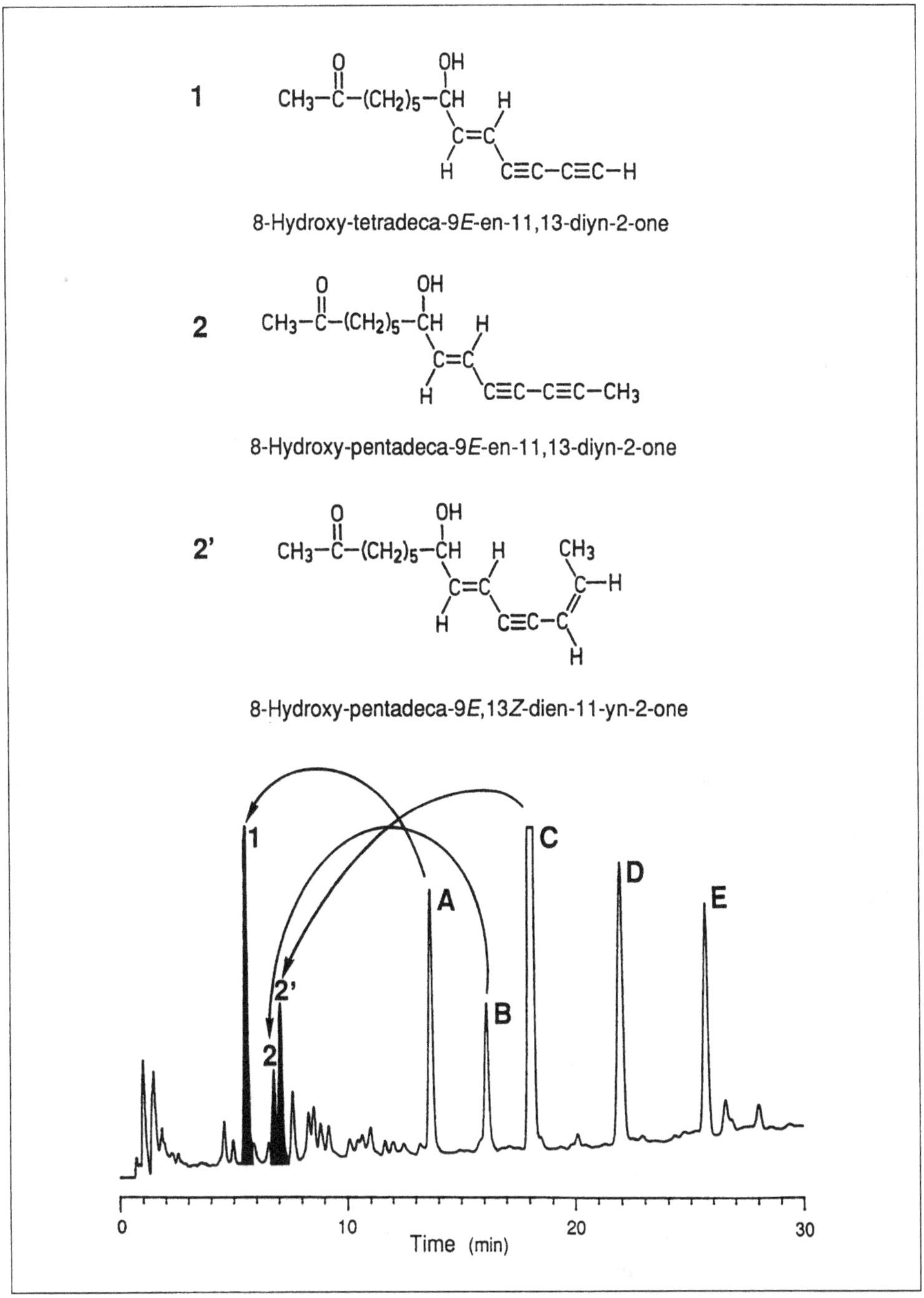

Figure 8
HPLC separation of a methanolic extract of stored powdered Echinacea pallida *roots with hydroxylated artifacts of ketoalkenyns. Separation parameters: see Fig. 2.*

Alkamides

The roots of *E. pallida* should contain 0.001% of echinacein (dodeca-2*E*,6*Z*,8*E*, 10*E*-tetraenoic acid isobutylamide) [23, 28], which, however, has never been confirmed since [29]. The absence of alkamides can be used for the discrimination of *E. angustifolia* roots.

Caffeic acid derivatives

Echinacoside has been found (0.3–1.7%) as a major polar compound in *E. pallida* roots [42]. In low quantity, 6-O-caffeoyl-echinacoside has also been detected [73]. 1,3- and 1,5-O-dicaffeoyl-quinic acid are missing, which is an identity criterion of *E. pallida* roots. Echinacoside is present in *E. angustifolia* as well [31].

Echinacoside is used as an analytical marker compound in the quality control of phytopreparations from *E. pallida* roots. It can be analysed by TLC or HPLC (see *E. angustifolia*, section on *caffeic acid derivatives*) [15, 31]. Recently, capillary electrophoresis (micellar electrokinetic chromatography, MEKC) has also been applied for the analysis of caffeic acid derivatives (see Fig. 5) [44].

Polysaccharides and glycoproteins

There is no information in the literature on polysaccharides from *E. pallida* roots. However, it may be suspected that research performed with *E. angustifolia* before 1985 may have erroneously used *E. pallida.*

Using an ELISA method which has been developed for the detection and determination of glycoproteins in *Echinacea* preparations [53], it was found that *E. pallida* roots contain less glycoproteins than *E. angustifolia* and *E. purpurea* roots [57].

Immunological effects

An ethanolic extract obtained from the roots of *E. pallida* (1:10) at a concentration of 10^{-2}% enhanced phagocytosis of yeast particles by human PMN *in vitro* by 23%. No activity was observed below a concentration of 10^{-6}%. The chloroform soluble part of the extract, which contained the full spectrum of genuine ketoalkenyns, stimulated phagocytosis by 39% at a concentration of 10^{-4}%, while the water soluble part, containing echinacoside, only stimulated by 14% at a concentration of 10^{-3}% [54]. Also *per os* administration of 10 ml/kg b.w./day of a solution of 0.5 ml of the ethanolic extract in 30 ml normal saline solution enhanced phagocytosis of carbon particles by a factor of 2.2 in mice [54]. The lipophilic fraction at the same dose enhanced phagocytosis in the carbon-clearance assay by a factor of 2.6. The water soluble fraction was not active (see Fig. 6) [54].

An alcoholic extract (30% ethanol), standardized on glycoproteins/polysaccharides by an ELISA method, was shown to enhance production of IgM, IL-1, IL-6, TNFα and IFNα,β in NMRI- and C3H/HeJ mouse spleen cell lines [57]. *In vivo* it increased IL-1 concentration in the serum of mice [57].

Echinacoside protected dose-dependently the free radical-induced degradation of Type III collagen by a reactive oxygen scavenging effect [60]. The authors conclude a protective activity of *Echinacea* polyphenols against photodamage of the skin.

Preparations from *Echinacea purpurea* roots

Chemical constituents and analysis

Essential oil

Roots of *Echinacea purpurea* contain up to 0.2% essential oil [4, 14, 15, 21, 67, 69, 74]. According to Becker [75] and Martin [76] it is composed of 2.1% caryophyllene, 0.6% humulene and 1.3% caryophyllene epoxide. Heinzer et al. [14] have analyzed the essential oil by gas chromatography-mass spectrometry (GC-MS) and found compounds of the type dodeca-2,4- dien-1-yl-isovalerate, as well as palmitic and linolenic acid, vanillin, p-hydroxycinnamic acid methyl ester and germacrene D, which had already been reported by Bohlmann and Hoffmann [27] for the aerial parts of the plant. Nevertheless, *E. purpurea* roots are not a typical essential oil drug, and therefore analysis of the essential oil has not been used often for standardization purposes of phytopreparations. However, gas chromatography of the essential oil can be used for the discrimination of the species (see Fig. 1) [14].

Alkamides

Eleven alkamides have beeen identified in *Echinacea purpurea* roots [24, 77]. In contrast to *E. angustifolia*, most of these alkamides possess a 2,4-diene moiety. Bohlmann and Grenz [24] isolated a mixture of two dodeca-2,4,8,10-tetraenoic acid-isobutylamides, whose stereochemistry was not determined, as well as undeca-2*Z*,4*E*-dein-8,10-diynoic acid-isobutylamide and dodeca-2*Z*,4*E*-dien-8,10-diynoic acid-isobutylamide. Bauer et al. [77] found a series of alkamides which were identified as the isobutylamides of undeca-2*E*,4*Z*-dien-8,10-diynoic acid, dodeca-2*E*,4*Z*-dien-8,10-diynoic acid, dodeca-2*E*,4*E*,10*E*-trien-8-ynoic acid and dodeca-2*E*,4*E*,8*Z*-trienoic acid, as well as the 2'-methyl-butylamide of dodeca-2*E*,4*Z*-dien-8,10-diynoic acid. The main compounds, already isolated by Bohlmann and Grenz [24], were shown to be the isomeric mixture of dodeca-2*E*,4*E*,8*Z*,10*E*/*Z*-tetraenoic acid isobutylamides. A further compound, undeca-2*E*,4*Z*-dien-8,10-diynoic acid-2'-methyl-butylamide had already been described as a constituent of *Acmella ciliata* [78]. Alkamides could also be produced in transformed callus and hairy roots of *E. purpurea* which therefore might be a promising source for continuous and standardized production of dodeca-2*E*,4*E*,8*Z*,10*E*/*Z*-tetraenoic acid isobutylamide and related amides [79].

With the aid of HPLC analysis and photodiode array detection (DAD), the different types of alkamides can easily be identified by their different UV-spectra [30]. Hence, the roots of *E. purpurea* and *E. angustifolia* can clearly be discriminated by DAD-HPLC of these lipophilic constituents (see Figs. 2 and 9). Quantitative determination in phytopreparations is also possible by HPLC. The roots of E *purpurea* were found to contain 0.004–0.039% dodeca-2*E*,4*E*,8*Z*,10*E*/*Z*-tetraenoic acid isobutylamide [30]. HPLC analysis of the alkamides in extracts of *Echinacea purpurea* roots would therefore be especially suitable for standardization purposes. An RPLC procedure published recently for the quantitative analyses of alkamide levels in *Echinacea purpurea* extracts [80] is suspected of leading to elevated levels of alkamides and should therefore only be applied after careful recalibration.

Echinacea purpurea roots have been substituted for a long time with *Parthenium integrifolium*. The sesquiterpene esters, echinadiol-, epoxyechinadiol-, echinaxanthol- and dihydroxy-nardol-cinnamate, described as constituents of *Echinacea purpurea* roots [81], were in fact derived from the adulterant *Parthenium integrifolium* which was mistakenly processed at that time. Since both species contain different constituents, HPLC and TLC methods have been developed to distinguish them [32]. *Parthenium integrifolium* is characterized by the sesquiterpene esters (Fig. 10) which cannot be found in *Echinacea* roots.

Caffeic acid derivatives

The roots of *E. purpurea* do not contain echinacoside, but cichoric acid (2*R*,3*R*-dicaffeoyl tartaric acid) and caftaric acid (monocaffeoyl tartaric acid) as shown in Figures 4 and 11. Cichoric acid was first found as a major constituent in the aerial parts of *Echinacea* species [82, 83]. Later it was found that it is abundant also in *Echinacea purpurea* roots and the content has been determined by HPLC to be 0.6–2.1% [84]. Schenk and Franke recently found 0.9% in cultivated material [15]. Cichoric acid undergoes rapid enzymatic degradation (see *Echinacea purpurea* aerial parts, section on *caffeic acid derivatives and phenolic acids*) [84]. Therefore, the quality of phytopreparations needs to be thoroughly checked. For analytical methods, see also *Echinacea purpurea* aerial parts.

Alkaloids

Röder et al. [36] and Hille [85] detected the pyrrolizidine alkaloids tussilagin and isotussilagin in *E. purpurea* roots and reported a content of 0.006% tussilagin for the dried drug. According to the structure-toxicity relationships elucidated by Mattocks [38], a 1,2-unsaturated necine ring system is necessary for the hepatotoxicity

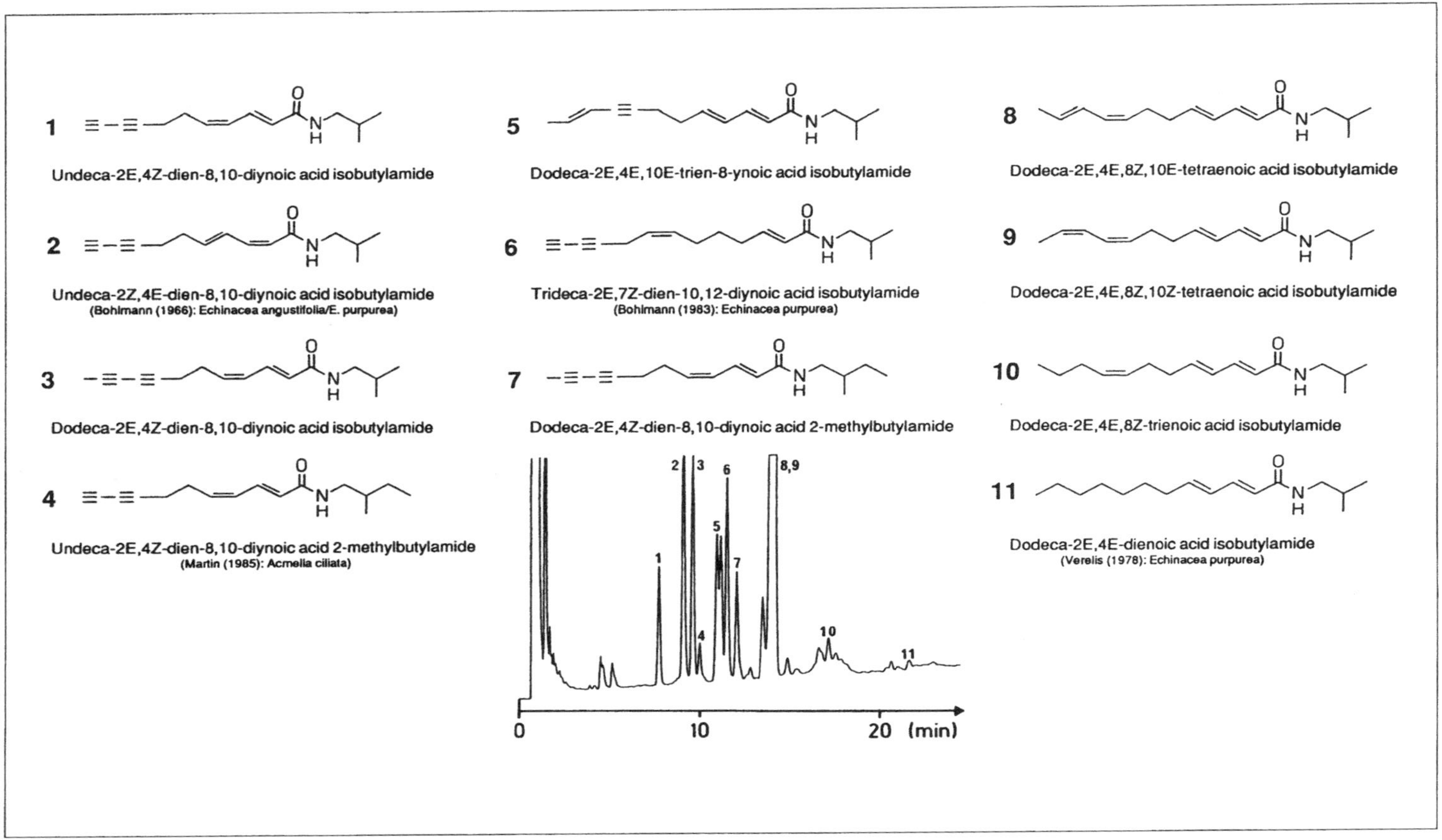

Figure 9
HPLC separation of an alcoholic extract from Echinacea purpurea *roots with alkamides. From [4]. Separation parameters: see Fig. 2.*

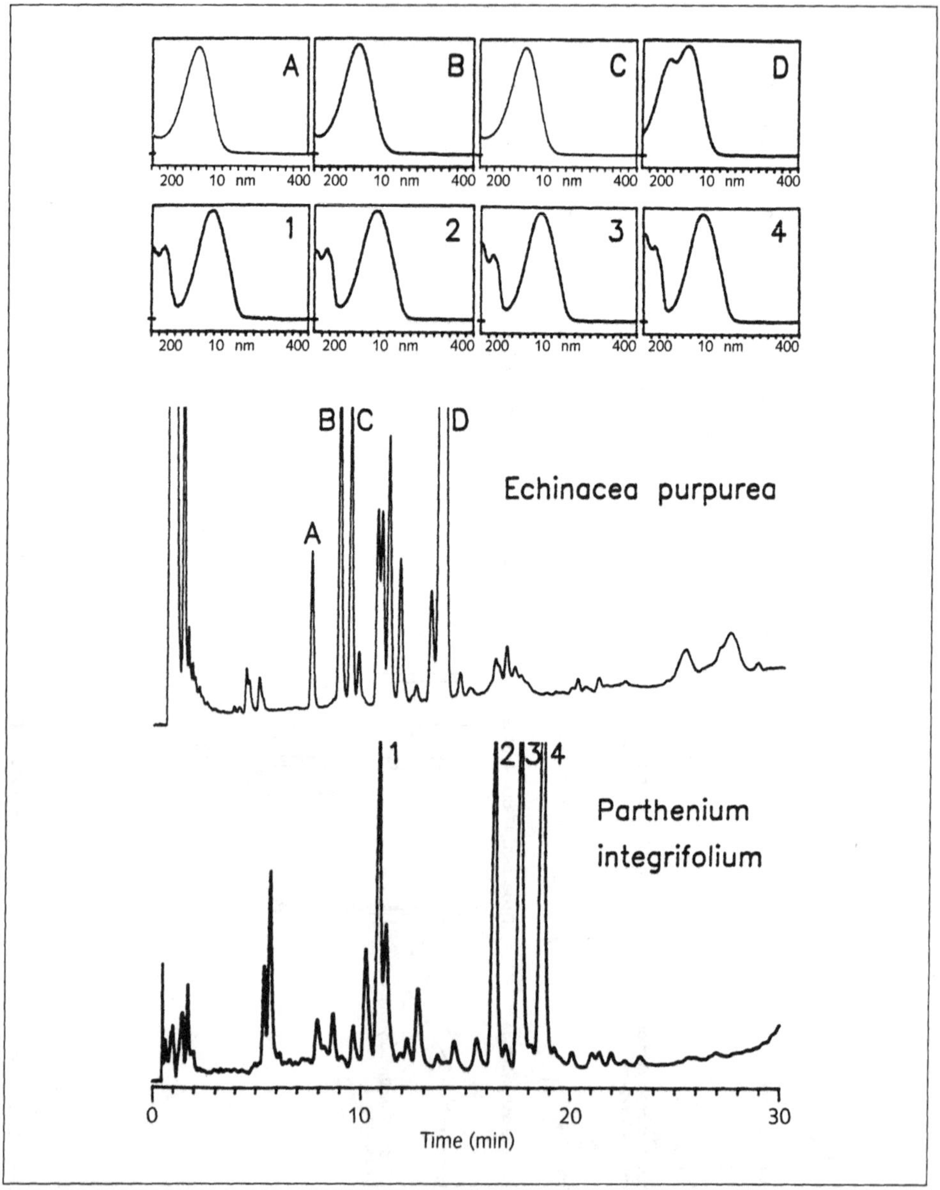

Figure 10

HPLC separation of a lipophilic extract from Parthenium integrifolium *roots, with UV-spectra of the main compounds. Separation parameters: see Fig. 2. From [32].*

A = undeca-2E,4Z-dien-8,10-diynoic acid-isobutylamide; B = undeca-2Z,4E-dien-8,10-diynoic acid-isobutylamide; C = dodeca-2E,4Z-dien-8,10-diynoic acid-isobutylamide; D = dodeca-2E,4E,8Z,10-tetraenoic acid-isobutylamide; 1 = epoxyechinadiol cinnamate; 2 = echinaxanthol cinnamate; 3 = dihydroxy-nardol cinnamate; 4 = echinadiol cinnamate.

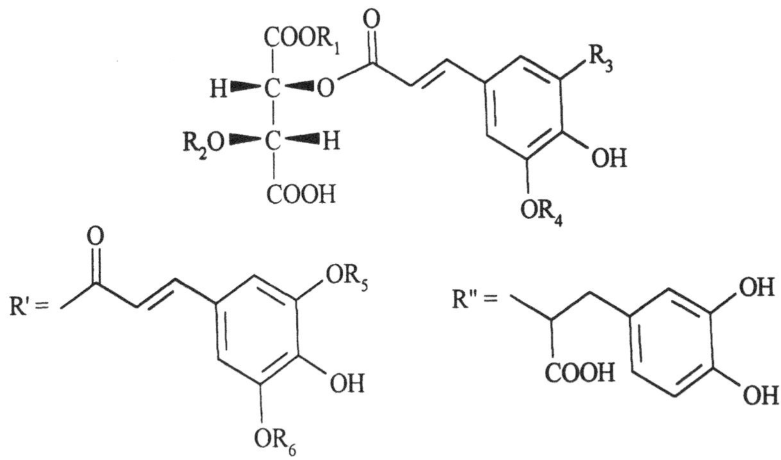

	R_1	R_2	R_3	R_4	R_5	R_6
2-O-Caffeoyl tartaric acid (Caftaric acid)	H	H	OH	H	-	-
2,3-O-Di-caffeoyl tartaric acid (Cichoric acid)	H	R'	OH	H	OH	H
2,3-O-Di-caffeoyl tartaric acid methyl ester	CH_3	R'	OH	H	OH	H
2-O-Feruloyl tartaric acid	H	H	OCH_3	H	-	-
2-O-Caffeoyl-3-O-cumaroyl tartaric acid	H	R'	H	H	H	H
2-O-Caffeoyl-3-O-feruloyl tartaric acid	H	R'	OH	H	OCH_3	H
2,3-O-Di-5-[α-carboxy-β-(3,4-dihydroxy-phenyl)-ethyl] tartaric acid	H	R'	OH	R"	OH	R"
2-O-Caffeoyl-3-O-{5-[α-carboxy-β-(3,4-dihydroxy-phenyl)-ethyl]-caffeoyl} tartaric acid	H	R'	OH	H	OH	R"

Figure 11
Tartaric acid derivatives from Echinacea purpurea.

of pyrrolizidine alkaloids. Since neither tussilagin nor isotussilagin contain this structure, they are unlikely to cause liver damage.

Polysaccharides and glycoproteins

A raw polysaccharide fraction from *E. purpurea* roots was isolated by Wagner et al. [50]. It has not yet been characterized in detail, but seems to be similarly composed as the polysaccharides from the aerial parts.

Giger et al. [51] investigated the fructan content of *Echinacea purpurea* and found that the total fructose in the roots was lowest in May, increasing during the summer and autumn. The formation of highly polymerized fructans occurred earlier in *Echinacea purpurea* than in *Echinacea angustifolia*. *Echinacea purpurea* was characterized by the accumulation of fructosans during the winter, mainly of polymerization grade 4 [51].

Three glycoproteins, MW 17,000, 21,000 and 30,000 Da, containing about 3% protein, have been isolated from *E. purpurea* and *E. angustifolia* roots. The dominant sugars were found to be arabinose (64–84%), galactose (1.9–5.3%) and glucosamines (6%). The protein moiety contained high amounts of aspartate, glycine, glutamate and alanine [52]. An ELISA method has been developed for the detection and determination of glycoproteins and polysaccharides in *E. purpurea* preparations [53]. It seems that *E. purpurea* and *E. angustifolia* roots contain similar amounts of glycoproteins, while *E. pallida* contains less [57]. Recently, lectins have also been described as biologically active substances in different parts of *Echinacea purpurea* [86].

Immunological investigations

First studies with alcoholic extracts of *E. purpurea* roots were undertaken by Vömel [87], who used isolated, perfused rat liver and tested the influence on the activity of Kupffer cells. It was shown that the phagocytosis of erythrocytes was improved significantly and that it influenced phagocytosis-dependent metabolism.

More intensive studies were performed by Bauer et al. [54]: An ethanolic extract obtained from the roots of *E. purpurea* (1:10) in a concentration of 10^{-3}% stimulated phagocytosis of yeast particles by human PMN *in vitro* by 33%. The chloroform soluble part of the extract, which contained the full spectrum of alkamides, stimulated phagocytosis by 37% at a concentration of 10^{-3}%, and also the water soluble part, containing cichoric acid, stimulated by 42% at a concentration of 10^{-3}% [54]. *Per os* administration of 10 ml/kg b.w./day of a solution of 0.5 ml of the ethanolic extract in 30 ml normal saline solution enhanced phagocytosis of carbon particles in mice by a factor of 3.1 [54]. The lipophilic alkamide fraction at the same dose enhanced phagocytosis in the carbon-clearance-assay by a factor of 1.7, and the polar fraction by 1.9 (see Fig. 6) [54, 55]. In tinctures made from *E. purpurea* roots, active compounds seem to be in the lipophilic as well as in the polar fraction.

A marked stimulatory effect was observed on the lysosomal and peroxidal activity of peritoneal macrophages and splenic cells after five days *in vivo* treatment of C57BL6 inbred mice with the ethanolic extract from the roots of *E. purpurea* (E. gloriosa) [62, 63].

Extracts of *Echinacea purpurea* and *Panax ginseng* were evaluated for stimulatory effects on cellular immune function by peripheral blood mononuclear cells (PBMC) from normal individuals and patients with either the chronic fatigue syndrome or the acquired immunodeficiency syndrome. PBMC isolated on a Ficoll-hypaque density gradient were tested in the presence or absence of varying concentrations of each extract for natural killer (NK) cell activity versus K562 cells and antibody-dependent cellular cytotoxicity (ADCC) against human herpesvirus six infected H9 cells. Both *Echinacea* and *Ginseng*, at concentrations $\geq$ 0.1 or 10 μg/kg, respectively, significantly enhanced NK-function of all groups. Similarly, the addition of either herb significantly increased ADCC of PBMC from all subject groups [88].

In a double blind study with 24 healthy humans, an ethanolic extract (1:5) of *E. purpurea* roots was tested for phagocytosis stimulatory effects *in vivo*. The extract or a placebo were administered orally at a dose of 3×30 drops daily for five days, representing about 1 mg cichoric acid and about 1 mg alkamides per day. Granulocyte phagocytosis was measured by the modified Brandt test. Maximal stimulation was found at day 5 with 120% of the starting value (Fig. 12). After discontinuation of the extract, phagocytosis activity decreased within three days to the normal level. The other immune parameter (IgA, IgG, IgM) used to monitor the course of immunoactivity, as well as leukocytes and the BKS values, remained within normal biological ranges. Tolerance was good in all cases. Only two subjects showed a slight temperature increase of about 0.5° C [89].

Besides the alkamides, cichoric acid exhibited phagocytosis stimulatory activity *in vitro* (40% stimulation at a concentration of 10^{-5} mg/ml), while echinacoside, verbascoside, and 2-caffeoyl-tartaric acid did not possess this activity [55]. Recently, cichoric acid was also shown to inhibit hyaluronidase (Fig. 13) [48] and to protect collagen type III from free radical-induced degradation [60]. Amongst the caffeic acid conjugates tested by Cheminat et al. [73], it was the only one active (50% inhibition at 125 μg/ml) against vesicular-stomatitis-virus (VSV) in L-929 mouse cells after 4 h incubation. Caffeic acid showed the same activity at 62.5 μg/ml. Recently it was found that cichoric acid selectively inhibits human immunodeficiency virus type 1 integrase [90–92]. However, cichoric acid is a rather labile compound and therefore bioavailability needs to be checked.

A raw polysaccharide fraction of *E. purpurea* roots stimulated phagocytosis in mice determined by the carbon-clearance assay at a dose of 10 mg/kg b.w. and also

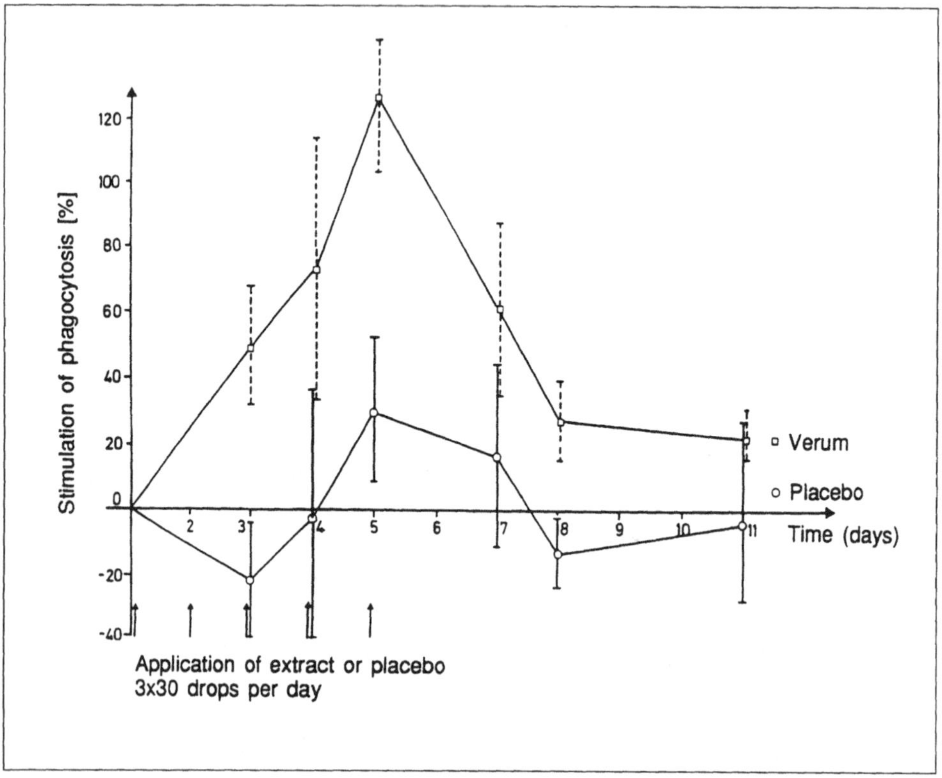

Figure 12
Double blind study with oral application of an ethanolic extract of Echinacea purpurea *roots. Stimulation of phagocytosis of granulocytes* ex vivo. *From [89].*

enhanced phagocytosis of human PMN *in vitro* by 27% at a concentration of 0.01 mg/ml [50].

A glycoprotein fraction (MW > 10000 Da) obtained from *E. purpurea* roots stimulated interleukin 1 secretion from murine macrophages *in vitro*, which was shown by the interleukin 1 dependent T-helper cell line D10G4.1 [93]. In mice, i.v. application of the fraction caused a significant and dose-dependent secretion of interleukin 1 and TNFα, which was comparable to the effect of LPS l-7136 (Fig. 14). A further purified fraction, which contained a high yield of glycoprotein (MW 40 kDa) induced secretion of interferon α and β, and IgM in cultured murine spleen macrophages. The retentate (200 μg/ml) also reduced the number of plaques in a plaque-reduction assay (VSV) by 80% [59, 93]. The lyophilisates and the retentates exhibited a mitogenic activity in NMRI- as well as in lipopolysaccharide (LPS)-non-sensitive C3H/HeJ-mice, which demonstrates that the effect is not due to contamination with LPS [94].

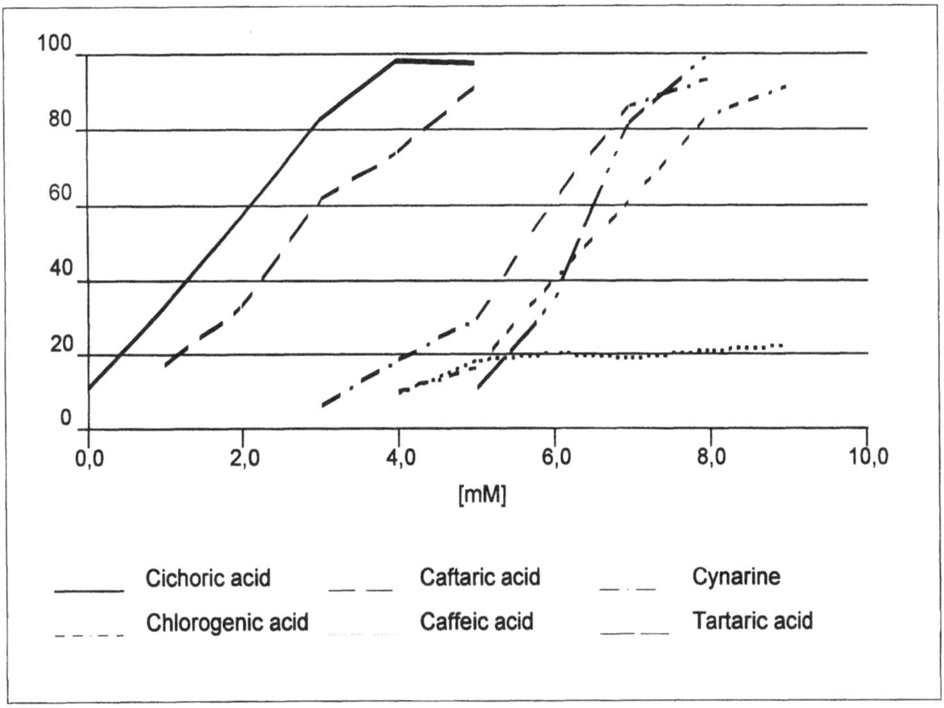

Figure 13
Inhibitory effects on hyaluronidase by caffeoyl esters, caffeic acid and tartaric acid [48].

An ethanolic extract of *E. purpurea* roots displayed a dose-dependant inhibition of the collagen gel contraction in collagen lattices populated with C3H10T1/2 fibroblasts. With increasing time elapsing between preparation of gel and addition of extract, less inhibition of elongation of fibroblasts and of processes leading to collagen linking were observed. Addition of the extract one hour after gel preparation had no effect [95].

Preparations from *Echinacea purpurea* aerial parts

Chemical constituents and analysis

Essential oil

Flowering aerial parts of *E. purpurea* contain less than 0.1% essential oil [14, 21, 67, 69, 74]. Bos et al. [96] showed that it contains borneol, bornyl acetate, pentadeca-8-en-2-one, germacrene D, caryophyllene, caryophyllene epoxide and palm-

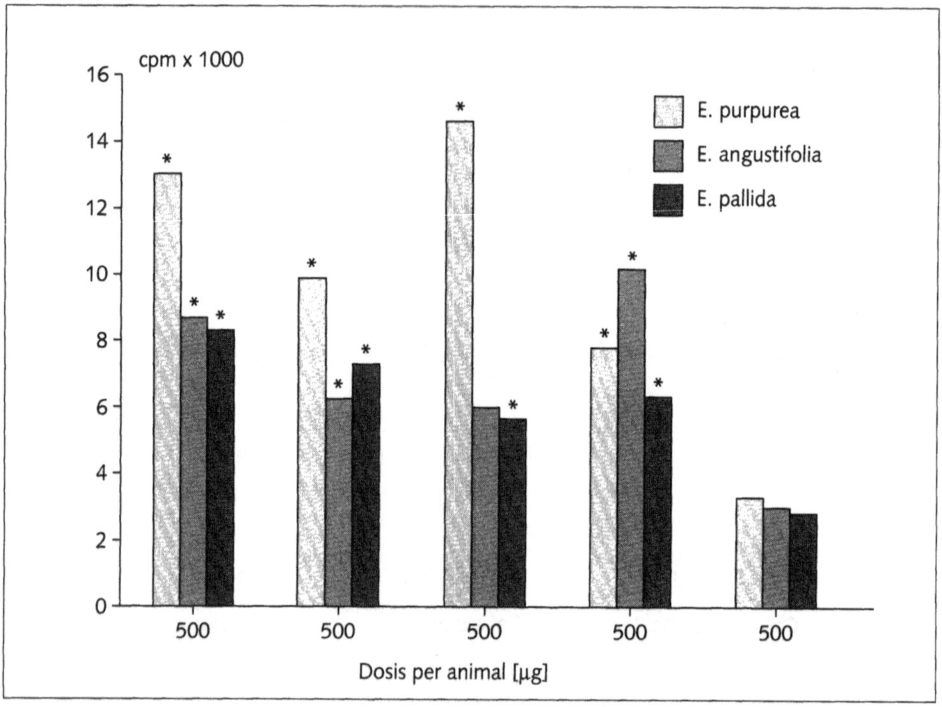

Figure 14
Effect of purified extracts (glycoproteins) of E. purpurea, E. angustifolia *and* E. pallida *roots on IL-1 production in mice. From [57].*

itic acid. *E. angustifolia* and *E. pallida* contain identical constituents. Therefore discrimination via the essential oil is difficult. Schulthess et al. [97] found α-pinene, β-farnesene, myrcene, limonene, carvomenthene, caryophyllene and germacrene D in the essential oil from the achenes of *Echinacea purpurea*. The germacrene alcohol, isolated by Bauer et al. [98] from the aerial parts of *E. purpurea*, is probably also a component of the essential oil. It has not been detected in the dried drug, and HPLC analysis shows that it is a characteristic indicator substance for fresh plant extracts and regularly present as a major component in homeopathic tinctures [84].

Alkamides

The aerial parts of *Echinacea purpurea* contain alkamides of the same 2,4-diene type as found in the roots. Main constituents are dodeca-2*E*,4*E*,8*Z*,10*E*/*Z*-tetraenoic acid isobutylamides [27, 82]. As minor constituents the isobutylamides of undeca-2*E*,4*Z*-dien-8,10-diynoic acid and dodeca-2*E*,4*E*-dienoic acid were found [82]. Alkamides can be detected in alcoholic tinctures of aerial parts of *Echinacea* (e.g. homeopathic mother tinctures) as well as in expressed juice preparations.

HPLC analysis with photodiode array detection is the best method for analysis of alkamides, because the different types can be identified via their UV-spectra. However, it is difficult to distinguish the aerial parts of the different *Echinacea* species, because they show no qualitative difference in the alkamide pattern (see Fig. 15) [30, 82]. HPLC is also useful for the determination of the contents of alkamides and was applied successfully for the analysis of fresh plant tinctures [99]. It could be shown that the yield in the aerial parts is 0.001–0.03% [30]. Small amounts of alkamides can also be found in the expressed sap of *E. purpurea* [100]. It could be shown that the content varies considerably between the different products on the market and even in between the batches of one product (Fig. 16) [100]. One reason may be the seasonal variation of the alkamide content, which is low at the beginning of the vegetation period and becomes high only in the middle of August (data of 1996, see Fig. 17) [101]. Another reason may be the different yields of alkamides in the various parts of the plant. Alkamides are especially accumulated in the flower heads in particular in the tubulous flowers and achenes (Fig. 18) [82, 101, 102]. Therefore the date and mode of harvest play an important role and standardization is urgently needed.

Flavonoids and anthocyanins

In the aerial parts of *E. purpurea*, flavonoids of quercetin and kaempferol type, such as rutoside, have been identified [103]. However, as seen by HPLC, the content is rather low [82]. They can also be analysed photometrically [104].

The major anthocyanins of *E. purpurea* (and *E. pallida*) have been identified as cyanidin-3-O-(β-D-glycopyranoside) and cyanidin-3-O-(6-O-malonyl-β-D-glycopyranoside) [105]. So far, they do not play any role for standardization purposes.

Caffeic acid derivatives and phenolic acids

The main caffeic acid derivative in the aerial parts of *Echinacea purpurea* is cichoric acid (2*R*,3*R*-O-dicaffeoyl-tartaric acid). It was first isolated from the leaves of *E. purpurea* by Becker and Hsieh [83]. Hsieh [106] reported no data on the optical activity of cichoric acid. The cichoric acid isolated later from *E. purpurea* by Remiger [84] and by Soicke et al. [107] had an optical rotation $[\alpha]_D^{20}$ of ca. –370°. In contrast, the cichoric acid first isolated by Scarpati and Oriente [108] from *Cichorium intybus* displayed a rotation of +383.5°. Cichoric acid from lettuce (*Lactuca sativa*) [109] and from endives (*Cichorium endivia*) [110] was also dextrorotatory. Synthetic studies by Scarpati and Oriente [108] showed that cichoric acid from *Cichorium intybus* contains a residue of (2*S*,3*S*)-(–)-tartaric acid. Conversely, that in

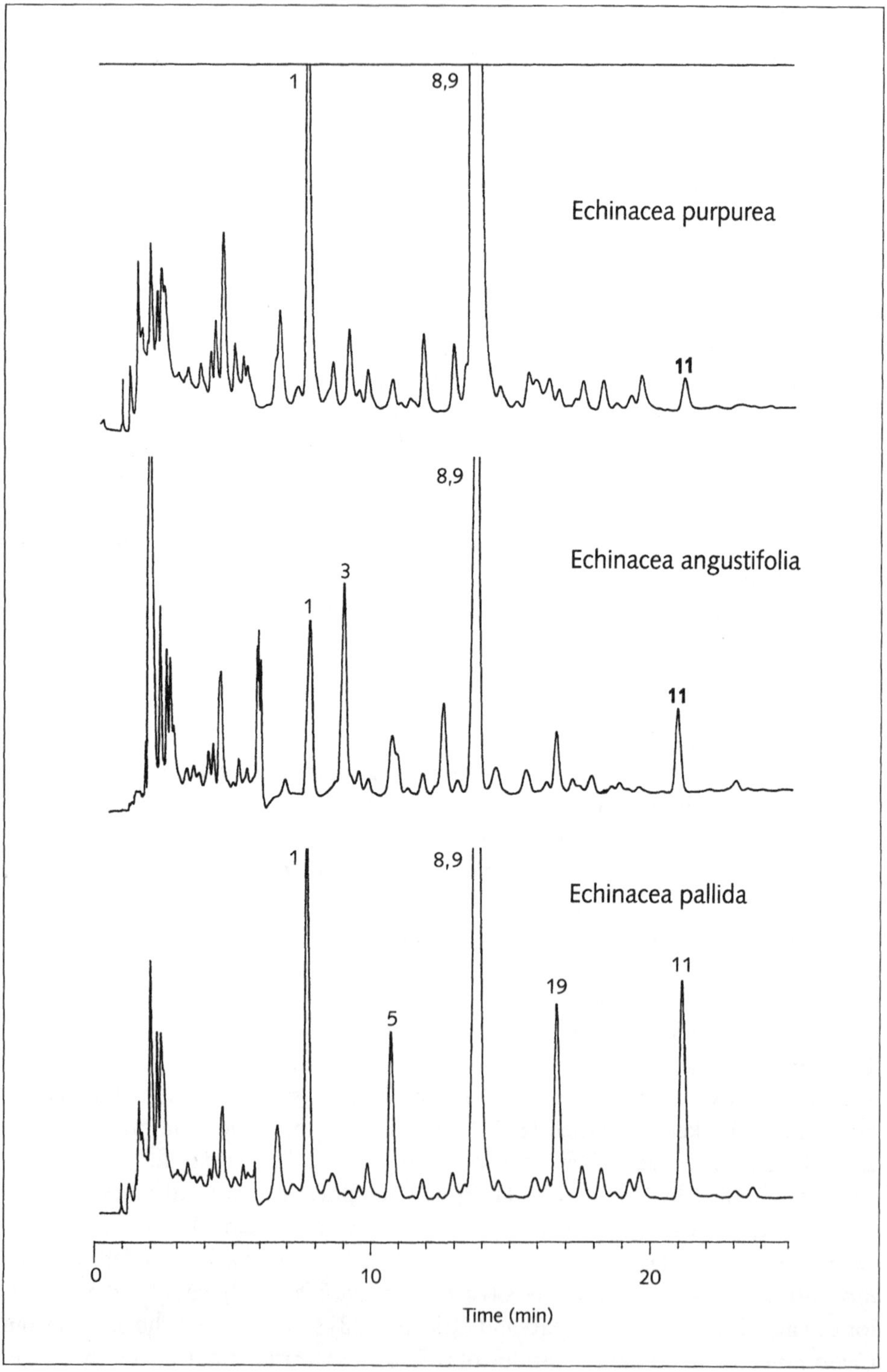
1
8,9
Echinacea purpurea
11
8,9
Echinacea angustifolia
3
1
11
1
8,9
Echinacea pallida
11
19
5
0
10
20
Time (min)

E. purpurea must contain a residue of (2*R*,3*R*)-(+)-tartaric acid. For standardization purposes, cichoric acid is now available by synthesis via a facile route [111].

From the leaves of *E. purpurea*, cichoric acid methyl ester, as well as 2-O-caffeoyl-3-O-feruloyl-tartaric acid and 2,3-O-diferuloyl-tartaric acid were isolated [83]. Later 2-O-feruloyl-tartaric acid and 2-O-caffeoyl-3-O-cumaroyl-tartaric acid were found [107].

Cichoric acid is especially abundant in the flowers of *E. purpurea* (1.2–3.1%), especially in the liguls (Fig. 18). Much less is present in the leaves and stems [82, 84]. The content, however, strongly depends on the season and the stage of development of the plant [104, 101]. The content is highest at the beginning of the vegetation period and decreases during the growth of the plant (Fig. 17). Cichoric acid (**14**) was also detected in tissue cultures of *E. purpurea* [112–114].

For the determination of cichoric acid and other caffeoylics present in *Echinacea* preparations, HPLC methods have been described (see Fig. 2) [82, 104]. Cichoric acid can also be determined by a recently-developed capillary zone electrophoresis (MEKC) method (see Fig. 5) [44].

When analyzing the maceration process of homeopathic mother tinctures, it was observed that cichoric acid undergoes degradation during preparation of the tinctures. During five days of 50% ethanol maceration of *E. purpurea* aerial parts, it was found that the content of cichoric acid decreased rapidly, although it was stable when the plant material was filtered off after the first day. Therefore, enzymatic degradation during the extraction process is likely [84]. Similar enzymatic degradation also occurs during the preparation of *E. purpurea* expressed sap [100]. When analyzing six different products containing the same amount of *E. purpurea* expressed sap, dramatically different contents of cichoric acid (0.0–0.4%), even within different batches of the same brand were found (Fig. 16). This mainly is due to different manufacturing processes which allow or inhibit enzymatic activity (e.g. by heating) [100].

HPLC has also been used for the analysis of phenolic acids in *Echinacea* preparations [115]. A validated HPLC method has been published for the determination

Figure 15
HPLC separation of the lipophilic fractions of the aerial parts of Echinacea purpurea, E. pallida *and* E. angustifolia. *From Bauer et al. [82].*
Separation parameters: Column: Hibar 125-4 with LiChrospher 100 CH-18 (2), 5 µm (Merck); solvents: A = water, B = acetonitrile, gradient: 40–60% B linearly in 30 min; flow rate: 1.0 ml/min; detection: 254 nm.
1 = undeca-2E,4Z-dien-8,10-diynoic acid-isobutylamide; 3 = dodeca-2E,4Z-dien-8,10-diynoic acid-isobutylamide; 5 = dodeca-2E,4E,10E-trien-8-ynoic acid-isobutylamide; 8/9 = dodeca-2E,4E,8Z,10E-tetraenoic acid-isobutylamide and dodeca-2E,4E,8Z,10Z-tetraenoic acid-isobutylamide; 11 = dodeca-2E,4E-dienoic acid-isobutylamide; 19 = hexadeca-2E,9Z-dien-12,14-dynoic acid-isobutylamide.

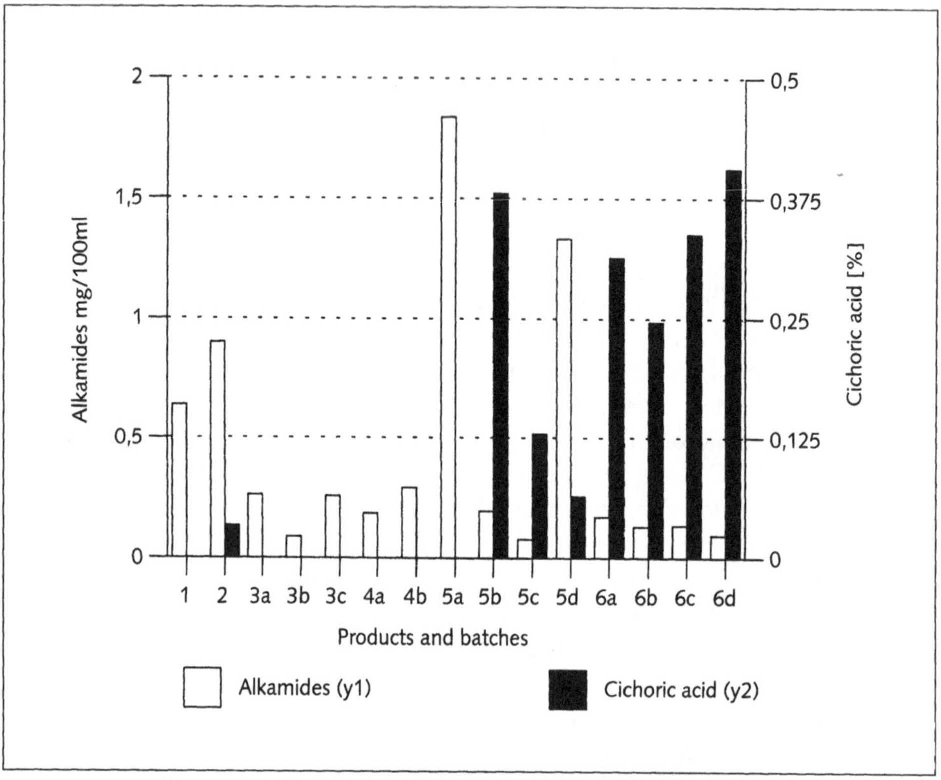

Figure 16
Content of cichoric acid and dodeca-2E,4E,8Z,10E,Z-tetraenoic acid-isobutylamide in different preparations containing the same amount of Echinacea purpurea *expressed sap [100].*

of *p*-coumaric acid and for the standardization of preparations of *E. purpurea* expressed sap [116]. However, *p*-coumaric acid is not a specific constituent of *E. purpurea* and, moreover, it has to be regarded as a hydrolysis product of *p*-coumaric acid esters present in *E. purpurea* [107].

Moreover, HPLC determination of glycin-betain has been suggested for the standardization of *Echinacea purpurea* expressed sap preparations [117]. However, glycin-betain is also an ubiquitous compound and therefore not specific for *Echinacea* preparations.

Polysaccharides

Systematic fractionation and subsequent pharmacological testing of the aqueous extracts of the aerial parts of *E. purpurea* led to the isolation of two polysaccharides (PS I and PS II) with immunostimulatory properties [118, 119]. Structural analysis

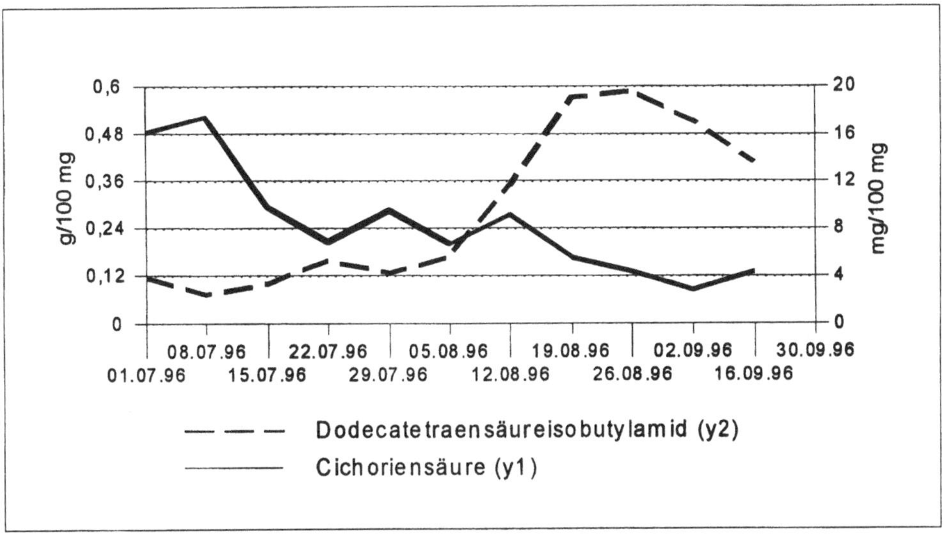

Figure 17
Seasonal variation of the content of cichoric acid and dodeca-2E,4E,8Z,10E,Z-tetraenoic acid-isobutylamide in aerial parts of Echinacea purpurea *[101].*

showed PS I to be a 4-O-methyl-glucuronoarabinoxylan with an average MW of 35,000 Da, while PS II was shown to be an acidic arabinorhamnogalactan of MW 450,000 Da [120, 121]. A xyloglucan, MW 79,500 Da, was isolated from the leaves and stems of *E. purpurea*, and a pectin-like polysaccharide from the expressed sap [122]. Recently, lectins have also been described as biologically active substances in different parts of *E. purpurea* [86].

Polysaccharides have also been obtained from cell cultures of *Echinacea purpurea*. From the growth medium of *E. purpurea* cell cultures, three homogeneous polysaccharides, i.e. two neutral fucogalactoxyloglucans with MW of 10,000 and 25,000 Da, and an acidic arabinogalactan, MW 75,000 Da, have been isolated [122–124]. The structure of these polysaccharides differs from those of the aerial parts, since cells in suspension culture possess exclusively primary cell wall components [125]. Detailed structural data on the immunomodulatory active polysaccharides from *Echinacea* are presented in the chapters by Wagner et al. [150] and Emmendörffer et al. in this volume [151].

So far, no routine analytical methods are available for the analysis of the polysaccharides in phytopreparations. An exact characterization can only be achieved by gas chromatographic determination of the sugar sequences and linkages after isolation and purification [120]. The identification and quantification of monosacharides after hydrolysis, recently suggested as a standardization method [126],

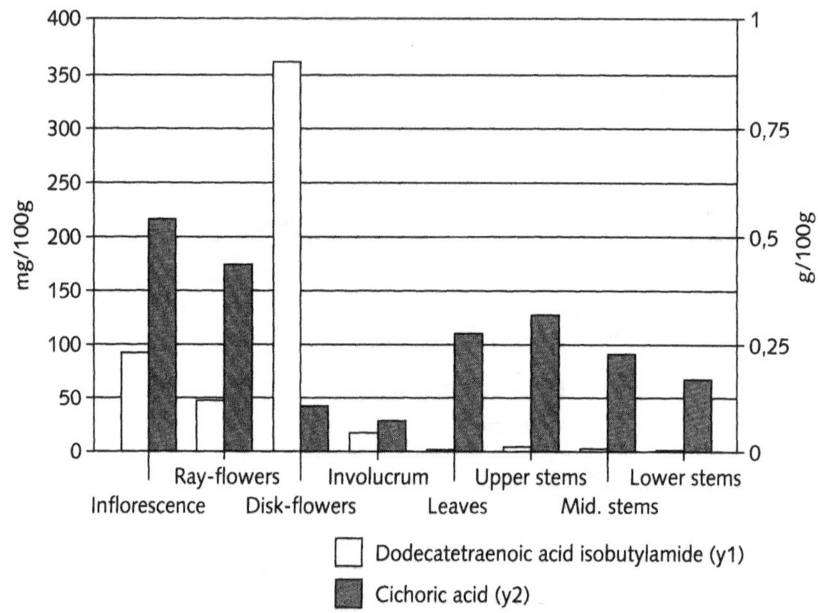

Figure 18
Yield of cichoric acid in the different parts of Echinacea purpurea *[101].*

still lacks a specificity for the active polysaccharides. It is more promising to develop fluorescence or radioactively labelled polysaccharides or antibodies for a specific assay [127].

From a theoretical point of view, the immunostimulatory polysaccharides can only be expected in phytopreparations which have been prepared with aqueous solvents. By 50% (V/V) ethanol the immunostimulatory active polysaccharides are precipitated, as can be seen from their isolation protocol [120]. Therefore, such preparations should be void of these polysaccharides. However, aqueous preparations and also expressed saps at least have the potential to contain them, and it would be desirable to establish corresponding standardization methods.

Giger et al. [51] investigated the fructan content of *Echinacea purpurea* and found that the aerial parts contained ten times less than the roots and that homeopathic tinctures contained fructans with polymerization grades up to 15. It has been suggested to standardize *Echinacea purpurea* fresh plant preparations on the content of β-1,2-fructofuranosides [128]. The method is based on enzymatic hydrolysis of the fructans by invertase and subsequent determination of fructose by HPLC. Since β-1,2-fructofuranosides are easily degraded enzymatically during the manufacturing process and since the yield varies over the vegetation period, their content is an indication of proper harvest and treatment of the plant material. However, the content lacks any pharmacological relevance since these components do not contribute to the immunostimulatory activity of *Echinacea.*

Immunological investigations

An immunostimulatory effect was observed on the phagocytic, metabolic and bactericidal activities of peritoneal macrophages, and the total weight of the spleens was increased when mice were treated for five days with the ethanolic extract of the aerial parts of *E. purpurea* and the activity was tested on day 7 [63, 129].

An extract prepared with 90% ethanol from fresh plants (final ethanol concentration 65%) inhibited significantly the contraction of collagen seeded with C3H10T1/2 fibroblasts. A corresponding amount of ethanol showed no effect. Depending on the time of addition of the extract, the elongation of fibroblasts and the processes leading to the linking of the collagen were inhibited. When adding the extract one hour after starting the collagen linking, no effect was observed. The authors conclude an influence on wound healing [95].

An ethanolic extract (1:10) of the dried aerial parts of *E. purpurea* stimulated carbon clearance in NMRI-mice by 40% when applied per os at a dose of 5 mg/kg b.w. daily for two days. The lipophilic fraction was even more potent (110% stimulation) while the polar fraction was less active (30%). A similar or even higher effect (110% stimulation) was achieved when a homeopathic mother tincture (prepared from fresh aerial parts) was applied at a dose of 0.17 ml/kg b.w. daily [55].

Most pharmacological investigations with the aerial parts of *E. purpurea* have been performed with a preparation containing the expressed sap of the fresh plant material (Echinacin®), which has been on the market in Germany for 60 years.

Dilutions of expressed sap (1:5 and 1:10) (Myo-Echinacin® 5%) improved granulocyte phagocytosis of yeast cells *in vitro* to the same intensity as identical dilutions of Intraglobin F [130, 131]. A lyophilisate of the expressed sap of *E. purpurea* at the concentration of 5.0 mg/ml increased the number of phagocyting human granulocytes from 79% to 95% ($p < 0.001$) and stimulated phagocytosis of yeast particles also significantly by more than 50% ($p < 0.01$). At the highest tested dose of 12.5 mg/ml the number of phagocyting granulocytes and the phagocytosis index decreased [132]. Stimulation of phagocytosis by the expressed sap of *E. purpurea* has been demonstrated in three further *in vitro* studies [133–135].

A preparation of *E. purpurea* expressed sap increased the *in vitro* phagocytosis of *Candida albicans* by granulocytes and monocytes from healthy donors by 30–45%. The chemotactic migration of granulocytes in the Boyden Chamber was increased by 45%. There was no effect in either direction on intracellular killing of bacteria or yeasts and the preparation did not induce *in vitro* transformation of lymphocytes [136].

The effect of an expressed sap preparation of *E. purpurea* on phagocytosis in granulocytes was measured by a chemiluminescence method. It was found that the reaction of the granulocytes depends on the dose and method applied. The authors conclude that standardized methods and investigations of various immunoparameters are necessary to prove the immunostimulatory effect of such preparations [137].

In vivo, phagocytosis of isolated peritoneal macrophages of mice and macrophages of the isolated perfunded rat liver have been stimulated by i.p. injection or oral application of *E. purpurea* expressed sap [138]. By low concentrations of expressed sap, an induction of TNF, IL-1 and IL-6 secretion has been observed [134, 135]. After application of 1 ml/kg b.w. to rabbits, a cold-defense-reaction has been described as a cytokine-mediated effect. Body temperature raised monophasic by 1° C after a lag time of 30 min [139].

With rabbits, 72 h after i.v. injection of ^{3}H-thymidine, 1.5 ml *E. purpurea* expressed sap preparation was injected i.v. and leukocytes were controlled until 6 h after injection. After a further 19 h animals were decapitated and comparative bone marrow smears were prepared. It became obvious, that 6 h after injection of the sap preparation, leukocytosis was observed with a relative decrease of lymphocytes and an increase of granulocytes in peripheral blood. The number of ^{3}H-labelled lymphocytes and granulocytes had increased 7–40% and 34–89% respectively [140]. Concentrations of expressed sap of 50 µg/ml and 5 µg/ml resulted in a 35–50% stimulation acting as a chemotactic and chemokinetic to polymorphonuclear neutrophiles (PMN) in comparison to CT-reference compound 10^{-6} mol N-f-Met-Leu-Phe (FMLP). FMLP stimulated PMNs possessed 24% lower CT-activity ($p = 0.005$) after 15 min preincubation at 37° C. Coincubation of 5 µg/ml expressed sap could antagonize this negative effect on activity ($p = 0.005$). Chemoluminescence (CL) of neutrophile granulocytes was stimulated from 6.1 to 6.9×10^3 cpm by 10 min preincubation with 5 µg/ml expressed sap compared to a control [142].

Cultures of bone marrow with cytologically unchanged bone marrow, as well as cultures with blood from chronic myeloic leukemia (CML), osteomyelosclerosis (OMS) and acute non-lymphatic lykemia (ANLL) patients have been treated over 72 h with expressed sap of *E. purpurea* at a concentration of 2.0 and 0.2 mg/ml culture suspension respectively. In the bone marrow cultures a highly significant enhancement of the mitosis index of the granulo- and monopoesis with accelerated differentiation from the staff cells to segmented granulocytes have been observed, and an increased number of macrophages within the CML and OMS blood cultures. In the ANLL cultures, the total number of mature granulocytes was enhanced. Stimulation of T-lymphocyte populations was observed in an *in vitro* experiment. In the T-Lymphocyte-Transformation-Test, the expressed sap of *E. purpurea* stimulated ^{3}H-thymidine incorporation at medium doses, while high concentrations showed a suppressive or cytotoxic effect [141].

Formation of oxygen radicals has been demonstrated with human granulocytes and macrophages from mice by the chemiluminescence method. After 60 min preincubation with 50 µg/ml expressed sap and suboptimal stimulation by Zymosan, a significant stimulation of granulocyte activity of 24% was observed [142, 143].

After activation by expressed sap of *E. purpurea*, macrophages showed cytotoxic effects to tumour cells *in vitro*. Cell-mediated cytotoxicity was observed in cocultures of tumour cells (ABLS-8.1, Yac-1, L12-10) with bone marrow macrophages and *E. purpurea* expressed sap [144]. An antitumour effect of the expressed sap has also been found *in vivo* after oral application to mice with Meth A tumour [143].

A lyophylisate of the expressed sap of *E. purpurea* in cultures of mice L-cells (clone 929) at a concentration of 10 µg/ml to 100 µg/ml exhibited no direct antiviral activity against encephalomyocarditis virus (EMC virus) or vesicular-stomatitis-virus (VSV). An antiviral effect was only observed when the sap was added together with DEAE dextran. DEAE dextran itself showed no effect. The authors concluded an interferon-like activity [145]. By the colorimetric assay according to Finter and by the Plaque-Reduction-Assay it could be shown, that mice L-929 cells or HeLa cells became resistant for 24 h against influenza-, herpes- and vesicular-stomatitis-virus by 50–80%, when the cells were pretreated 4–6 h with 20 µg/ml of an *E. purpurea* expressed sap preparation. Together with hyaluronidase, no effect was observed. The active component could not be inactivated by heat (60–80° C) [146].

Eichler and Krüger [147] showed by tissue culture experiments, that various viral antigens related to virus replication and to the synthesis of structural components appear earlier in cells stimulated with *E. purpurea* expressed sap, timunox and TP-1, but not following the stimulation with isoprinosine. Similarly, virus genome containing cells increased after stimulation with thymic preparations (thymostimulin and thymopentin), but not with *E. purpurea* expressed sap and isoprinosine. The authors conclude that the synthesis of proteins or DNA of lymphotropic viruses may be transiently enhanced when lymphoid cells are stimulated by certain non-specific immunostimulants. There was no evidence, however, of increased virus replication.

In the modified Spreading-Test with rats, spreading of a s.c.-applied mixture of colours has been measured under the simultanous s.c. application of 0.04 ml of 1/7 concentrated *E. purpurea* expressed sap. By simultaneous application of hyaluronidase and by 0.04 ml of the genuine expressed sap, stimulated spreading could be inhibited. The effect correlates to the activity of 1 mg cortison s.c. For 0.04 ml s.c. of the concentrated (factor 7:1) expressed sap, the effect of hyaluronidase could be antagonized [148]. Pretreatment with 2 × 0.3 ml of an expressed sap preparation s.c. within 24 h before infection reduced spreading and intensity of artificial *Streptococcus* infection of guinea pigs. In contrast to the non-treated control group, no lethality was observed in the treated group (10 animals/group). In addition, s.c. application of 0.3 ml of the preparation at days 3,

5, 7 and 10 after infection reduced intensity of the infection. Lethality was not observed in the treated group. In the non-treated group, six of 16 animals died from sepsis. The authors discuss an activity related to hyaluronidase [149].

As already outlined in the chapter on *E. purpurea* roots (5.2), cichoric acid was recently shown to inhibit hyaluronidase (Fig. 13) [48] and to protect collagen type III from free radical-induced degradation [60]. Cichoric acid also exhibited phagocytosis stimulatory activity *in vitro* [55] and showed some effect against VSV in L-929 mouse cells [73]. Therefore, pharmacologically it is an interesting compound. However, it is rather labile and bioavailability needs to be checked.

Since alkamides are also present in preparations of *E. purpurea* expressed sap and have shown phagocytosis stimulatory and anti-inflammatory effects (see *E. angustifolia* and *E. purpurea* roots) [54–56], they have also to be discussed as one of the active principles.

Immunomodulatory active polysaccharides have been isolated from the aerial parts of *E. purpurea* [118, 123]. Their pharmacological activity is well documented and will be reviewed in the chapters by Wagner et al. and Emmendörffer et al. in this volume [150, 151]. Lectins from *Echinacea purpurea* have been shown to possess agglutinative properties and it is argued that they may also have adaptogenic effects [86].

Conclusions and considerations for standardization of *Echinacea* phytopreparations

From pharmacological investigations it is obvious that not a single, but several constituents like the alkamides, cichoric acid, glycoproteins and polysaccharides, contribute to the immunostimulatory activity of *Echinacea* extracts (for summary see Tab. 1) [152, 153]. Therefore the application of extracts is still reasonable and hence the native extract is regarded as "the active principle" for regulatory purposes by the health authorities [154]. However, standardization of these extracts is a must for a rational therapeutic application of phytopreparations [155, 156], and reproducible quality needs also to be documented from a regulatory point of view [157, 158].

Since the variability of the plant material is due to different growth, harvest, drying and storage conditions, cultivation of *Echinacea* under standardized conditions is desirable and has already been achieved for the three main species [159, 160]. Nevertheless, *E. pallida* and *E. angustifolia* roots are still collected partially from the wild. A test for adulterations (e.g. *Parthenium integrifolium*) therefore still is necessary.

The polarity of the solvent, the mode of extraction, and the instability of constituents also influence the composition and quality of the extracts, as was shown for the ketoalkenyns present in *Echinacea pallida* or for cichoric acid in *Echinacea*

Table 1 - Constituents which contribute to the immunostimulatory activity of Echinacea *extracts*

Species and plant part	Constituents	Activity
Echinacea purpurea		
Roots and aerial parts	Polysaccharides	Stimulation of phagocytosis
		Induction of cytokine production
	Glycoproteins	Induction of cytokine production
		Mitogenic activity
	Cichoric acid	Stimulation of phagocytosis
		Inhibition of hyaluronidase
	Alkamides	Stimulation of phagocytosis
		Inhibition of PG- and LT synthesis
Echinacea pallida		
Roots	Polysaccharides	Stimulation of phagocytosis
	Glycoproteins	Induction of cytokine production
		Mitogenic activity
Echinacea angustifolia		
Roots	Alkamides	Stimulation of phagocytosis
		Inhibition of PG and LT synthesis
	Glycoproteins	Induction of cytokine production
		Mitogenic activity

purpurea. The manufacturing procedure therefore needs to be kept absolutely constant. Buying extracts or expressed saps from different sources may lead to an inconsistency in the batches of a product.

For standardization purposes, adequate marker compounds need to be selected in order to base quality control on therapeutically relevant constituents. Compounds which specifically occur in *Echinacea* should be preferred. Accordingly, glycin-betain, coumaric acid or fructofuranosides may not be well suited for a specific characterization of *Echinacea* products.

Echinacoside is a typical and major compound of *E. angustifolia* and *E. pallida* roots. It may be used as a marker compound, but as far as we know, it does not possess any immunomodulatory relevance. Nevertheless, it may be the best suited constituent in *E. pallida* roots for standardization purposes. However, ketoalkenyns should not be neglected and a constant pattern of these compounds should be guaranteed as well. Determination of two compounds (one polar and one lipophilic) would also demonstrate that the extract has been properly prepared.

In the case of *E. angustifolia* roots, the alkamides are best suited as markers, because they enable identification of the species. They are also related to activity since they have exhibited anti-inflammatory and immunomodulatory effects [55, 56]. They are present in alcoholic extracts and tinctures and studies are in progress to determine their bioavailability.

Alkamides are also typical and relevant constituents of *E. purpurea* roots and aerial parts. They should be used for quality control besides the determination of cichoric acid. While absorbtion of alkamides can be suspected from their lipophilic nature and from the fact that they are responsible for the local anaesthetic effect ("tingling sensation") on the tongue [28], bioavailability of cichoric acid still needs to be determined. Nevertheless, both compounds are good markers for a reproducible manufacturing process, because they readily undergo degradation when extraction and storage parameters are not optimal.

Expressed saps of *E. purpurea* aerial parts are per se highly diluted preparations, compared to alcoholic tinctures. Lipophilic constituents like alkamides are present only in the mg scale. However, polar phenolic compounds like cichoric acid may also not be contained since they undergo rapid enzymatic degradation. Cichoric acid can only be preserved by denaturation of the enzymes, e.g. by heat, before or during the pressing process. Then expressed saps with high cichoric acid content can be obtained. However, the influence of heat etc. on other constituents still needs to be investigated.

Since no routine method is available for the determination of polysaccharides, standardization on these pharmacologically relevant compounds is not yet possible. In addition, standardization on glycoproteins via the published ELISA method can, unfortunately, not be performed by most of the companies because the antibodies are not freely available.

Standardization via biological activity has been discussed, but it is difficult to agree on an appropriate assay and *in vivo* assays are not acceptable to the public opinion.

In summary, there is still a need for more research in *Echinacea*, especially on the active components and the mode of action. *Echinacea* will be accepted as a rational drug only on the basis of more valid pharmacological and clinical data, obtained with standardized preparations.

References

1 Bauer R (1998) Pflanzliche Immunstimulanzien in der Selbstmedikation. *Pharmazie in unserer Zeit* 27: 144–157

2 Brevoort P (1996) The U.S. Botanical Market – an Overview. *Herbalgram* 36: 49-57

3 Richman A, Witkowski JP (1997) Herbs by the numbers. *Whole Foods* October 1997: 20–28

4 Bauer R, Wagner H (1990) *Echinacea – Ein Handbuch für Ärzte, Apotheker und andere Naturwissenschaftler*. Wissenschaftliche Verlagsgesellschaft, Stuttgart

5 Bauer R, Liersch R (1993) *Echinacea.* In: R Hänsel, K Keller, H Rimpler, G Schneider (eds): *Hagers Handbuch der Pharmazeutischen Praxis.* Springer-Verlag, Berlin, Heidelberg, New York, Vol. 5, 1–34

6 Melchart D, Linde K (1999) Clinical investigations of *Echinacea* phytopharmaceuticals. In: H Wagner (ed): *Immunomodulatory agents from plants.* Birkhäuser Verlag, Basel, 105–118

7 Bauer R, Wagner H (1991) *Echinacea* species as potential immunostimulatory drugs. In: H Wagner, NR Farnsworth (eds): *Economic and medicinal plant research*, Vol. 5, Academic Press, London, 253–321

8 McGregor RL (1968) The taxonomy of the genus *Echinacea* (Compositae). *The University of Kansas Science Bulletin* 48: 113–142

9 Lloyd JU (1904) History of *Echinacea angustifolia. Pharm Review* 22: 9–14

10 Moerman DE (1986) Medicinal Plants of Native America, *Res Rep Ethnobotany*, Contrib 2, Technical Reports No 19, University of Michigan Museum of Anthropology

11 Schindler H (1940) Geschichte, Systematik und Verbreitung der therapeutisch wichtigen *Echinacea* Arten: *E. angustifolia* DC, *E. pallida* Nutt und *E. purpurea* Moench. *Pharm Zentralhalle* 81: 579–583

12 Bauer R, Khan IA, Wagner H (1988) TLC and HPLC analysis of *Echinacea pallida* and *E. angustifolia* roots. *Planta Med* 54: 426–430

13 Madaus G (1939) *Echinacea purpurea* Moench, *Med Biol Schriftenreihe*, Issue 13, Verlag Rohrmoser, Radebeul/Dresden

14 Heinzer F, Chavanne M, Meusy J-P, Maitre H-P, Giger E, Baumann TW (1988) Ein Beitrag zur Klassifizierung der therapeutisch verwendeten Arten der Gattung *Echinacea. Pharm Acta Helv* 63:132–136

15 Schenk R, Franke R (1996) Content of echinacoside in *Echinacea* roots of different origin. *Beitr Züchtungsforsch* 2: 64–67

16 Bischoff F (1924) Oil of *Echinacea angustifolia. J Am Pharm Assoc* 13: 898–902

17 Voaden DJ, Jacobson M (1972) Tumor Inhibitors 3. Identification and Synthesis of an Oncolytic Hydrocarbon from American Coneflower Roots. *J Med Chem* 15: 619–623

18 Jacobson M, Redfern RE, Mills GDjr (1975) Naturally occurring insect growth regulators. – III. Echinolone, a highly active juvenile hormone mimic from *Echinacea angustifolia* roots. *Lloydia* 38: 473–476

19 Schulte KE, Rücker G, Perlick J (1967) Das Vorkommen von Polyacetylen-Verbindungen in *Echinacea purpurea* MOENCH und *Echinacea angustifolia* DC. *Arzneim-Forsch* 17: 825–829

20 Verelis CD (1978) *Untersuchung der lipophilen Inhaltsstoffe von Radix Echinaceae angustifoliae DC.*, Dissertation, Universität Heidelberg

21 Neugebauer H (1949) Zur Kenntnis der Inhaltsstoffe von *Echinacea. Pharmazie* 4: 137–140

22 Bohlmann F, Burkhardt T, Zdero (1973) *Naturally occurring acetylenes.* Academic Press, London, New York

23 Jacobson M (1967) The structure of echinacein, the insecticidal component of American coneflower roots. *J Org Chem* 32: 1646–1647
24 Bohlmann F, Grenz M (1966) Über die Inhaltsstoffe aus *Echinacea*-Arten. *Chem Ber* 99: 3197–3200
25 Bauer R, Remiger P, Wagner H (1989) Alkamides from the Roots of *Echinacea angustifolia*. *Phytochemistry* 28: 505–508
26 Martin R, Becker H (1984) Spilanthol-related amides from *Acmella ciliata*. *Phytochemistry* 23: 1781–1783
27 Bohlmann F, Hoffmann H (1983) Further amides from *Echinacea purpurea*. *Phytochemistry* 22: 1173–1175
28 Jacobson M (1954) Occurrence of a pungent insecticidal principle in American coneflower roots. *Science* 120: 1028–1029
29 Greger H (1988) Comparative Phytochemistry of the Alkamides. In: J Lam, H Breteler, T. Arnason, L Hansen (eds) *Chemistry and biology of naturally-occurring acetylenes and related compounds*. Elsevier, Amsterdam, 159–178
30 Bauer R, Remiger P (1989) TLC and HPLC analysis of alkamides in *Echinacea* drugs. *Planta Med* 55: 367–371
31 Bauer R, Khan IA, Wagner H (1988) TLC and HPLC analysis of *Echinacea pallida* and *E. angustifolia* roots. *Planta Med* 54: 426–430
32 Bauer R, Khan IA, Wagner H (1987) *Echinacea* – Nachweis einer Verfälschung von *Echinacea purpurea* (L.) MOENCH mit *Parthenium integrifolium L. Dtsch Apoth Ztg* 127: 1325–1330
33 Lloyd JU (1897) Empiricism – *Echinacea. Eclect Med J* 57: 421–427
34 Heyl FW, Staley JF (1914) Analyses of two *Echinacea* roots. *Am J Pharm* 86: 450–455
35 Heyl FW, Hart MC (1915) Some Constituents of the Root of Brauneria *angustifolia. J Am Chem Soc* 37: 1769–1778
36 Röder E, Wiedenfeld H, Hille T, Britz-Kirstgen R (1984) Pyrrolizidine in *Echinacea angustifolia* DC und *Echinacea purpurea* MOENCH – Isolierung und Analytik. *Dtsch Apoth Ztg* 124: 2316–2318
37 Britz-Kirstgen R (1985) *Phytochemische Untersuchungen an Senecio cacallaster L., Echinacea angustifolia DC und Pulmonaria officinalis L.* PhD thesis, Universität Bonn
38 Mattocks AR (1986) *Chemistry and toxicology of pyrrolizidine alkaloids*. Academic Press, London
39 Stoll A, Renz J, Brack A (1950) Isolierung und Konstitution des Echinacosids, eines Glykosids aus den Wurzeln von *Echinacea angustifolia* D.C. *Helv Chim Acta* 33: 1877–1893
40 Bauer R, Remiger P (1989) Der Einsatz der HPLC bei der Standardisierung von *Echinacea*-Drogen. *Arch Pharm* 322: 324
41 Becker H, Hsieh WC, Wylde R, Laffite C, Andary C (1982) Struktur von Echinacosid. *Z Naturforsch* 37: 351–353
42 Bauer R, Wagner H (1987) Neue Ergebnisse zur Analytik von *Echinacea*-Wurzeln. *Sci Pharm* 55: 159–161

43 Berkulin W, Honerlagen H, Schilling HJ (1984) Isolierung von Echinacosid durch präparative Gelchromatographie an Fractogel TSK HW 40. *Farm Tijdschr Belg* 61: 359

44 Pietta P, Mauri P, Bauer R (1998) MEKC Analysis of Different *Echinacea* Species. *Planta Med; in press*

45 Trypsteen MFM, Van Severen RGE, De Spiegeleer BMJ (1989) Planar chromatography of *Echinacea* species extracts with automated multiple development. *Analyst* 114: 1021–1024

46 Gocan S, Cimpan G, Muresan L (1996) Automated multiple development thin layer chromatography of some plant extracts. *J Pharm Biomed Anal* 14: 1221–1227

47 Facino RM, Sparatore A, Carini M, Gioia B, Arlandini E, Franzoi L (1991) Field desorption mass spectrometry, fast atom bombardment mass spectrometry and fast atom bombardment tandem mass spectrometry of echinacoside, the main caffeoyl-glycoside from *Echinacea angustifolia* roots (Asteraceae). *Org Mass Spectrom* 26: 951–955

48 Facino RM, Carini M, Aldini C, Marinello C, Arlandini E, Franzoi L, Colombo M, Pietta P, Mauri, P. (1993) Direct characterization of caffeoyl esters with antihyaluronidase activity in crude extracts from *Echinacea angustifolia* roots by fast atom bombardment tandem mass spectrometry. *Farmaco* 48: 1447–1461

49 Bonadeo I, Botazzi G, Lavazza M (1971) Echinacin B, an active polysaccharide from *Echinacea. Riv Ital Essenze – Profumi – Piante offic – Aromi – Saponi – Cosmetici – Aerosol* 53: 281–295

50 Wagner H, Proksch A, Riess-Maurer I, Vollmar A, Odenthal S, Stuppner H, Jurcic K, LeTurdu M, Fang JN (1985) Immunstimulierend wirkende Polysaccharide (Heteroglykane) aus höheren Pflanzen. *Arzneim-Forsch* 35: 1069–1075

51 Giger E, Keller F, Baumann TW (1989) Fructans in *Echinacea* and in its phytotherapeutic preparations. *Planta Med* 55: 638–639

52 Beuscher N, Kopanski L, Ernwein C (1987) Modulation der Immunantwort durch polymere Substanzen aus *Baptisia tinctoria* und *Echinacea angustifolia. Adv Biosci* 68: 329–336

53 Egert D, Beuscher N (1992) Studies on antigen specifity of immunoreactive arabinogalactan proteins extracted from *Baptisia tinctoria* and *Echinacea purpurea. Planta Med* 58: 163–165

54 Bauer R, Jurcic K, Puhlmann J, Wagner H (1988) Immunologische *in vivo*- und *in vitro*-Untersuchungen mit *Echinacea*-Extrakten. *Arzneim-Forsch* 38: 276–281

55 Bauer R, Remiger P, Jurcic K, Wagner H (1989) Beeinflussung der Phagozytose-Aktivität durch *Echinacea*-Extrakte. *Z Phytother* 10: 43–48

56 Müller-Jakic B, Breu W, Pröbstle A, Redl K, Greger H, Bauer R (1994) *In vitro* inhibition of cyclooxygenase and 5-lipoxygenase by alkamides from *Echinacea* and *Achillea* species. *Planta Med* 60: 37–40

57 Beuscher N, Bodinet C, Willigmann I, Egert D (1995) Immunmodulierende Eigenschaften von Wurzelextrakten verschiedener *Echinacea*-Arten. *Z Phytother* 16: 157–166

58 Beuscher N, Beuscher HN, Bodinet C (1989) Enhanced release of Interleukin-1 from

mouse macrophages by glycoproteins and polysaccharides from *Baptisia tinctoria* and *Echinacea* species. *Planta Med* 55: 660

59 Bodinet C, Beuscher N (1991) Antiviral and immunological activity of glycoproteins from *Echinaceae purpureae* radix. *Planta Med* 57, Suppl 2: A33–A34

60 Facino RM, Carini M, Aldini G, Saibene L, Pietta P, Mauri P (1995) Echinacoside and caffeoyl conjugates protect collagen from free radical-induced degradation: A potential use of *Echinacea* extracts in the prevention of skin photodamage. *Planta Med* 61: 510–514

61 Li J, Wang PF, Zheng R, Liu ZM, Jia Z (1993) Protection of phenylpropanoid glycosides from *Pedicularis* against oxidative hemolysis *in vitro*. *Planta Med* 59: 315–317

62 Bukovsky M, Vaverkova S, Kostalova D, Magnusova R (1993) Immunomodulating activity of ethanol-water extracts of the roots of *Echinacea gloriosa* L., *Echinacea angustifolia* DC. and *Rudbeckia speciosa* Wenderoth tested on the immune system in C57BL6 inbred mice. *Cesk Farm* 42: 184–187

63 Bukovsky M, Vaverkova S, Kostalova D (1995) Immunomodulating activity of *Echinacea gloriosa* L., *Echinacea angustifolia* DC. and *Rudbeckia speciosa* Wenderoth ethanol-water extracts. *Pol J Pharmacol* 47: 175–177

64 Wild J (1991) *Beeinflussung der Phagozytose humaner Granulozyten durch echinaceahaltige Präparate, sowohl mikroskopisch als auch druchflußzytometrisch bestimmt.* MD Thesis, Universität München

65 Schumacher A, Friedberg KD (1991) Untersuchungen zur Wirkung von *Echinacea angustifolia* auf die unspezifische zelluläre Immunantwort der Maus. *Arzneim-Forsch* 41(I): 141–147

66 Schranner I, Würdinger M, Klumpp N, Lösch U, Okpanyi SN (1989) Beeinflussung der aviären humoralen Immunreaktion durch Influex und *Echinacea angustifolia* Extrakt. *Zbl Vet Med* B36: 353–364

67 Schindler H (1953) Die Inhaltsstoffe von Heilpflanzen und Prüfungsmethoden für pflanzliche Tinkturen – 58. *Echinacea. Arzneim-Forsch* 3: 485–488

68 Stawowczyk A, Karkoszka A (1959) Some chemical properties of *Echinacea purpurea* and *Echinacea pallida* and the alcoholatures from these plants. *Dissertationes Pharm* 11: 183–190; ref. *Chem Abstr* (1959) 53: 22750h

69 Bomme U (1981–1987) *Versuchsergebnisse der Bayerischen Landesanstalt für Bodenkultur und Pflanzenbau, Heil- und Gewürzpflanzen.* Freising-München

70 Oniga I, Popescu H, Verite P, Oprean R (1997) Research on the chemical constituents of essential oils from *Echinacea pallida* (Nutt.). *Clujul Med* 70: 304–308

71 Khan IA (1987) *Neue Sesquiterpenester aus Parthenium integrifolium L. und Polyacetylene aus Echinacea pallida NUTT.* PhD thesis, Universität München

72 Bauer R, Khan IA, Wray V, Wagner H (1987) Two acetylenic compounds from *Echinacea pallida* roots. *Phytochemistry* 26: 1198–1200

73 Cheminat A, Zawatzky R, Becker H, Brouillard R (1988) Caffeoyl conjugates from *Echinacea* species: Structures and biological activity. *Phytochemistry* 27: 2787–2794

74 Kuhn A (1939). In: G Madaus (ed): *Echinacea purpurea Moench. Med Biol Schriftenreihe*, Vol 13. Verlag Rohrmoser, Radebeul/Dresden

75 Becker H (1982) Gegen Schlangenbiß und Grippe – Verwendung und Inhaltsstoffe von *Echinacea angustifolia* und *Echinacea purpurea. Dtsch Apoth Ztg* 122: 2320–2323

76 Martin R (1985) *Säureamide und andere lipophile Inhaltsstoffe aus Acmella ciliata (H.B.K.) CASS.* PhD Thesis, Heidelberg

77 Bauer R, Remiger P, Wagner H (1988) Alkamides from the Roots of *Echinacea purpurea. Phytochemistry* 27: 2339–2342

78 Martin R, Becker H (1985) Amides and other constituents from *Achmella ciliata. Phytochemistry* 24: 2295–2300

79 Trypsteen M, Van Lijsebettens M, Van Severen R, Van Montagu M (1991) Agrobacterium rhizogenes-mediated transformation of *Echinacea purpurea. Plant Cell Rep* 10: 85–89

80 Perry NB, Van Klink, JW, Burgess EJ, Parmenter GA (1997) Alkamide levels in *Echinacea purpurea.* A rapid analytical method revealing differences among roots, rhizomes, stems, leaves, and flowers. *Planta Med* 63: 58–62

81 Bauer R, Khan IA, Lotter H, Wagner H, Wray V (1985) Structure and stereochemistry of new sesquiterpene esters from *Echinacea purpurea* (L.) MOENCH. *Helv Chim Acta* 68: 2355–2358

82 Bauer R, Remiger P, Wagner H (1988) *Echinacea* – Vergleichende DC- und HPLC-Analyse der Herba-Drogen von *Echinacea purpurea, E. pallida* und *E. angustifolia. Dtsch Apoth Ztg* 128: 174–180

83 Becker H, Hsieh WCh (1985) Chicoree-Säure und deren Derivate aus *Echinacea*-Arten. *Z Naturforsch* 40c: 585–587

84 Remiger P (1989) *Zur Chemie und Immunologie neuer Alkylamide und anderer Inhaltsstoffe aus Echinacea purpurea, Echinacea angustifolia und Echinacea pallida.* PhD Thesis, Universität München

85 Hille Th (1985) *Zur Isolierung, Strukturaufklärung und Analytik der Pyrrolizidinalkaloide aus Senecio sylvaticus L., Echinacea purpurea MOENCH und einige Partialsynthesen.* PhD Thesis, Universität Bonn

86 Pogorelaja N F, Menshova VO, Brajon AV, Voevodina, OV, Pogorelaja ZA, Brodovskaya NV (1997) Lectins – biologically active substances of *Echinacea purpurea. Farm Zh* (Kiev) (4): 80–83

87 Vömel Th (1985) Der Einfluß eines pflanzlichen Immunstimulans auf die Phagozytose von Erythrozyten durch das retikulohistozytäre System der isoliert perfundierten Rattenleber. *Arzneim-Forsch* 35: 1437–1439

88 See DM, Broumand N, Sahl L, Tilles JG (1997) In vitro effects of *Echinacea* and *Ginseng* on natural killer and antibody-dependent cell cytotoxicity in healthy subjects and chronic fatigue syndrome or acquired immunodeficiency syndrome patients. *Immunopharmacol* 35: 229–235

89 Jurcic K, Melchart D, Holzmann M, Martin P, Bauer R, Doenicke A, Wagner H (1989)

Zwei Probandenstudien zur Stimulierung der Granulozytenphagozytose durch *Echinacea*-Extrakt-haltige Präparate. *Z Phytother* 10: 67–70
90 Robinson WE Jr, Reinecke MG, Abdel-Malek S, Jia Q, Chow SA (1996) Inhibitors of HIV-1 replication [corrected, erratum to be published] that inhibit HIV integrase. *Proc Natl Acad Sci USA* 93: 6326–6331
91 Neamati N, Hong H, Sunder S, Milne GW, Pommier Y (1997) Potent inhibitors of human immunodeficiency virus type 1 integrase: identification of a novel four-point pharmacophore and tetracyclines as novel inhibitors. *Mol Pharmacol* 52: 1041–1055
92 McDougall B, King PJ, Wu BW, Hostomsky Z, Reinecke MG, Robinson WE Jr (1998) Dicaffeoylquinic and dicaffeoyltartaric acids are selective inhibitors of human immunodeficiency virus type 1 integrase. *Antimicrob Agents Chemother* 42: 140–146
93 Beuscher N, Scheit K-H, Bodinet C, Egert D (1991) Modulation der körpereigenen Immunabwehr durch polymere Substanzen aus *Baptisia tinctoria* und *Echinacea purpurea*. In: KN Masihi, W Lange (eds): *Immunotherapeutic prospects of infections diseases*. Springer Verlag, Berlin Heidelberg
94 Schaper and Brümmer, personal communication
95 Zoutewelle G, Van Wijk R (1990) Effects of *Echinacea purpurea* extracts on fibroblast populated collagen lattice contraction. *Phytotherapy Res* 4: 77–84
96 Bos R, Heinzer F, Bauer R (1988) Volatile constituents of the leaves of *Echinacea purpurea, E. pallida* and *E. angustifolia*. Poster at the 19. International Symposium on Essential Oils and Other Natural Substrates, 7.–10.9.1988 in Zürich.
97 Schulthess BH, Giger ER, Baumann TW (1991) *Echinacea*: anatomy, phytochemical pattern, and germination of the achene. *Planta Med* 57: 384–388
98 Bauer R, Remiger P, Wray V, Wagner H (1988) A germacrene alcohol from fresh aerial parts of *Echinacea purpurea. Planta Med* 54: 478–479
99 Tobler M, Krienbühl H, Egger M, Maurer C, Bühler U (1994) Charakteristik von Frischpflanzengesamtextrakten. Teil 1: Ergebnisse analytischer Untersuchungen. *Schweiz Zschr Ganzheitsmedizin* 257–266
100 Bauer R (1997) Standardisierung von *Echinacea purpurea*-Preßsaft auf Cichoriensäure und Alkamide. *Z Phytother* 18:270–276
101 Bauer R, vom Hagen-Plettenberg F (1997) Gehalt an Cichoriensäure und Alkamiden in *Echinacea purpurea*-Kraut und daraus hergestellten Preßsäften. Poster auf dem 8. Kongreß der Gesellschaft für Phytotherapie, Würzburg
102 Giger E (1990) *Echinacea purpurea und Echinacea angustifolia – Biomasse, Alkamide und Fructane in Abhängigkeit von Jahreszeit, Alter und Nachbarschaftssituation.* PhD Thesis, Universität Zürich
103 Malonga-Makosi J-P (1983) *Untersuchung der Flavonoide von Echinacea angustifolia DC und Echinacea purpurea MOENCH.* PhD Thesis, Universität Heidelberg
104 Alhorn R (1992) *Phytochemische und vegetationsperiodische Untersuchungen von Echinacea purpurea (L.) MOENCH unter Berücksichtigung der Kaffeesäurederivate.* PhD Thesis, Universität Marburg/Lahn

105 Cheminat A, Brouillard R, Guerne P, Bergmann P, Rether B (1989) Cyanidin 3-malonylglucoside in two *Echinacea* species. *Phytochemistry* 28: 3246–3247
106 Hsieh WCh (1984) *Isolierung und Charakterisierung von Kaffeesäurederivaten aus Echinacea-Arten*. PhD Thesis, Universität Heidelberg.
107 Soicke H, Al-Hassan G, Görler K (1988) Weitere Kaffeesäure-Derivate aus *Echinacea purpurea*. *Planta Med* 54: 175–176
108 Scarpati ML, Oriente G (1958) Chicoric acid (dicaffeoyltartaric acid): Its isolation from chicory (*Cichorium intybus*) and synthesis. *Tetrahedron* 4: 43–48
109 Feucht G, Herrmann K, Heimann W (1971) Über das Vorkommen der Hydroxyzimtsäuren im Gemüse – III. Über die im Kopfsalat hauptsächlich vorkommende Kaffeesäure-Verbindung. *Z Lebensm Unters Forsch* 145: 206–212
110 Wöldecke M, Hermann K (1974) D-(+)-Dikaffeoyl-Weinsäure aus Endivien (*Cichorium endivia* L.). *Z Naturforsch* 29c: 360–361
111 Zhao H, Burke TR (1998) Facile syntheses of (2R, 3R)-(–)- and (2S, 3S)-(+)-chicoric acids. *Synthetic Commun* 28: 737–740
112 Sicha J, Hubik J, Dusek J (1989) Production of phenylpropanes by tissue cultures of the genus *Echinacea*. *Cesk Farm* 38: 124–129
113 Sicha J, Becker H, Dusek J, Hubik J, Siatka T, Hrones I (1991) Callus cultures of the genus *Echinacea*. II. Effect of phenylalanine on the growth of cultures and the production of cinnamic acids. *Pharmazie* 46: 363–364
114 Sicha J, Dusek J, Hubik J, Siatka T, Hrones I (1993) Production of phenylpropanes in the callus cultures of the plants of the genus *Echinacea* and the possibilities of its influencing. *Folia Pharm Univ Carol* 17: 75–96
115 Glowniak K, Zgorka G, Kozyra M (1996) Solid-phase extraction and reversed-phase high-performance liquid chromatography of free phenolic acids in some *Echinacea* species. *J Chromatogr* A 730: 25–29
116 De Swaef SI, De Beer JO, Vlietinck AJ (1994) Quantitative determination of *p*-coumaric acid in *Echinacea purpurea* press juice and Urgenin. A validated method. *J Liquid Chrom* 17: 4169–4183
117 Soicke H, Görler K, Krüger D (1988) Glycine-Betaine in *Echinacea* species and their preparations. *Fitoterapia* 59: 73–75
118 Wagner H, Proksch A (1981) Über ein immunstimulierendes Wirkprinzip aus *Echinacea purpurea* MOENCH. *Z angew Phytother* 2: 166–171
119 Stimpel M, Proksch A, Wagner H, Lohmann-Matthes M-L (1984) Macrophage Activation and Induction of Macrophage Cytotoxicity by Purified Polysaccharide Fractions from the Plant *Echinacea purpurea*. *Infect Immun* 46: 845–849
120 Proksch A, Wagner H (1987) Structural Analysis of a 4-O-Methylglucuronoarabinoxylan with Immuno-Stimulating Activity from *Echinacea purpurea*. *Phytochemistry* 26: 1989–1993
121 Proksch A (1982) *Über ein immunstimulierendes Wirkprinzip aus Echinacea purpurea (L.) MOENCH*. PhD Thesis, Universität München
122 Stuppner H (1985) *Chemische und immunologische Untersuchungen von Polysacchari-*

den aus der Gewebekultur von Echinacea purpurea (L.) MOENCH. PhD Thesis, Universität München

123 Wagner H, Stuppner H, Puhlmann J, Jurcic K, Zenk MA, Lohmann-Matthes M-L (1987) Immunstimulierend wirkende Polysaccharide aus Zellkulturen von *Echinacea purpurea* (L.) Moench. *Z Phytother* 8: 125–126

124 Wagner H, Stuppner H, Schäfer W, Zenk MA (1988) Immunologically Active Polysaccharides of *Echinacea purpurea*-Cell Cultures. *Phytochemistry* 27: 119–126

125 McNeil M, Darvill AG, Albersheim P (1979) In: W Herz, H Grisebach, GW Kirby (eds): *Progress in the chemistry of organic natural products.* Springer Verlag, Wien, New York, 37: 191–249

126 Wagner H (1997) *Echinacea*-Polysaccharide und immunologische Wirkung. In: Bauer R (1997) *Echinacea* – Pharmazeutische Qualität und therapeutischer Wert. *Z Phytother* 18: 207–214

127 Kraus S, Wagner H, Liptak A (1996) Labelling of bioactive polysaccharides for resorption studies. Abstract of the 2nd International Congress on Phytomedicine, Munich

128 Giger E, Ramp T, Kreuter MH (1995) β-1,2-fructofuranosides in preparations of *Echinacea purpurea* (L.) Moench. Abstract of Poster K17 at the 43th Annual Congress of the Society for Medicinal Plant Research, Halle

129 Bukovsky M, Kostalova D, Magnusova R, Vaverkova S (1993) Testing for immunomodulating effects of ethanol-water extracts of the above-ground parts of the plants *Echinacea* (Moench) and *Rudbeckia* L. *Cesk-Farm* 42: 228–231

130 Tympner KD (1981) Der immunbiologische Wirkungsnachweis von Pflanzenextrakten. *Z angew Phytother* 2:181–184

131 Fanselow G (1981) *Der Einfluß von Pflanzenextrakten (Echinacea purpurea, Aristolochia clematitis) und homöopathischen Medikamenten (Acidum formicicum, Sulfur) auf die Phagozytoseleistung humaner Granulozyten in vitro.* MD thesis, Universität München

132 Stotzem CD, Hungerland U, Mengs U (1992) Influence of *Echinacea purpurea* on the phagocytosis of human granulocytes. *Med Sci Res* 20: 719–720

133 Bittner E (1969) *Die Wirkung von Echinacin auf die Funktion des Retikuloendothelialen Systems.* MD Thesis, Universität Freiburg

134 Fontana A (1998) De Gruyter; *in press*

135 Miller K et al (1998) De Gruyter; *in press*

136 Wildfeuer A, Mayerhofer D (1994) The effects of plant preparations on cellular functions in body defense. *Arzneim-Forsch* 44: 361–366

137 Gaisbauer M, Schleich T, Stickl HA, Wilczek I (1990) The effect of *Echinacea purpurea* Moench on phagocytosis in granulocytes measured by chemiluminescence. *Arzneim-Forsch* 40: 594–598

138 Leng-Peschlow et al (1998) De Gruyter; *in press*

139 Riedel W (1998) De Gruyter; *in press*

140 Choné B (1965) Gezielte Steuerung der Leukozyten-Kinetik durch Echinacin. *Ärztl Forsch* 19: 611–612

141 Krause M (1984) *Die Wirkung von Echinacin auf Knochenmarkkulturen bei zytologisch unverändertem Knochenmark sowie Blutkulturen bei chronisch-myeloischer Leukämie, Osteomyeolo-sklerose und akuter nicht lymphatischer Leukämie.* MD Thesis, Freie Universität Berlin

142 Krause W (1986) *Untersuchungen zur Wirkung von Ascorbinsäure und Echinacin auf die Funktion neutrophiler Granulozyten.* MD Thesis, Universität Tübingen

143 Hoh K (1990) *Untersuchungen über immunmodulierende Wirkungen von Echinacea-purpurea-Preßsaft und dafür verantwortliche Inhaltsstoffe.* MD Thesis, Universität Freiburg

144 Mantovani A (1981) *In vitro* effects on tumor cells of macrophages isolated from an early-passage chemically-induced murine sarcoma and from its spontaneous metastases. *Int J Cancer* 27: 221–228

145 Wacker A, Hilbig W (1978) Virushemmung mit *Echinacea purpurea. Planta Med* 33: 89–102

146 Orinda D, Diederich J, Wacker A (1973) Antivirale Aktivität von Inhaltsstoffen der Composite *Echinacea purpurea. Arzneim-Forsch* 23: 1119–1120

147 Eichler F, Krüger GRF (1994) Effects of non-specific immunostimulants (Echinacin, isoprinosine and thymus factors) on the infection and antigen expression in herpesvirus-6 exposed human lymphoid cells. *In Vivo* 8: 565–576

148 Koch FE, Haase H (1952) Eine Modifikation des Spreading-Tests im Tierversuch – gleichzeitig ein Beitrag zum Wirkungsmechanismus von Echinacin. *Arzneim-Forsch* 2: 464–467

149 Koch FE, Uebel H (1954) Experimentelle Untersuchungen über die lokale Beeinflussung der Gewebsresistenz gegen Streptokokkeninfektion durch Cortison und Echinacin. *Arzneim-Forsch* 4: 551–560

150 Wagner H, Kraus S, Jurcic K (1999) Search for potent immunostimulating agents from plants and other natural sources. In: H Wagner (ed): *Immunomodulatory agents from plants.* Birkhäuser Verlag, Basel, 1–39

151 Emmendörffer AC, Wagner H, Lohmann-Matthes ML (1998) Immunologically active polysaccharides from Echinacea purpurea plant and cell cultures. In: H Wagner (ed) *Immunomodulatory agents from plants.* Birkhäuser Verlag, Basel, 89–104

152 Bauer R (1993) *Echinacea*-Drogen – Neue Ergebnisse zur Frage der Wirksubstanzen. *Natur und Ganzheitsmedizin* (6): 13–22

153 Bauer R (1994) *Echinacea* – Eine Arzneidroge auf dem Weg zum rationalen Phytotherapeutikon. *Dtsch Apoth Ztg* 134: 94–103

154 Bauer R, Czygan F-C, Franz G, Ihrig M, Nahrstedt A, Sprecher E (1994) Pharmazeutische Qualität, Standardisierung und Normierung von Phytopharmaka. *Z Phytother* 15: 82–91

155 Bauer R (1998) Quality criteria and standardization of phytopharmaceuticals: Can acceptable drug standards be achieved? *Drug Information Journal* 32: 101–110

156 Bauer R, Tittel G. (1996) Quality assessment of herbal preparations as a precondition of pharmacological and clinical studies. *Phytomedicine* 2: 193–198

157 Feiden K (ed) (1997) *Arzneimittelprüfrichtlinien*. Wissenschaftliche Verlagsgesellschaft, Stuttgart
158 EEC Notes for Guidance "Quality of Herbal Remedies" CD 75/318 EEC and CD 91/507 EEC
159 Bomme U (1987) Sonnenhut – Pflanze mit Marktchancen? *DLZ* 38: 384–386
160 Shalaby A, Angina E.A, El-Gengaihi SE, El-Khayat AS (1997) Response of *Echinacea* to Some Agricultural Practices. *J Herbs Spices & Medicinal Plants* 4: 59–67

Immunologically active polysaccharides from *Echinacea purpurea* plant and cell cultures

Andreas C. Emmendörffer[1], *Hildebert Wagner*[2], *Marie-Luise Lohmann-Matthes*[1]

[1]Department of Immunobiology, Fraunhofer Institute of Toxicology and Aerosal Research, Hannover; [2]Institute of Pharmaceutical Biology, Ludwig-Maximilians-Universität München, Karlstrasse 29, D-80333 Munich, Germany

Introduction

The use of extracts of *Echinacea angustifolia* and *E. purpurea* by the American Indians and later in the Traditional medicine of Europe against wounds, burns, swellings of the lymph glands (mumps), measles and various infections has initiated a thorough chemical and pharmacological search for the active components of the drugs. Since the weak antimicrobial activity found for the extract and the isolated caffeic acid derivative echinacoside, isolated from the root of *Echinacea angustifolia*, could not explain the therapeutic efficacy of the drug, *in vitro* and *in vivo* immunological investigations were started. They resulted in the isolation of several low and high molecular weight compounds such as caffeic acid derivatives, poly-acetylenes, alkylamides, and polysaccharides (see chapter by R. Bauer, this volume). Among them the 2,3-O dicaffeoyl tartaric acid (cichoric acid) and the polysaccharides, a 4-O-methylglucuronoarabinoxylan (EPS-XG) (MW ≅ 35 kDa) and an acidic arabinorhamnogalactan (EPS-AG) (MW ≅ 50 kDa) turned out to be the most active compounds in several *in vitro* and *in vivo* immunological assays [1, 2] (Fig. 1). The expensive isolation procedure of the polysaccharides in a pure form and the difficulty of obtaining them with reproducible activity prompted one of us to produce them from tissue cultures of *Echinacea purpurea* leaves. From the growth medium two homogeneous polysaccharides, i.e. a neutral fucogalactoxyloglucan (MW ≅ 25 kDa) and an acidic arabinogalactan (MW ≅ 75 kDa) could be isolated [3] (Fig. 2a, b).

As expected, the structure of the tissue culture polysaccharides differed from those of the aerial parts, since cells cultured in suspension culture possess exclusively primary cell wall components. In Table 1 the molar sugar composition of both polysaccharides compared with those isolated from the plant are listed.

In the first experiments a polysaccharide mixture from the plant was investigated (EPS). During this time we succeeded in producing a polysaccharide mixture on an industrial scale in 75,000 l-fermenters, from which a pure arabinogalactan (EP-AG) was isolated. This made it possible to repeat and extend the earlier investigations with pure arabinogalactan. The homogeneity of EP-AG was assessed by

Immunomodulatory Agents from Plants, edited by H. Wagner

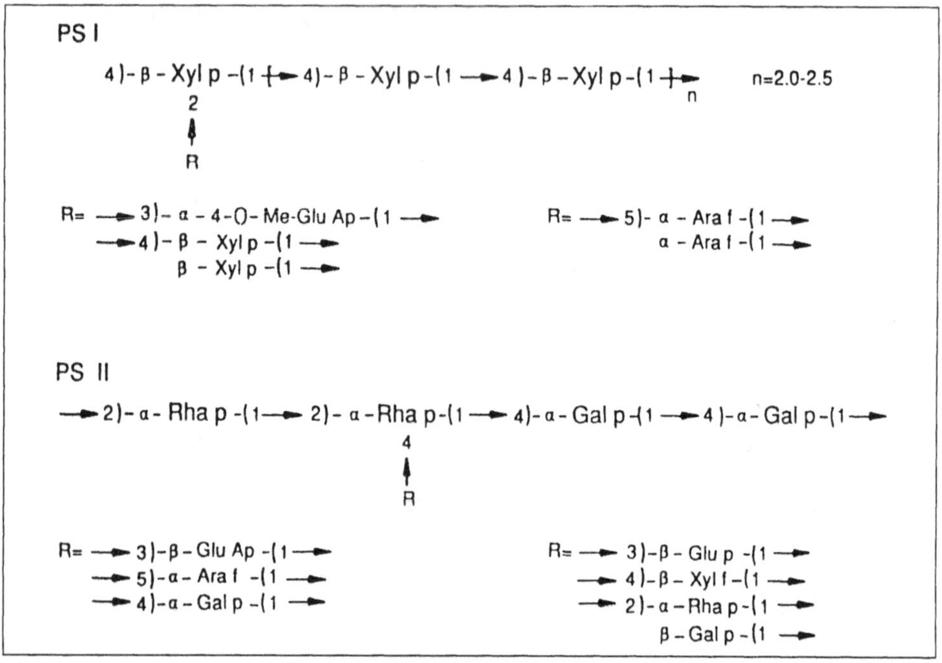

Figure 1
Structures of polysaccharides EPS-XG (PS I) and EPS-AG (PS II) isolated from the herb of Echinacea purpurea.

HPGGP (high pressure gel permeation chromatography), ultracentrifugation, optical rotation and other parameters. The structure elucidation was performed by qualitative and quantitative sugar analysis, permethylation analysis, ^{13}C-NMR- and 500 MHz ^{1}HNMR-spectroscopy and partial acidic as well as enzymatic hydrolysis. In addition, process controls were performed to assure the lack of bacterial contamination, especially the absence of bacterial LPS. As shown later, the marginal inducing effect of EP-AG on the B cell proliferation effectively distinguished EP-AG from bacterial lipopolysaccharides, which are potent B cell mitogens.

Immunological *in vitro* studies

T and B cell-proliferation

Employing the conventional proliferation assay using lymphocytes isolated from spleen (mouse, rat), lymph nodes (mouse, rat), or peripheral human blood and

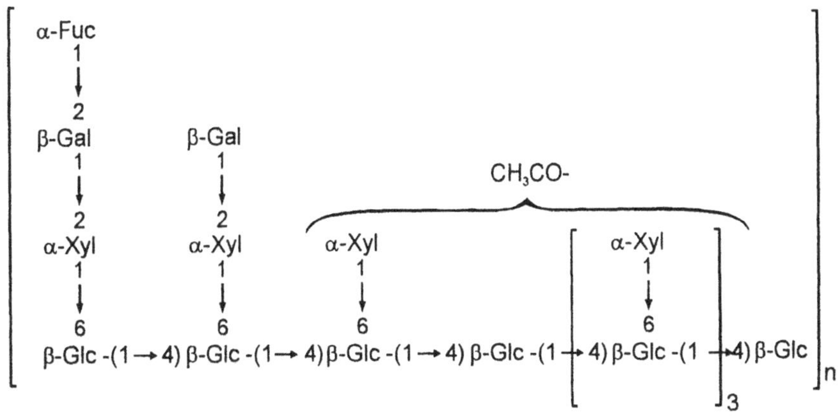

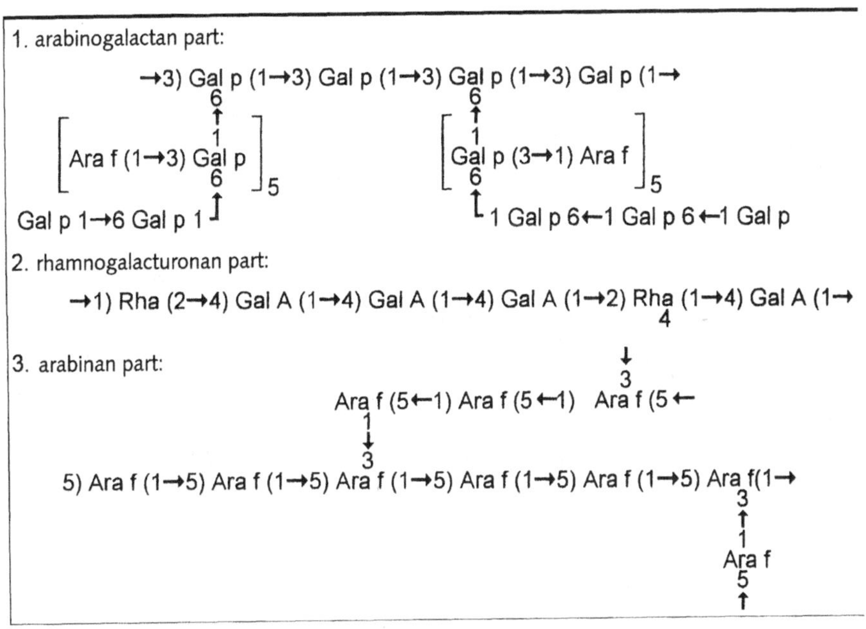

Figure 2a + b
Structures of polysaccharides EP-XG and EP-AG isolated from tissue cultures of Echinacea purpurea.

Table 1 - Molecular sugar composition of polysaccharides from Echinacea purpurea *herb and tissue culture*

Polysaccharides: herb						
PS I:	Xy	Ar	Ga	4-O-Me-Gls	Glu	Rha
	4.9 :	1.0 :	0.9	0.9 :	0.4 :	0.3 mol
PS II:	Ar	Rha	Ga	Gls		
	1.0 :	0.8 :	0.6 :	0.6 mol		
Polysaccharides: tissue culture						
AG:	Ga	Ar	Rha	Ma	Uronic acid	
	1.0 :	1.04 :	0.02 :	0.03 mol	16 %	
Fucogalactoxyloglucan:	Fu	Ga	Xy	Glu		
	0.1 :	1.5 :	1.0 :	0.27 mol		

ConA as reference compound no significant effect of EPS could be found with respect to the induction of T cell proliferation [4–6].

When T cells were incorporated with arabinogalactan and the supernatants tested on the IL-2-dependent cell line CTLL, even after 48 h of stimulation with 500 µg AG, no significant IL-2 production was observed. T lymphocytes stimulated with ConA (1 µg/ml) secreted 13 U of IL-2/ml. Addition of EP-AG during ConA stimulation of T cells or during the CTLL assay had no effect [4, 5, 7].

A similar result was obtained in the B lymphocyte proliferation assay. B lymphocytes were isolated from spleen of NMRI nu/nu mice by using the indirect rosetting method for depleting the cell suspension of macrophages. B cells did not proliferate in response to 500 µg EP-AG. The incorporated radioactivity of the non-activated rosetting cells was higher than that of the non-activated original spleen cell suspension because of the anti-IgM antibody, which slightly activated B-lympho-cytes. These rosetting cells however could be stimulated by 10 µg LPS to incorporate six times more radioactivity than the cells cultured with medium or EP-AG.

Granulocyte and macrophage phagocytosis

Using neutrophils (PMN) isolated from the peripheral blood, either by density centrifugation or in a whole blood assay, EPS and EP-AG were screened for their potential to enhance phagocytosis. Similar experiments were also carried out with bone marrow and peritoneal macrophages of rodents. The phagocytosis assays were carried out by the microscopy smear test according to Brandt [8] and from 1992 on, by flow cytometry [9]. EPS and EP-AG directly enhanced, without the presence of lymphocytes, the *in vitro* phagocytosis of granulocytes as well as the *in vivo* phagocytosis of macrophages by 30 to 50 % in a concentration range of 0.01 to 0.001 mg/ml [10].

Chemiluminescence induction

200 μg EPS were able to enhance the reactive oxygen intermediates (ROI) producing capacity of J 774 mouse macrophages by about 270%, as compared to untreated cells, in a lucigenin/zymosan chemiluminescence assay but were less effective than 100 U/ml IFNγ. Higher concentrations of EPS demonstrated the tendency to suppress ROI production. Incubation of macrophages for 24 h with 20 μg EP-AG was followed by a dose-dependent increase in chemiluminescence, i.e. a two-fold and four-fold increase, respectively, compared with the controls [11].

Induction of cytokine production

Incubation of macrophages with EP-AG resulted in an enhanced production of cytokines. As shown in Table 2, EP-AG was able to induce peritoneal macrophages,

Table 2 - TNFα production by arabinogalactan-activated macrophages [7]*

Incubation of macrophages with	TNF secretion (U/ml)
Medium	< 4
Arabinogalactan (μg/ml)	
500	> 5.000
250	2,560
125	1,280
62.6	644
15.5	320
7.8	160
3.7	80

**2 × 10^5 thioglycollate-induced peritoneal macrophages were incubated with arabinogalactan or medium for 18 h at 37°C in 5% CO_2. Supernatants were collected and serially diluted onto 2 × 10^4 L929 cells treated with 2.5 μg of actinomycin/ml.*

Table 3 - Activation of macrophages to cytotoxicity by EPS [6]

Activation with	**Specific ^{51}Cr release from P815 tumor cells (%) by 2×10^5 of the following macrophage effector cells:**		
	Starch induced peritoneal	**Bone marrow induced**	**Thioglycolate induced**
Medium	28 ± 3	29 ± 4	31 ± 4
100 µg of EPS	62 ± 4	58 ± 5	64 ± 5
10 U of MAF	68 ± 3	60 ± 4	72 ± 5

Macrophages were incubated for 24 h with medium. EPS or MAF. After activation, macrophages were washed and tested for cytotoxicity against labeled P815 cells. The percent spontaneous ^{51}Cr release from P815 was 28 ± 4. Data are given as mean ± standard deviations.

1 U of MAF is the smallest amount of MAF required to render macrophages fully cytotoxic.

in a dose-dependent manner, to produce tumor necrosis factor (TNFα), as measured by the lysis of TNF sensitive L-929 target cells (indicator cells). Even a very small concentration of EP-AG (2.5 µg/ml) showed a stimulatory effect [7, 11].

Bone marrow macrophages were incubated with EP-AG, and for comparison with LPS, and the cytoprotective effect of secreted IFNβ_2 (IL-6) was measured using vesicular stomatitis virus to induce cytolysis. 250 µg EP-AG showed the same activity as 10 µg LPS, causing the release of 150 units of IFNβ-2 [7].

During incubation of resident peritoneal macrophages with EP-AG, the secretion of IL-1 was three times higher than that spontaneously secreted. By far the highest amount of secreted IL-1, however, was induced by LPS. When LPS and arabinogalactan were incubated with macrophages, the results were similar to those with LPS alone. Addition of AG to the supernatant containing LPS-induced IL-1 had no effect, indicating that EP-AG had no effect on the IL-1-induced proliferation [6].

Induction of tumor cytotoxicity and intracellular killing

Incubation of peritoneal macrophages with 100 µg EPS, followed by cocultivation with ^{51}Cr-labeled TNFα-sensitive tumor cells (WEHI 164-tumor cells) resulted in a degree of cytotoxicity equivalent to about 10 U MAF (macrophage activating factor) (Tab. 3).

Table 4 - Intracellular killing of Leishmania enriettii parasites by thioglycollate-induced peritoneal macrophages activated by IFNγ or arabinogalactan [7]*

Incubation of macrophages with	^{3}H-thymidine incorporation (cpm) into released parasites	% intracellular lysis
Medium	6.750 ± 430	–
Arabinogalactan (250 mg/ml)	915 ± 272[2]	86.4
IFNγ (1,000 U/mL)	620 ± 65[2]	90.8

** Macrophages were first parasitized at an effector to target ratio of 1:10 for 24 h. Effector-cells were then activated overnight, and after this incubation period parasites were set free, macrophages were lysed by 0.01% sodium dodecyl sulfate, and parasites were cultured in adequate growth medium in the presence of ^{3}H-thymidine for 48 h. Incorporated radioactivity was measured in scintillation counter. Values = means ± SD.*

[2] $p < 0.001$ for activated vs. nonactivated macrophages.

Peritoneal macrophages were parasitized with ^{3}H-thymidine-labeled *Leishmania enriettii* promastigotes, followed by activation with EP-AG. The macrophages were lysed and the number of released viable parasites was quantified [7] (Tab. 4).

In a similar experiment, EP-AG-activated Kupffer cells (liver macrophages) were cocultivated with *Candida albicans* cells and the *Candida* cells released from the lysed macrophages counted. 100 μg of EP-AG turned out to be as effective in activating the macrophages to inhibit growth of *C. albicans* as the maximal activation obtained by LPS and IFNγ together [11].

In order to investigate whether EPS was able to activate the macrophage transcription factor NFκB, which after translocation to the nucleus controls the transcription of several genes, mouse peritoneal macrophages were cultivated with two different EPS preparations (1 μg/ml) and LPS for comparison. The activation of NFκB was measured by an electromobility shift assay (Fig. 3).

Immunological *in vivo* investigations

Based on the promising *in vitro* results, several *in vivo* studies were performed in rodents to further substantiate the immunostimulatory activity of EPS and EP-AG.

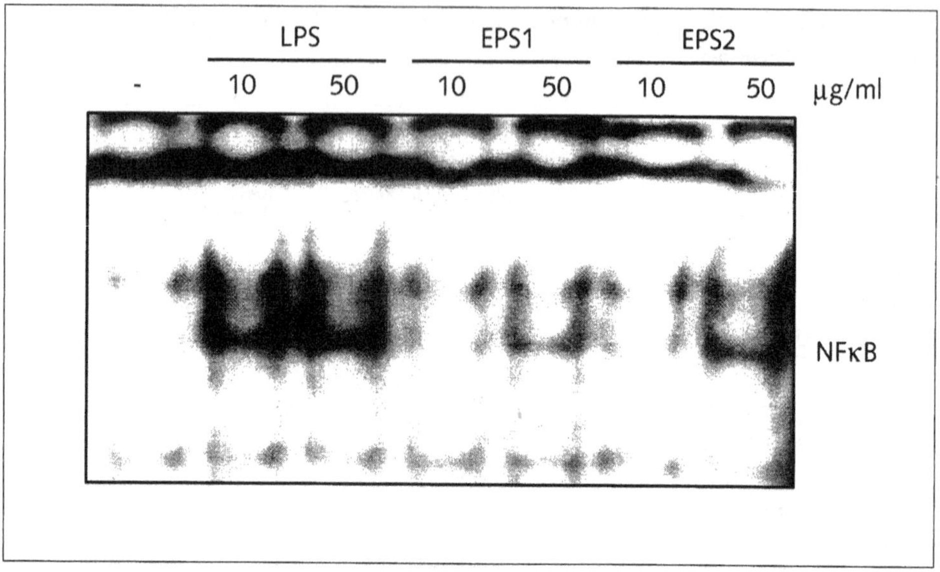

Figure 3
EPS induces activation of NFκB.
Mouse peritoneal macrophages were cultivated for 120 min either in medium alone or medium containing LPS (100 ng/ml) and two different EPS preparations (1 µg/ml). The activation of NFκB was measured by an electromobility shift assay.

Induction of leucocytosis

EPS induced, 3–4 h after i.v. application of 200 µg/mouse, a high increase in the number of peripheral blood leucocytes preceded by a slight, but reproducible, fall. Both the initial decrease and the following increase in the leucocyte number, were due to changes in the numbers of polymorphonuclear cells (PMN) as demonstrated by the differential blood count. The absolute number of lymphocytes remained more or less constant. The initial fall in the number of PMN may indicate their adherence to endothelial cells whereas the subsequent appearance of immature PMN indicates migration of cells from the bone marrow into the peripheral blood [4].

Phagocytosis enhancement

In the carbon clearance assay carried out with mice according to Biozzi et al. [12], 10 mg/kg EPS enhanced the clearance two- to three fold compared to the control [10].

Induction of CSF

200 µg EP i.v. administered to mice, resulted in a significant induction of CSF (colony stimulating factor) as measured by the bone marrow proliferation assay. A further experiment showed that the augmentation of serum-CSF parallels the increase of progenitor cells of macrophages in the bone marrow [11].

Protection against systemic infections

Mice i.v. pretreated with 10 mg/kg EP-AG were infected 24 h later with *Listeria monocytogenes* and treated at the same time with a second dose of EP-AG. After 48 h, the number of colony-forming *Candida* cells (CFU) in the liver and spleen showed a highly significant decrease. 500 µg/kg EP-AG was able to protect mice 100% against the otherwise fatal consequences of an LD_{50} dose of *L. monocytogenes* [11] (Fig. 4).

In another infection load test using *Candida albicans* cells, 10 mg/kg of EG-AG, i.v. administered, was also able to reduce the number of colony-forming *Candida* cells in the kidney. Both protective experiments were repeated with cyclophosphamide and cyclosporin pretreated mice. They also resulted in a significant reduction in the counts of CFU of *Candida* and *Listeria* in the organs and a 75–90% survival rate of the mice [13]. These studies clearly showed that EPS and EP-AG are able to restore the resistance against lethal infections even in an immune-compromized T cell system. In this context it has to be emphasized that *Listeria monocytogenes* infection is a predominantly macrophage-dependent model, while the infection load with *Candida albicans* is primarily controlled by granulocytes [4, 11].

Toxicological investigations

Toxicological data are available for the *Echinacea* polysaccharides. Using the method of Lorke [14] on mice, Lenk [15] found a LD_{50} value of > 2500 and > 5000 mg/kg respectively, for a polysaccharide mixture from the aerial part of *E. purpurea* and ≥ 4000 mg/kg for EPS-AG after i.p. administration. Therefore, according to Loomis [16], it can be assumed that the two pure polysaccharides (fucogalactoxyloglucan and acidic arabinogalactan) are non-toxic. The lungs of the animals that died within 24 h of the intraperitoneal injection of 5000 mg/kg displayed marked interstitial and interalveolar edema with localized leukodiapedesis, indicating an acute circulatory failure. It could be suggested that the animals in the acute experiment died from non-compensated shock, which was not due to the polysaccharide per se, but to the hyperosmolar and syrupy nature of their solutions.

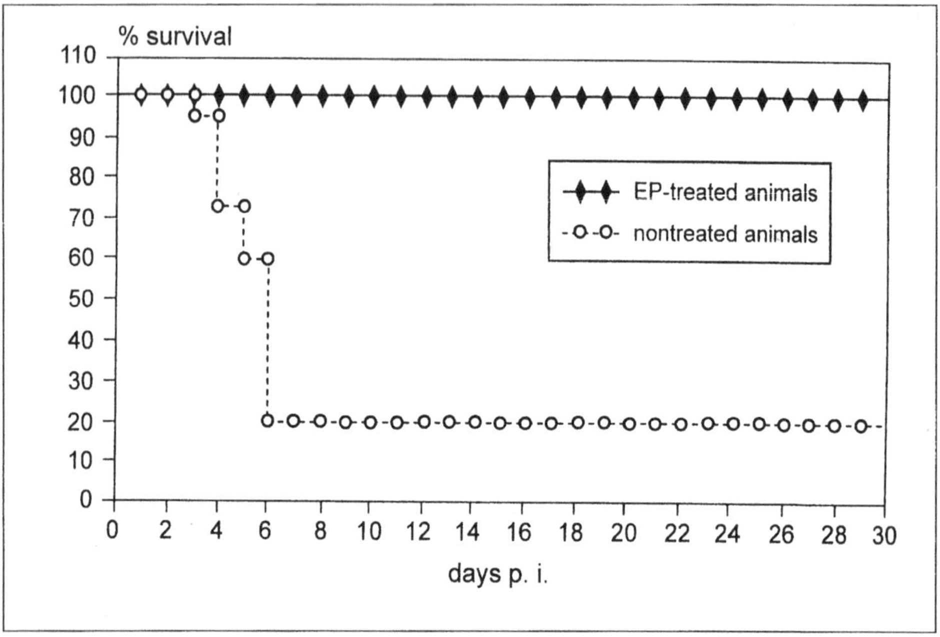

Figure 4
Survival rates of Listeria *infected mice with and without EPS-pretreatment.*
The mice were infected i.v. with 2 × 10^4 Listeria monocytogenes. *EPS-treatment was carried out with 0.2 mg i.v. on days –1, 0 and +1.*

Results from sub-chronic 28-days toxicity of EPS in rats (i.v. administration) showed no toxic effects up to 144-fold of the human dose. The same holds true for chronic 3-months toxicity of EPS-AG in beagle dogs up to 190-fold of the human dose.

Local tolerance after different parenteral administrations in rabbits and tests on hemocompatibility were excellent.

The neutral polysaccharide, NFA10, from *E. purpurea* tissue cultures was tested by Schimmer et al [17] for possible gene toxicity in human lymphocyte cultures. Sister chromatid exchange (SCE) and structural chromosome aberrations (CA) were monitored as criteria of genetic damage. To determine the SCE rate, 25 complete second metaphases were evaluated in each test series, while 100 metaphases per test series were monitored for the determination of CA. No significant dose-dependent increase in SCE or CA was observed, either in short-term or long-term experiments, up to a polysaccharide concentration of 500 µg/ml. In view of these *in vivo* results and since a high correlation of negative results has been shown for the *in vitro*/*in vivo* comparison of cytogenetic test methods, a gene toxicity for *Echinacea* polysaccharides *in vivo* is very unlikely.

Since the *Echinacea* polysaccharides induce several immunological functions in macrophages it was investigated whether EP also induces MHC class II antigens, as characteristic for IFNγ. By using two human cell lines, the human monocyte-line U937 and the human tumor cell line Colo 205, and IFNγ as positive control, neither 0.1 mg nor 1.0 mg EP/ml resulted in the expression of MHC, whereas human INFγ (100 U/ml) showed a very high antigen expression. The expression was determined by staining the macrophages with FITC-labeled anti-HLA DR antibodies and using flow cytometry.

Clinical studies with EPS and EP-AG

Clinical phase I studies/side effects

The trials in healthy volunteers, performed in two centers (Fraunhofer Institute for Toxicology and Aerosol Research, Hannover; Institute of Experimental Anesthesiology, University of Munich) using EPS as a mixture of AG and XG, showed after i.v. injection an increase in the number of neutrophils and a significant release of cytokines from granulocytes and macrophages. Figure 5 shows that 4, 6 and 8 mg of EPS-AG and EPS increased the granulocyte count more than three fold, whereas after a single dose of 8 mg EPS-AG and EPS a significant serum level of interleukin-6 could be observed [18].

At that time a significant rise in the CRP-level (acute phase protein = C-reactive protein) was also seen. After repeated doses of EPS the level of CRP remained constantly increased. According to new findings, the concentration of CRP correlates with the macrophage activity, i.e. release of IL-6. Repeated i.v. administration of EPS-AG (up to five injections) with different time intervals between the injections has led to reproducible effects following each single injection with respect to all parameters of a differential blood count. The time course for granulocyte count (increase 3.5-fold) is shown in Figure 6. In all phase I studies the equipotency of EPS-AG and EPS could be demonstrated.

Side effects

Slight and transitory unwanted side effects occurred only at high doses of 5 mg per injection: muscular soreness-like findings, influenza-like symptoms, and headaches. Allergic reactions and sensibilisations have not occurred.

The second series of phase I studies in healthy volunteers were performed using EPS-AG in comparison with EPS and EPS-XG (45–50). The equipotency of EPS-AG and EPS could again be demonstrated in comparative trials.

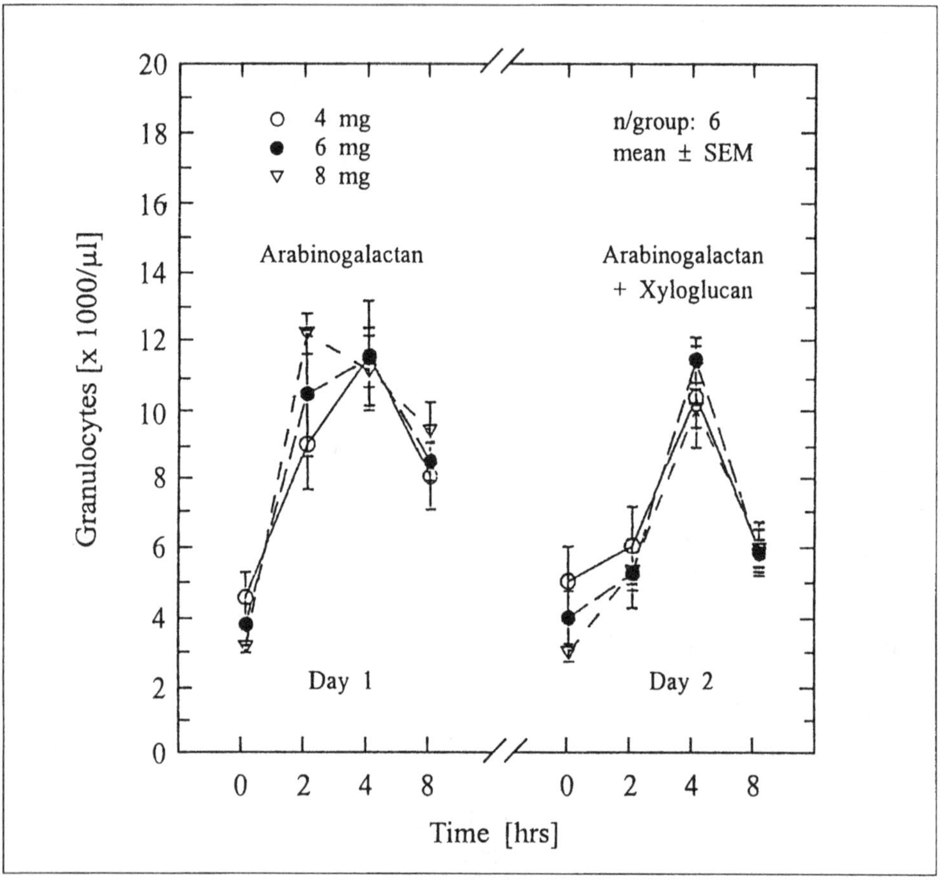

Figure 5
Time course of granulocyte counts [10^3 cells/µl] in healthy volunteers after different doses of EPS-AG and EPS.

Clinical trials, phase II/III [19, 20]

Since in preceding studies a dose of 1 mg/ml per day was found to be equipotent with 4 or 6 mg/ml doses, this dose was used for the first clinical trial with patients through a period of two weeks or 2 × 4 days, respectively.

The following pilot studies were completed:

I. AIDS: 7 HIV-infected patients with oral candidosis; treatment: 2 × 4 days (2 days break) with 1 mg/ml i.v. daily at the University Hospitals of Dermatology, Frankfurt/M. and Munich.

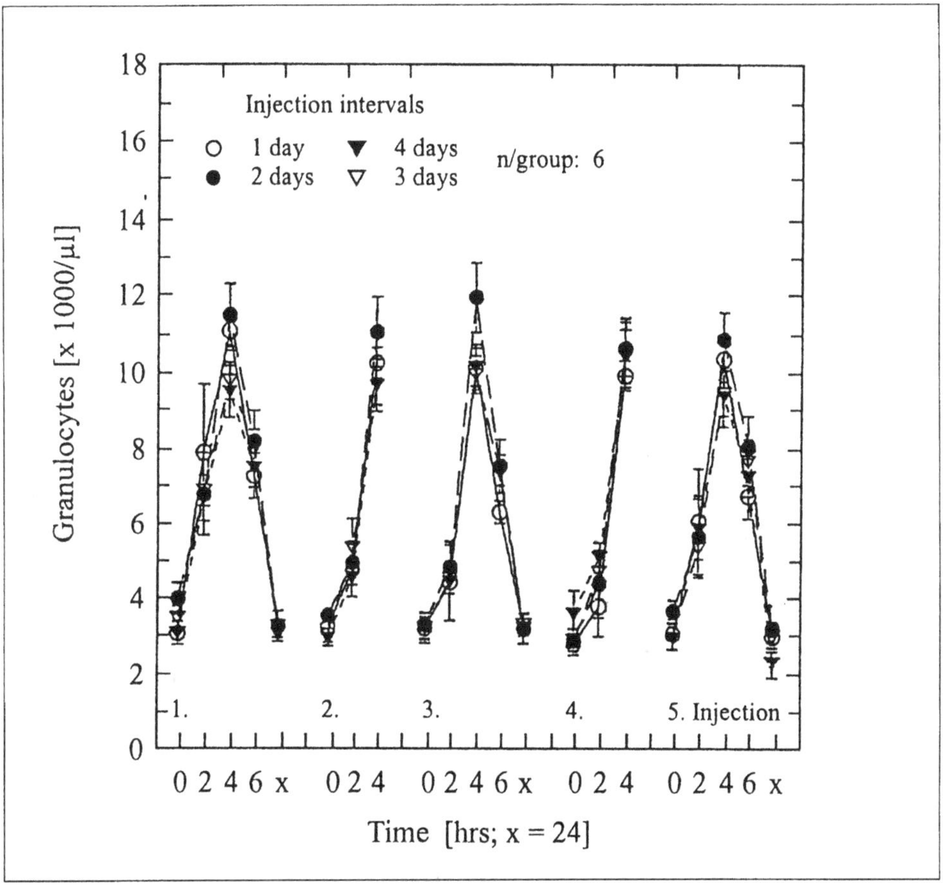

Figure 6
Time course of granulocyte counts [$10^3/\mu l$] in healthy volunteers after five injections given daily, every other day, or longer intervals.

II. Melanoma: Treatment of immunodeficiency in nine patients with melanoma;
treatment: 2 × 4 days (2 days break) with 1 mg/ml i.v. daily at the Hospital of Dermatology of the Technical University, Munich.

III. Leukemia: Treatment of immunodeficiency following chemotherapy in acute leukemia or cellular immunodeficiency, 11 patients;
treatment: 2 weeks with 1 mg/ml i.v. p.d. at Children's Hospital of Harlaching, Munich.

These three studies have demonstrated, that

(i) in HIV-infected persons with oral candidosis, redness and white furrings of the tongue and check receded, although no antimycotic treatment was performed during the trial. In addition, the colonization of the mouth decreased from10^5 to 10^2 germs/ml;

(ii) in melanoma patients the activity of the NK cells was increased;

(iii) in children with cellular immunodeficiency (acute leukemia) the number of leukocytes and the CRP-level was increased significantly (n = 8). Moreover, the platelet count, which generally decreases during chemotherapy, was stabilized or slightly increased.

Three further cases of children with untreatable, chronic infections showed surprising recoveries: a boy suffering from osteomyelitis (entire tibia) was released from the hospital after two weeks therapy with EPS; an otherwise necessary amputation of the leg was avoided.

An open, necrotizing ulcer with extreme aggravation of wound healing at the big toe could be markedly improved, an amputation was also avoided. Last but not least the course of the disease in a girl with agranulocytosis and a vulvar abscess could be improved.

Clinical trials, phase III

After completing these clinical pilot studies, comparative trials with a statistically sufficient number of patients are planned (in part under the auspices of the WHO; indications: neutropenia following chemotherapy; AIDS). Adequate comparator drugs have yet to be defined.

Moreover, it is planned to investigate possible synergistic effects in treatments with antibiotics in combination with EPS-AG.

References

1 Wagner H, Proksch A (1981) Über ein immunstimulierendes Wirkprinzip aus *Echinacea purpurea* MOENCH. *Z angew Phytother* 2: 166–171

2 Proksch A, Wagner H (1987) Structural analysis of a 4-O-Methylglucurono-arabinoxylan with immunostimulating activity from *Echinacea purpurea*. *Phytochemistry* 26: 1989–1993

3 Wagner H, Stuppner, H, Schäfer W, Zenk MA (1988) Immunologically active polysaccharides of *Echinacea purpurea* cell cultures. *Phytochemistry* 27: 119–126

4 Roesler J, Steinmueller C, Kiderlen A, Emmendoerffer A, Wagner H, Lohmann-Matthes M-L (1991) Application of purified polysaccharides from cell cultures of the plant *Echinacea purpurea* to mice mediates protection against systemic infections with *Listeria monocytogenes* and *Candida albicans. Int J Immunopharmac* 13: 27–37

5 Elsasser-Beile U, Willenbacher W, Bartsch HH, Gallati H, Schulte Monting J, von Kleist S (1996) Cytokine production in leukocyte cultures during therapy with *Echinacea* extract. *J Clin Lab Anal* 10: 441–445

6 Stimpel M, Proksch A, Wagner H, Lohmann-Matthes M-L (1984) Macrophage activation and induction of macrophage cytotoxicity by purified polysaccharide fractions from the plant *Echinacea purpurea. Infect Immun* 46: 845–849

7 Luettig B., Steinmüller C, Gifford GE, Wagner H, Lohmann-Matthes M-L (1989) Macrophage activation by the polysaccharide arabinogalactan isolated from plant cell cultures of *Echinacea purpurea. J Nat Cancer Inst* 81: 669–675

8 Brandt L, (1967) Studies on the phagocytic activity of neutrophilic leucocytes. *J Hematol* (Suppl 2)

9 Wagner H, Jurcic K (1996) A new flowcytometric assay for measuring the leukocyte phagocytosis activity of immunostimulating plant extracts, polysaccharides and various low molecular weight compounds. *Phytomedicine* 3 (Suppl 1): 31

10 Wagner H, Proksch A, Riess-Maurer I, Vollmar A, Odenthal S, Stuppner H, Jurcic K, Le Turdu M, Fang IN (1985) Immunstimulierend wirkende Polysaccharide (Heteroglykane) aus höheren Pflanzen. *Arzneim-Forsch* 35: 1069–1075

11 Lohmann-Matthes M-L, Wagner H, (1989) Aktivierung von Makrophagen durch Polysaccharide aus Gewebekulturen von *Echinacea purpurea. Z Phytother* 10: 52–59

12 Biozzi G, Benacerraf B, Stiffel C, Halpern BN (1954). Etude quantitative de l'activité granulopectique du système réticuloendothelial chez la souris. *R.C. Soc Biol Paris* 148: 431

13 Steinmueller C, Roesler J, Gröttrup, Franke G, Wagner H, Lohmann-Matthes M-L (1993) Polysaccharides isolated from plant cell cultures of *Echinacea purpurea* enhance the resistance of immunosuppressed mice against systemic infections with *Candida albicans* and *Listeria monocytogenes. Int J Immunopharmac* 15: 605–614

14 Lorke D (1983) A new approach to practical acute toxicity testing. *Arch Toxicol* 54: 275–287 (1983)

15 Lenk M (1989) Die akute Toxizität von verschiedenen Polysaccharid-Fraktionen aus *Echinacea purpurea* an der Maus. *Z Phytother* 10: 49–52

16 Loornis TA (1978) *Essentials of toxicology,* 3rd ed. Lea & Felbiger, Philadelphia

17 Schimmer O, Abel G, Behringer C (1989) Untersuchungen zur gentoxischen Potenz eines neutralen Polysaccharids aus *Echinacea*-Gewerbekulturen in menschlichen Lymphocytenkulturen. *Z Phytother* 10: 39–42

18 Doenicke A (1992) Wirksamkeit und Verträglichkeit des Immunodulators EPS bei Probanden nach verschiedenen Applikationsformen. *Medical Report (unpublished)*

19 Vogt HJ, Schöfer H, Kaiser PM (1990) Wirksamkeit und Verträglichkeit des neuen

Immunmodulators EPS bei HIV-infizierten Patienten mit oraler Candidose. Abstract 3, *Deutscher AIDS-Kongreß*, Nov. 1990
20 Tympner KD, Klose PK (1991) Wirksamkeit und Verträglichkeit von EPS bei Tumorpatienten. Explorative Studie mit 11 Patienten, *Medical Report (unpublished)*, January 1991

Clinical investigations of *Echinacea* phytopharmaceuticals

Dieter Melchart and Klaus Linde

Münchener Modell – Centre for Complementary Medicine Research, Technical University/
Ludwig-Maximilians-University, Kaiserstr. 9, D-80801 München, Germany

Introduction

Preparations containing extracts of the plant *Echinacea* (family *Compositae*) are widely used by patients and practitioners in some European countries for preventing and treating upper respiratory tract infections as well as more generally for "stimulating the body's own defense mechanisms." At present, about 1000 preparations are obtainable which contain extracts of *Echinacea* alone or in combination with other plant extracts [1]. In 1993 German physicians prescribed over 3 million daily doses of the five leading preparations with a cost of 50 million DM [2]. As these preparations are often sold over the counter the actual overall use is probably much more widespread. Despite this frequent use, there is considerable debate about the effectiveness of *Echinacea* extracts, and doubts have been raised about safety in the (relatively rare) case of parenteral application [3,4].

Echinacea was first used as a medicinal plant by North American Indians for a large range of indications. In the late 19th century it became very popular also among the non-Indian North American population and was widely used until the early nineteen-thirties. While its use then declined in North America, the interest in Europe rose [5].

Three species of *Echinacea* are in medicinal use: *Echinacea* (*E.*) *purpurea*, *E. angustifolia* and *E. pallida*. Depending on the species, the part of the plant (roots, herb) and the method of extraction (hydrophilic, lipophilic), the commercially available preparations of *Echinacea* contain varying concentrations of flavonoids, essential oils, polysaccharides, derivates of caffeic acid, polyacetylenes, alkylamides and alkaloids. Apart from a very few exceptions these preparations are not standardized in their content of any of these substances. The evidence available so far indicates that it is not a single component but the mixture of various groups of substances which is responsible for the observed immunomodulatory effects [5].

The chemical heterogeneity and lacking standardization of the commercially available preparations make a valid scientific assessment very problematic. Furthermore, in a number of the most frequently prescribed preparations other plant ex-

Immunomodulatory Agents from Plants, edited by H. Wagner

tracts are added. For example, three of the five preparations prescribed most often in 1993 in Germany were combinations. Still, many practitioners and patients consider all these preparations to be "Echinacea" and more or less equivalent.

Only for two extracts of *Echinacea* has the Commission E of the German Federal Institute for Drugs (BPharm), which is responsible for the assessment of phytopharmaceuticals, published positive monographs regarding a limited number of indications (see Tab. 1). For other extracts and further illnesses the evidence is considered insufficient.

The following review of the available randomized, controlled trials in humans is not restricted to preparations containing only *Echinacea* extracts (monopreparations) but includes also combinations of *Echinacea* extracts with other plant extracts or homeopathic remedies. Table 2 gives a short overview of the number of trials of monopreparations and combinations for various conditions; Table 3 gives more detailed information on the single trials and their results.

Table 1 - Indications for Echinacea

Extracts and indications acknowledged by the Commission E for Phytopharmaceuticals of the German Federal Institute for Drugs (BPharm) • *Echinaceae pallidae* radix: treatment of common cold/influenza-like syndroms • *Echinaceae pupureae* herba: adjuvant treatment of recurrent respiratory and urinary tract infections (systemic use); healing of wounds (local use)
Other claimed indications • prevention and treatment of infections • adjuvant cancer treatment (decreasing side effects of cancer therapy) • non-specific immunostimulation

Table 2 - Randomized or quasi-randomized controlled clinical trials of preparations containing extracts of Echinacea

Indication	**Mono-preparations**	**Combinations**
Treatment of common cold/influenza-like syndromes	2	5
Prevention of common cold/influenza-like syndromes	2	5
Early treatment of common cold	1	
Treatment of other respiratory tract infections		3
Other indications		8
Trials in patients measuring only laboratory variables		2
Trials in healthy volunteers	3	2
Total	8	25

Table 3 - Randomized clinical trials of preparations containing extracts of Echinacea

first author	patients n	indication	intervention preparation	*Echinacea*	control	design blinding	results/comments results	comments
Bräunig [6, 7]	160	upper respiratory tract infection	mono	*pallida* root	placebo	double	duration and symptoms significantly better in treatment group	insufficient details in publication
Bräunig [8]	180	upper respiratory tract infection	mono	*purpurea* root (2 dosages)	placebo	double?	symptoms better in high dosage group, low dose without significant effect	blinding of high-dose group inadequate
Vorberg [9]	100	upper respiratory tract infection	combination	*angustifolia*	placebo	double	attenuation of symptoms better in treatment group	
Dorn [10]	100	upper respiratory tract infection	combination	*angustifolia*	placebo	double	improvement of some symptoms better in treatment group	relevant differences between groups at baseline
Vorberg [11]	100	upper respiratory tract infection	combination	*angustifolia* + *pallida* root	placebo	double	attenuation of symptoms better in treatment group	insufficient details in publication
Reitz [12]	150	upper respiratory tract infection	combination	*angustifolia* + *pallida* root	placebo	double	attenuation of some symptoms better in treatment group	insufficient details in publication
Melchart [43]	302	prevention of infections	mono	1) *pallida* root 2) *purpurea* root	placebo	double	1) RRR = 12% (95%CI 30–41%) 2) RRR = 20% (95%CI 21–47%)	insufficient sample size
Schoeneberg [14]	302	prevention of infections	mono	*purpurea herba*	placebo	double	RRR = 13% (95%CI 13–32%)	insufficient sample size
Schmidt [15]	646	prevention of infections	combination	*angustifolia*	placebo	double	RRR = 14% (95%CI 2–27%)	

RRR, relative risk reduction

Table 3 (continued)

first author	patients n	indication	intervention preparation	*Echinacea*	control	design blinding	results/comments results	comments
Forth [16]	95	prevention of infections	combination	*angustifolia* + *pallida* root	placebo	partly	RRR = 49% (95%CI 22–67%)	inadequate analysis
Reitz [12]	150	prevention of infections	combination	*angustifolia* + *pallida* root	placebo	double	no data presented	
Hoheisel [20]	120	early treatment of beginning common cold	mono	*purpurea herba*	placebo	double	40% developed a "full" common cold in the treatment group vs. 60% with placebo; duration of illness shorter	
Freitag [21]	52	pertussis (basic treatment) erythromycin)	combination	*angustifolia* + *pallida* root	untreated	open	duration of illness better in trreatment group	no blinding, unclear operationalization of outcomes
Blumröder [22]	50	angina lacunaris (erythromycin)	combination	*angustifolia* + *pallida* root	untreated	open	duration of illness better in treatment group	no blinding, unclear operationalization of outcomes
Zimmer [23]	30	acute sinusits (doxycyclin)	combination	*angustifolia* + *pallida* root	untreated	open	x-ray and global assessment much better in treatment group	no blinding, unclear operationalization of outcomes
Bendel [28]	70	toxicity of radio-chemotherapy	combination	*angustifolia* + *pallida* root	untreated	open	protection against hemato-toxic effect only in case of limited prior damage	
Bendel [29]	50	toxicity of radio-therapy	combination	*angustifolia* + *pallida* root	untreated	open	no protective effects observed observed	
Sartor [30]	50	prevention of leuco-penia after radion	combination	*angustifolia* + *pallida* root	untreated	open	stat. significant less radion days lost in treatment group	assessment difficult due to insufficient reporting

Table 3 (continued)

Hill [31]	20	mosquito bites	combination (topical)	*angustifolia*	placebo	double	erythema reduction better in treatment group	pilot trial with small sample size
Hill [32]	68	mosquito bites	combination	*angustifolia*	placebo	double	better erythma reduction in	rigorous trial
Hill [33]	100	mosquito bites	combination (topical)	*angustifolia*	placebo	double	erythema slightly better in treatment group ($p = 0.1$), no difference for itching	rigorous trial
Qadripur [36]	43	skin infections	combination	*angustifolia* + *pallida* root	placebo	double	statistically significantly higher phagocytosis in treatment group	insufficient reporting; no clinical outcome measures
Cubasch [37]	43	recurrent infections	combination	*angustifolia*	placebo	double	changes in a number of immune parameters	
Wagner [38]	25		combination	*angustifolia*	placebo	single	significant stimulation of phagocytosis in treatment group	
Jurcic [39]	24		mono	*purpurea* root	placebo	double	significant stimulation of phagocytosis in treatment group	
Melchart [40]	36		mono	1) *purpurea* 2) *pallida* roots	placebo	double	no difference between groups in a range of immune parameters	
Melchart [40]	24		mono	*purpurea* root	placebo	double	no difference between groups in a range of immune parameters	
Melchart [40]	24		combination	*angustifolia* (homeop.D4)	placebo	double	no difference between groups in a range of immune parameters	

Treatment of non-specific upper respiratory tract infections

A total of seven placebo-controlled, double blind, randomized clinical trials are available which have investigated the efficacy of two different mono-preparations and three combinations in the treatment of non-specific upper respiratory tract infections.

Bräunig and Knick ([6], see also [7]) tested if 900 mg extract of *Echinaceae pallidae radix* taken orally had a beneficial effect over placebo in 160 patients with upper respiratory tract infections. For inclusion, patients had to have a certain degree of severity (at least 15 points on a scale with a maximum of 24) and a duration of symptoms of less than three days. The duration of the illness was significantly shorter and the severity of symptoms after three and nine days significantly less in the treatment group. This study seems to provide good evidence that *Echinaceae pallidae radix* has a beneficial effect in the treatment of upper respiratory tract infections. Unfortunately, although the study has been published twice, the two reports lack a number of relevant details. For example, it remains unclear as to how the length of the illness has been measured and if all patients randomized actually completed the study. Furthermore, the results are presented in insufficient detail which makes an independent assessment difficult.

The same group also investigated the efficacy of *Echinaceae purpureae radix* [8]. 180 patients with upper respiratory tract infections were randomized to receive either placebo, 450 mg (90 drops) or 900 mg (180 drops) extract per day. Results on the length of illness were not reported (although listed as a primary outcome measure) but both patient- and physician-rated symptoms were statistically and clinically significantly better in the group treated with the high dose of *Echinaceae purpureae radix* while there was no difference between the lower dose and placebo. The results of this study look quite convincing; however, it has a relevant shortcoming: although the study was described as double-blind, personal communication with the author revealed that all placebo patients received only 90 drops. Thus, the treating physician knew which patients were in group three (the high dosage group).

Two trials have investigated the efficacy of a combination of *Echinacea angustifolia* with *Eupatorium perfoliatum*, *Baptisia tinctoria* and *Arnica montana* in non-specific upper respiratory tract infections [9,10]. Vorberg and Schneider [9] found that in the treatment group most symptoms were significantly better than in the placebo group at control visits after two to three and eight to ten days after inclusion. Dorn [10] presented an apparently well done study; however, the trial is difficult to interpret as there were relevant random differences at baseline between the two groups for a number of symptoms indicating more severe infections in the treatment group.

Vorberg [11] tested a combination of *Echinaceae angustifoliae* and *E. pallidae radix* with *Baptisia*, *Thuja* and four homeopathic remedies in potencies D4 and D6 in 100 patients. In the treatment group symptoms were attenuated significantly faster than in the placebo group. Unfortunately, the report lacks detail in the presentation of results. The preparation tested in this trial has been investigated in a number of other trials too; however, in the newer trials a modified version of the preparation without homeopathic additions is used.

The study of Reitz and Hergarten [12] is of special interest, but again, reporting is insufficient. 150 persons with acute viral upper respiratory tract infections (true influenza excluded) and a history of recurrency of such infections were randomized to receive the combination of *Echinaceae angustifoliae* and *E. pallidae radix*, *Baptisia* and *Thuja* (without homeopathic additions) or placebo (containing a low dose of vitamin C) for eight weeks. Attenuation of symptoms and a number of laboratory parameters were assessed after seven and 14 days as well as the number of recurrencies within the treatment period. Furthermore, patients were monitored for ten months for the occurrence of new infections. After seven and 14 days patients in the treatment groups had less severe symptoms (statistical significance was achieved in only a part of the symptoms). Within the treatment period four patients in the treatment group and six patients in the placebo group had a second episode of infection. It is reported that the number of infections in the post-treatment phase was generally low, but data is not reported.

Scaglione and Lund [13] tested a combination of *Echinacea purpurea* root extract, vitamin C, rosemary leaf extract, eucalyptus leaf extract, and fennel seed extract vs. placebo in 32 subjects suffering from a common cold. The duration of the illness (based on the rhinorrhea) was 3.37 ± 1.25 days in the treatment group and 4.37 ± 1.57 days in the placebo group ($p < 0.01$). Patients in the treatment groups also used a significantly lower number of paper tissues. No adverse effects were observed.

In conclusion, the available data suggests that some preparations containing extracts of *Echinacea* might in fact be effective in attenuating the symptoms of non-specific upper respiratory tract infections. However, convincing, independently reproduced evidence for a single preparation or a defined extract is still lacking.

Prevention of non-specific upper respiratory tract infections

Five randomized, placebo-controlled trials have been performed which investigated if preparations containing extracts of *Echinacea* prevent the occurence of non-specific upper respiratory tract infections [12, 14–16, 43].

Our own research group randomized 302 healthy volunteers to receive, for three months, either an extract of *Echinaceae purpureae radix*, of *Echinaceae angustifoliae radix*, or placebo [43]. 37% of the volunteers in the placebo group, 32% in the *Echinacea angustifolia* group, and 29% in the *Echinacea purpurea* group experienced at least one episode of infection. This corresponds to a reduction in the relative risk of getting an infection of 13% (95% confidence interval: –30 to 41%), and 20% (–21 to 47%) respectively, compared to placebo. These reductions are far from having statistical significance.

The two other available double-blind trials on *Echinaceae purpureae herba* [14] and on a combination of *Echinacea angustifolia* with *Eupatorium perfoliatum*, *Baptisia tinctoria* and *Arnica montana* [15] yielded very similar rates of relative risk reduction: 12% (95% CI: –13 to 32%), and 14% (95% CI: –2 to 27%) respectively. In the second trial [15] which included more than 600 volunteers the difference just missed statistical significance.

A fourth trial by Forth and Beuscher [16] on the combination of *Echinaceae angustifoliae* and *E. pallidae radix* with *Baptisia*, *Thuja* (with homeopathic additions) found a much larger relative risk reduction (49%, 95% CI: 22 to 67%). However, this trial was not fully double-blind and inadequately analyzed (an unclear but probably large number of patients not complying with the protocol were excluded). The trial by Reitz and Hergarten [12] (reported in the section on the treatment of upper respiratory tract infections) which included a post-treatment observation period of ten months looking for the occurrence of infections does not provide any results on this part of the study. Three older trials with alternate (not truly randomized) allocation to treatment, comparing the combination used by Forth and Beuscher and no treatment, report positive effects [17–19].

Although all available trials show at least some reduction in the risk of getting an infection, the evidence for a preventive effect of preparations containing extracts of *Echinacea* is insufficient to allow for reliable conclusions. If the size of the relative risk reduction is – as the newer, more reliable trials suggest – in fact in the range of 12 to 20%, the statistical power of the available trials is insufficient (the number of patients included in the trials has been too small to confirm statistically a potential effect of this size).

Early treatment of upper respiratory tract infections

In self-medication, the application of *Echinacea* preparations is very often started when patients experience the very first symptoms of a common cold. The objective of this early treatment is either to prevent that the common cold symptoms fully develop (some form of prevention) or to decrease the duration and the severity of the illness (in the sense of a typical treatment). In this early stage patients rarely consult a physician; consequently, it is not easy to study this type of use. Only recently a first study investigating this early treatment has been published [20]. The employees of a Swedish industrial plant were informed of the study and asked to consult the company physician in the case of the very first symptoms of a common cold. A total of 120 employees presenting during the recruitment period were then randomized to receive, in a double-blind manner, the pressed juice of *Echinacea purpureae herba* or placebo. 40% of the patients in the treatment group and 60% in the placebo group developed a "full" common cold (p = 0.044). The duration of the infections was also significantly shorter among the patients in the treatment group.

This apparently rigorous study yielded very promising results. Independent replications of this study approach seem highly desirable for the tested preparation as well as for other products.

Treatment of other infectious diseases

Three randomized trials have been published which have investigated the effectiveness of the combination of *Echinaceae angustifoliae* and *E. pallidae radix* with *Baptisia*, *Thuja* [21–23]. Freitag and Stammwitz randomized 52 children with pertussis to receive either erythromycin only, erythromycin and the *Echinacea* combination orally, or erythromycin and the *Echinacea* combination injected intramuscularly [21]. The duration of the illness was significanly shorter in the group which received intramuscular injections in addition to antibiotic treatment, while there was no signficant effect obtained from the oral application of the combination.

Blumroeder randomized 50 patients with angina lacunaris to receive either erythromycin alone or together with the *Echinacea* combination. The duration of the disease was significantly shorter in the group with the additional treatment and the symptoms subsided quicker [22].

Zimmer treated 30 patients with acute sinusitis with doxycyclin alone while 30 patients also received the *Echinacea* combination. X-ray assessment and symptoms were more favorable in the latter group [23].

Despite the positive results, these trials as well as four further non-randomized, controlled clinical studies [24–27] provide only limited evidence for the effectiveness of the tested preparations as methodological shortcomings cast some doubts on the reliability of the findings. Lack of blinding, unclear operationalization of clinical measurements and insufficient reporting make an independent judgement difficult. No trial on infectious diseases other than non-specific upper respiratory tract infections has been published since 1988.

Other conditions

There are at least eight randomized or possibly randomized controlled trials in which combinations containing *Echinacea* have been used in other conditions [28–35]. In three trials it was tested if the combination of *Echinaceaea angustifoliae* and *E. pallidae radix* with *Baptisia*, *Thuja* decreases undesired effects of anti-cancer treatments such as leukopenia or infections. The results suggest that there might be some beneficial effects, but these are insufficient for clear conclusions [28–30].

The effect of a topically applied homeopathic combination of the mother tinctures of *Echinacea angustifolia*, *Ledum palustrae*, and *Urica urens* on erythema and itching after mosquito bites has been investigated in three rigorous placebo-controlled trials [31–33]. Again, the results show a trend in favour of the *Echinacea* combination, but statisical significance is reached for some symptoms only and the clinical relevance is unclear.

Finally, two possibly randomized trials have tested other combinations for the treatment of incontinence and venous insufficiency [34, 35].

Clinical trials measuring laboratory parameters only and trials in healthy volunteers

Two randomized, placebo-controlled trials have been performed in patients which, however, evaluated laboratory outcome measures only. Qadripur [36] found that the granulocytes isolated from the blood of patients with bacterial skin infections receiving the combination of *Echinaceaea angustifoliae* and *E. pallidae radix* with *Baptisia*, *Thuja* had significantly higher phagocytosis rates than those receiving placebo. Cubasch and Stocksmeier [37] reported a modulation of a number of immune parameters after applying another combination to patients with recurrent infections.

The influence of various *Echinacea* extracts alone and in combination with other components on a number of immune parameters with a focus on the phagocytosis of polymorphonuclear neutrophile granulocytes has been investigated in five placebo-controlled trials in healthy volunteers with conflicting results [38–40]. While in two trials an immunostimulative effect could be shown, this was not the case in the three remaining studies.

Safety

The safety of *Echinacea* preparations has repeatedly stimulated polemic public discussions. Large-scale drug-monitoring studies which would allow a reliable estimate of the occurrence and frequency of side-effects do not exist. Cases of severe anaphylactic reactions, mainly after parenteral application, have been reported [1, 3]; however, in some of the cases a causality seems highly questionable. Nevertheless, there can be little doubt that the parenteral application of *Echinacea* extracts or combinations containing *Echinacea* bears some risk in susceptible individuals. Therefore, the majority of the manufacturers in Germany have withdrawn the preparations for parenteral use from the market. Given the widespread use for many years the oral preparations of *Echinacea* are likely to have only very minor risks.

Conclusion

This and other published overviews of the randomized clinical trials [41, 42] illustrate the complexity of the problem of how to assess the clinical value of preparations containing extracts of *Echinacea*. The huge variety of preparations available and the lack of replications of studies investigating a specific extract in a defined sample of patients make clinically valid and reliable conclusions difficult. Furthermore, from communications with experts in the field we have reasons to assume that a number of – possibily negative – trials remain unpublished.

Based on the available evidence for randomized trials the following conclusions can be drawn:

- although only very few trials provide convincing evidence there is a consistent trend in almost all studies which makes it likely that at least some preparations containg extracts of *Echinacea* have effects over placebo;
- the magnitude of the clinical effects is likely to be moderate at best;
- the evidence is insufficient to make clear recommendations as to which preparations to use and in which way;
- given the widespread use of *Echinacea* further clinical trials are needed; however, as long as the comparability of different extracts is completely unclear the results of such trials obtained with a defined preparation cannot be extrapolated onto others;
- trials on early treatment of upper respiratory tract infections as the one by Hoheisel et al. [20] should be a preference;
- the degree of publication bias regarding clinical trials of *Echinacea* preparations is a matter of concern. As long as health care researchers do not have access to all available data, all assessment of the literature implies a non-negligible degree of uncertainty.

References

1 Bauer R, Wagner H (1996) Wirbel um *Echinacea*-Präparate. *Ztschr Phytother* 17: 249–252

2 Haustein KO (1994) Immuntherapeutika. In: Schwabe U, Paffrath D (eds): *Arzneiverordnungsreport '94*. Gustav Fischer, Stuttgart, 245–250

3 Schoenhoefer PS, Schulte-Sasse H (1989) Sind pflanzliche Immunstimulantien wirksam und unbedenklich? *Dtsch med Wschr* 114: 1804–1806

4 Dorsch W (1996) Klinische Anwendung von Extrakten aus *Echinacea purpurea* oder *Echinacea pallida*. Klinische Wertung kontrollierter klinischer Studien. *Z ärztl Fortbild* 90: 117–122

5 Bauer R, Wagner H (1990) *Echinacea – Handbuch für Ärzte, Apotheker und andere Naturwissenschaftler*. Wissenschaftliche Verlagsgesellschaft, Stuttgart

6 Braeunig B, Knick E (1993) Therapeutische Erfahrungen mit *Echinaecae pallidae* bei grippalen Infekten. *Naturheilpraxis mit Naturmedizin* 1: 72–75

7 Dorn M, Knick E, Lewith G (1997) Placebo-controlled, double-blind study of *Echinaceae pallidaee radix* in upper respiratory tract infections. *Compl Ther Med* 5: 40–42

8 Braeunig B, Dorn M, Knick E (1992) *Echinaceae purpureae radix*: zur Stärkung der körpereigenen Abwehr bei grippalen Infekten. *Z Phytother* 13: 7–13

9 Vorberg G, Schneider B (1989) Pflanzliches Immunstimulans verkürzt grippalen Infekt. Doppelblindstudie belegt die Steigerung der unspezifischen Infektabwehr. *Ärztl Forsch* 36: 3–8

10 Dorn M (1989) Milderung grippaler Infekte durch ein pflanzliches Immunstimulans. *Natur- und Ganzheitsmedizin* 2: 314–319

11 Vorberg G (1984) Bei Erkältung unspezifische Immunabwehr stimulieren. *Ärztliche Praxis* 36: 97–98

12 Reitz HD, Hergarten H (1990) Immunmodulatoren mit pflanzlichen Wirkstoffen. 2. Teil: eine wissenschaftliche Studie am Beispiel *Esberitox N. Notab med* 20: 304–306, 362–366

13 Scaglione F, Lund B (1996) Efficacy in the treatment of the common cold of a preparation containing an *Echinacea* extract. *Int J Immunotherapy* 11: 163–166

14 Schoeneberger D (1992) Einfluß der immunstimulierenden Wirkung von Preßsaft aus *Herba Echinaceae purpureae* auf Verlauf und Schweregrad von Erkältungskrankheiten. *Forum Immunologie* 2(8): 18–22

15 Schmidt U, Albrecht M, Schenk N (1990) Pflanzliches Immunstimulans senkt Häufigkeit grippaler Infekte. Plazebokontrollierte Doppelblindstudie mit einem kombinierten *Echinacea*-Präparat mit 646 Studenten der Kölner Universität. *Natur- und Ganzheitsmedizin* 3: 277–281

16 Forth H, Beuscher N (1981) Beeinflussung der Häufigkeit banaler Erkältungsinfekte durch Esberitox. *Ztschr Allg-Med* 57: 2272–2275

17 Freyer HU (1974) Häufigkeit banaler Infekte im Kindesalter und Möglichkeiten der Prophylaxe. *Fortschr Med* 92: 165–168

18 Helbig G (1961) Unspezifische Reizkörpertherapie zur Infektionsprophylaxe. *Med Klin* 56: 1512–1514

19 Kleinschmidt H (1965) Versuche zur Herabsetzung der Infektneigung bei Kleinkindern mit Esberitox. *Ther d Gegenw* 104: 1258–1262

20 Hoheisel O, Sandberg M, Bertram S, Bulitta M, Schäfer M (1997) Die Behandlung mit

Echinagard verkürzt den Verlauf einer unkomplizierten Erkältung: Ergebnisse einer doppelblinden, placebokontrollierten klinischen Prüfung. *Eur J Clin Res* 9: 261–269.
21 Freitag U, Stammwitz U (1984) Reduzierte Krankheitsdauer bei Pertussis durch unspezifisches Immunstimulans. *Kinderarzt* 15: 1068–1071
22 von Blumroeder WO (1985) Angina lacunaris. Eine Untersuchung zum Thema "Steigerung der körpereigenen Abwehr". *Z Allg-Med* 61,8: 271–273
23 Zimmer M (1985) Gezielte konservative Therapie der akuten Sinusitis in der HNO-Praxis. *Therapiewoche* 35, 36: 4024–4028
24 Stolze H, Forth H (1983) Eine Antibiotikabehandlung kann durch zusätzliche Immunstimulierung optimiert werden. *Der Kassenarzt* 23: 43–48
25 Baetgen D (1984) Erfolge in der Keuchhusten-Behandlung mit Echinacin. *Therapiewoche* 1984;34: 5115–5119
26 Baetgen D (1988) Behandlung der akuten Bronchitis im Kindesalter. *Therapiewoche Pädiatrie* 1: 66–70
27 Coeugniet E, Kuehnast R (1986) Rezidivierende Candidiasis. Adjuvante Immuntherapie mit verschiedenen *Echinacea*-Darreichungsformen. *Therapiewoche* 36: 3352–3358
28 Bendel R, Bendel V, Renner K, Carstens V, Stolze K (1989) Zusatzbehandlung mit Esberitox N bei Patientinnen mit chemo-strahlentherapeutischer Behandlung eines fortgeschrittenen Mammakarzinoms. *Onkologie* 12, 3 (suppl): 32–38.
29 Bendel R, Renner K, Stolze K (1988) Zusatzbehandlung mit Esberitox bei Patientinnen mit kurativer adjuvanter Bestrahlung nach Mammakarzinom. *Strahlenther u Onkol* 164, 5: 278–283.
30 Sartor KJ (1972) Zur Wirksamkeit von Esberitox in der Behandlung strahlenbedingter Leukopenien. *Ther d Gegenw* 111, 8: 1147–1150
31 Hill N, van Haselen RA (1993) Clinical trial of a homeopathic insect after-bite treatment. *HomInt R&D Newsletter* 3/4: 4–5
32 Hill N, Stam C, Tuinder S, van Haselen RA (1995) A placebo-controlled trial investigating the efficacy of a homeopathic after-bite gel in reducing mosquito-bite induced erythema. *Eur J Clin Pharm* 49: 103–108
33 Hill N, Stam C, van Haselen RA (1996) The efficacy of Prrrigweg gel in the treatment of insect bites: a double-blind, placebo-controlled clinical trial. *Pharm World Sci* 18: 35–41
34 Timmermanns LM, Timmermanns LG (1990) Mesure de l'activité des extraits d'*Echinaceae* et de Sabal dans le traitement des mégavessies idiopathiques chez la femme. *Acta Urol Belg* 58, 2: 43–59
35 Ehringer H (1968) Objektivierbare Venentonisierung nach oraler Gabe eines Kombinationspräparates mit Roßkastanienextrakt. *Arzneim Forsch* 18: 432–434
36 Quadripur SA (1976) Medikamentöse Beeinflussung der Phagozytosefähigkeit der Granulozyten. *Ther d Gegenw* 115: 1072–1078
37 Cubasch H, Stocksmeier U (1992) Deutliche Zunahme der T-Helferzellen. *Therapiewoche* 42: 990–1000
38 Wagner H, Jurcic K, Doenicke A, Rosenhuber E, Behrens N (1986) Die Beeinflussung

der Phagozytosefähigkeit von Granulozyten durch homöopathische Arzneipräparate. *In vitro*-Tests und kontrollierte Einfachblindstudien. *Arzneim-Forsch/Drug Res* 36(II): 1421–1425

39 Jurcic K, Melchart D, Holzmann M, Martin P, Bauer R, Doenicke A, Wagner H (1989) Zwei Probandenstudien zur Stimulierung der Granulozytenphagozytose durch *Echinacea*-extrakthaltige Präparate. *Z Phytother* 10: 67–70

40 Melchart D, Linde K, Worku F, Sarkady L, Holzmann M, Jurcic K, Wagner H (1995) Results of five randomized studies on the immunomodulatory activity of preparations of *Echinacea. J Alternat Compl Med* 1: 145–160

41 Melchart D, Linde K, Worku F, Bauer R, Wagner H (1994) Immunomodulation with *Ech*inacea – a systematic review of controlled clinical trials. *Phytomedicine* 1: 145–254

42 Schneider B (1992) Probleme des Wirksamkeitsnachweises bei immunstimulierenden Arzneimitteln, dargestellt am Beispiel eines pflanzlichen Immunmodulators. *Erfahrungsheilkunde* 6: 396–400

43 Melchart D, Walther E, Linde K, Brandmaier R, Lersch C (1998) *Echinacea* root extracts for the prevention of upper respiratory tract infections – a double-blind, placebo-controlled randomized trial. *Arch Fam Med 7; in print*

Benefit and risks of the squeezed sap of the purple coneflower (*Echinacea purpurea*) for long-term oral immunostimulant therapy*

Michael J. Parnham

Institute of Pharmacology for the Natural Sciences, Goethe University Frankfurt, D-60439 Frankfurt am Main, Germany
Present address: PLIVA d.d., Research Institute, Prilaz baruna Filipovića 25, HR-10 000 Zagreb, Croatia

Background

Plant extracts have been used for their therapeutic properties for thousands of years. Many of the well known drugs still in widespread use today, such as morphine, digoxin or salicylic acid, were originally isolated from plants such as the poppy, the foxglove and the willow [1–3]. Yet plant extracts, as such, still have a place in therapy alongside synthetic chemical products. With increasing concern among both practising physicians and the lay public about the possible risks associated with drug treatment, there is an understandable desire to treat with traditionally well-tolerated drugs. Over-the-counter medicines are being used increasingly in the developed countries, particularly for children, and concern has been expressed as to whether parents are sufficiently well-informed about the benefits and risks of the products they keep at hand in the kitchen cupboard [4]. Many plant-derived products are regarded as well-tolerated by their proponents and ridiculed as inefficacious by their critics. In this controversial atmosphere, it is important to assess objectively the facts about individual therapeutic products.

The purple coneflower (Genus *Echinacea*), indigenous only to North America, was widely used for many medicinal purposes by the American Indians of the Great Plains and subsequently adopted by white settlers. An extract of *E. angustifolia* (narrow-leaved purple coneflower) was made available to medical practitioners by Lloyd Brothers Pharmacists Inc., at the end of the nineteenth century, and became widely used in the USA by eclectic physicians for infectious and inflammatory diseases [5]. With the introduction by the FDA of stricter requirements for testing of drugs, the use of *Echinacea* declined in the 1930's, but its use in self-medication has seen a renaissance in recent years. Since 1994, herbal remedies have been defined as dietary supplements in the USA which has allowed manufacturers to make general claims about their efficacy.

* This chapter is an updated version of a review article which appeared in *Phytomedicine* 3: 95–102 (1996).

In Europe, *Echinacea* was introduced into homeopathic practice in the late 19th century, but its increasing use for this purpose led to a severe shortage of the plant. To overcome this problem, Dr. Gerhard Madaus of Madaus & Co. bought seed in the US and started cultivating what turned out to be *Echinacea purpurea* (common purple coneflower) in Cologne. It is predominantly the squeezed sap of flowering *E. purpurea* planted, grown and processed under standardized conditions and prepared by Madaus (Echinacin®) which has been subjected to detailed pharmacological and clinical investigations [6]. Squeezed sap of *Echinacea purpurea* is approved in Germany for the supportive treatment of respiratory and urinary infections and the external treatment of wounds [7]. The extracts of the roots of the various *Echinacea* species are approved for homeopathic uses.

Mechanism of action

The squeezed sap of *E. purpurea* exerts a mild, non-specific immunostimulant action. In early clinical studies, on parenteral administration, a consistent acute leukocytosis was observed [7–9], which led to the introduction in Germany of the "Echinacin® leucocyte provocation test", in which Echinacin® was administered to test whether the hematopoetic system was sufficiently intact to withstand radiation therapy [10]. This test has also been applied to children with viral hepatitis as a test for reversible bone marrow suppression [11]. Subsequent experimental investigations demonstrated that Echinacin® enhances phagocytosis by human neutrophils *in vitro* [12], a property shared by various alcoholic root extracts of different *Echinacea* species [6]. In the latter extracts, alkylamide and chicoric acid fractions appear to be the main active principles [13]. Recent investigations indicate that the squeezed sap of the fresh flowers contains particularly high concentrations of alkylamides, while the concentration of chicoric acid varies markedly, depending on the manufacturing process used [14]. Dodeca-2*E*,4*E*,8*Z*,10*E*/*Z*-tetraenoic acid butylamide is a major constituent of the flowers, but while alkamides have been shown to enhance leucocyte phagocytosis, the constituents responsible for the therapeutic activity of the product remain unclear. For this reason, it is essential to define the source and standardization process for the preparation of treatment forms of *E. purpurea*.

The squeezed sap of the flowers of *E. purpurea* (Echinacin®) has been shown to contain a 75,000 Dalton acidic arabinogalactan. As shown in Table 1, this polysaccharide generates the oxidative burst and selective cytokine production in mouse macrophages, leading to specific toxicity to tumor cell lines, including the TNFα-selective WEHI 164 line, *Leishmania* parasites, and *Candida albicans*, the latter being shown *in vivo* [15–17]. Cytotoxicity was specific, since at concentrations of 0.1–10 mg/ml, the arabinogalactan caused no toxicity to lymphocytes. A slight proliferative action on B cells was observed, but no direct stimulatory effect on T lym-

Table 1 - Macrophage stimulating activity of the arabinogalactan (AG) isolated from Echinacea purpurea *[15–17]*

System	Dose of AG	Response
Mouse bone marrow macrophages macrophages	20–200 µg 8–250 µg	Oxidative burst activation. Interferon β release
Mouse bone marrow or peritoneal macrophages	100 µg	P815 tumor cell cytotoxicity
Mouse peritoneal macrophages	3–500 µg	TNFα (not IL1) release, *Leishmania* and WEHI 164 tumor cell toxicity
Mouse B cells	100 µg	Weak proliferation
Candida albicans-infected mice (± immunosuppressive pretreatment)	10 mg/kg i.v.	Reduced colonization of internal organs, increased survival

phocytes. Polysaccharides from cell cultures of *E. purpurea* have also been reported to stimulate phagocytosis in human polymorphonuclear leucocytes and to stimulate release of TNFα, interleukin 1 (IL-1), and IL-6 from human monocytes *in vitro* [18]. The molecular site of action of the polysaccharide remains to be established and it is unclear whether the same principle(s) is (are) responsible for both neutrophil and macrophage stimulation. Intravenous administration of *E. purpurea* polysaccharides to human volunteers resulted in a transient fall in circulating leucocyte count followed by a leucocytosis [18]. While the latter response reflects stimulation of leucocyte production, the fall in cell counts was considered to reflect adherence of leucocytes to the endothelium as a result of increased cytokine production.

The capability of Echinacin® to stimulate neutrophil phagocytosis *in vivo* has been demonstrated in two volunteer studies. In the first open study, in 12 healthy males, Echinacin® administered i.m. on 4 consecutive days significantly increased by 20–30% the ability of neutrophils to phagocytose *Candida albicans ex vivo* [19]. In a second double-blind study on 24 male volunteers, Echinacin® Liquidum was administered orally (30 drops, three times a day) for five days to 12 subjects, the other 12 received placebo [20]. By the fifth day of treatment, the phagocytic activity of isolated neutrophils was significantly higher (+ 120%) in the Echinacin® group in comparison to placebo.

In a recent randomized, placebo-controlled, double-blind study in 42 triathletes, oral administration of Echinacin® (120 drops daily in three divided doses) for the four weeks prior to a competition, led to a decrease in urinary soluble IL-2 receptor concentration before the competition and an increase in the serum IL-6 concentration immediately after the competition [21]. This finding was interpreted as reflecting activation of macrophages by the *E. purpurea*. Extreme exercise is well known to cause immunosuppression and the Echinacin® was proposed to counteract this effect. It is worth noting that while 4/13 subjects in the placebo group suffered from respiratory infections, none did in the active treatment group (n = 13), suggesting that the treatment had exerted an immunostimulating effect.

Despite the fact that extracts of *Echinacea purpurea* do not appear to exert direct stimulatory effects on T lymphocytes *in vitro*, reports have been published on clinical responses of lymphocytes to treatment [22, 23]. Neither of these were controlled studies and both included mixed populations of patients who were treated i.m. or s.c. for seven days with squeezed sap of *Echinacea purpurea*. In both reports a marked increase in mean total lymphocyte count in the peripheral blood was observed after seven days treatment, but this was not compared with the effects of placebo treatment. In the nine patients with "acute viral and bacterial infections" (not further defined) [22] as well as the 18 patients with *Candida* or *Herpes simplex* infections and ten patients with atopic or contact eczema [23], the investigators found a transient tendency towards a decrease in the ratio of T helper (CD4) : T suppressor/cytotoxic (CD8) cells immediately after treatment. After a further seven days, this ratio in the latter study was higher than normal. In the light of other mechanistic studies, such changes are likely to be related to acute changes in cytokine release by macrophages. The slight fall in the blood CD4/CD8 ratio may be attributable to adherence and/or migration and accumulation of activated CD4 cells at local sites of infection or in other lymphoid organs, similar to redistribution effects seen experimentally with other immunostimulants, such as thymic peptides [24].

Despite the uncontrolled nature of the studies, the possibility has been suggested that these effects of *E. purpurea* extract on lymphocytes could be interpreted as adverse events [6]. In contrast to the studies on arabinogalactan, discussed above, very high concentrations of *E. purpurea* extract were reported to inhibit T cell proliferation *in vitro* [20]. This is not entirely surprising since stimulation of macrophages *in vitro*, as would occur with *E. purpurea* extract, is frequently associated with the release of large amounts of prostaglandin E_2, a physiological inhibitor of T cell proliferation [25]. While extracts of *E. purpurea* and some of its purified constituents show clear non-specific immunostimulatory properties, the relevance of these mechanistic studies for the clinical safety of such preparations needs to be placed in perspective.

Benefit and risks in clinical studies

Following the application of industrial pharmaceutical methods to the preparation and clinical use of the squeezed sap of *E. purpurea* by Madaus in Germany in the

1940's, many publications on this product have appeared, as reviewed in two recent monographs [5, 6]. However, no comprehensive analysis of the benefit: risk relationship has been made. Since adverse events in clinical reports are usually just listed, the studies which are reviewed here are those in which the treatment protocol and number of subjects are clearly defined and an assessment of safety in relation to the dose, route of administration and indication is included.

Respiratory infections

Early studies on parenteral treatment

The major clinical indication for Echinacin® in Germany is as a supportive immunostimulant therapy for respiratory infections. In the 1950's and 1960's a series of publications appeared on the use of intramuscularly administered Echinacin® for the treatment of whooping cough in children. The dose administered was 1–2 ml of a squeezed aqueous extract of *Echinacea purpurea* (0.1 g/2 ml) given twice daily for periods of 3 to 21 days [9, 26, 27]. These studies involved a total of 257 children, from infants to 14 year olds, who were suffering from severe cough with vomiting of 1–2 weeks duration. Recovery in the majority of cases occured within 5-14 days. In the study of Zimmermann [9], in 91 children (including two infants and 67 small children), the immunostimulatory action was also assessed by measurement of blood lymphocyte counts. In 88 cases (94%) an increase of more than 29% in blood lymphocyte counts was observed and it was stated that no adverse events were observed. Volz [26] also saw no adverse events in the 45 children he treated. Baetgen [27] confirmed that no adverse events could be observed, not even in infants, and that the children often slept well the night after the first injection. In a few cases, a slight reddening at the injection site, lasting for 1–2 days, was seen and in one infant of nine months an increase in temperature from 40° C to 40.6° C occurred which lasted 12 h. Similarly, in their experience with nearly 300 small children with whooping cough, treated i.m. with 1–2 ml of Echinacin® for three days, followed by treatment three times a week for two weeks, Heesen and Orzechowski [28] only observed transient pain at the injection site and an associated increase in temperature (1–2° C) without any other adverse events.

Twenty-years after his first report, Baetgen [29] reported on a further 170 children with whooping cough, 77 of whom were treated concomitantly with antibiotics, 63 with Echinacin® alone, and 30 with antibiotics alone. In each case in which it was administered, Echinacin® (1–2 ml i.m.) was given at least three times over periods of 3–10 days, and in 83 patients it was administered on three consecutive days. Apart from the surprising finding that improvement was more rapid with Echinacin treatment alone, recurrence of infectious symptoms arose in only one of 63 cases with Echinacin alone and in three of 77 with combined treatment. No adverse events were reported.

These findings show that even given to very young children by parenteral administration, which will provide higher peak plasma concentrations than those achieved by oral administration, Echinacin® is very well tolerated during short-term administration. The slight increase in temperature observed in some cases can be attributed to the stimulation of phagocytes/accessory cells and the associated production of cytokines – a therapeutic goal. This is confirmed in a report by Heesen [8] on the treatment of more than 500 children with tuberculosis. The Echinacin® was given i.v. at doses increasing from 0.5 ml to 5 ml within two days and repeated up to 15 times over several weeks. Improvement in the general condition of some children was associated with acute signs of immunostimulation by Echinacin® such as shivering, headache, vomiting and fever within 2–4 h of the injection. After a further 1–2 h these symptoms disappeared in association with a 40–100% increase in blood leucocyte count, which decreased within 6–8 h.

Long-term oral therapy

Oral administration of drugs is simpler and results in a slower absorption and lower peak plasma levels than those obtained following parenteral administration. Consequently, it is possible to continue oral treatment for longer periods than is common by parenteral administration. In keeping with the lower peak plasma concentrations, tolerability in the short-term is usually greater on oral than on parenteral administration, but in the long-term, specific adverse events may arise.

Several investigations have been carried out recently to study the efficacy and safety of long-term treatment with oral Echinacin® in the prophylaxis and therapy of respiratory infections. They include double-blind, placebo-controlled studies, as well as general practice investigations. One of the double-blind studies has been published, the remainder are on file at Madaus AG, Cologne, Germany.

Double-blind studies

In Germany in 1989 the then Federal Institutes of Health (BGA) approved the oral use of the squeezed sap of *Echinacea purpurea* (2.5 : 1 dilution, Echinacin® Liquidum) for "the supportive treatment of recurrent infections of the respiratory tract and the urinary tract" given for continual periods of administration of up to eight weeks [7].

Following this official approval, an eight-week double-blind, placebo-controlled study of oral Echinacin® Liquidum was carried out during the winter of 1990/91 in 109 subjects at risk of respiratory infection, i.e. they had had more than three colds during the previous winter [30]. Treatment with Echinacin® or placebo (n = 54 each) was given twice daily, physical examinations with blood sampling being carried out immediately before, and after four and eight weeks of treatment. As far as efficacy was concerned, there was a tendency for Echinacin® to reduce the incidence of pronounced respiratory infections (requiring absence from work or bed rest), 16 cases (32%) being reported in the placebo group and eight cases (19%) in the Echinacin® group. Before treatment, 29 subjects in the Echinacin® group and 37 in the placebo group had a CD4/CD8 ratio in the blood of < 1.5, which was taken as an indication of a raised risk of infection. Among these subjects at risk, only 17% of Echinacin®-treated subjects, as opposed to 37% of placebo-treated subjects had pronounced colds during treatment. The average duration of cold symptoms was 5.34 days/patient in the Echinacin® group and 7.54 days/patient in the placebo group. The overall condition of the Echinacin®-treated subjects was, therefore, somewhat healthier than that of the placebo-treated subjects.

The tolerability of the treatment was assessed in terms of a score (very good, good, satisfactory, poor), recorded after four and eight weeks. In this respect, Echinacin® did not differ from placebo, 88.9% of subjects on Echinacin® reporting the tolerability as good to very good, as opposed to 94.4% on placebo. Drop-outs from the study (n = 4 for Echinacin®, n = 3 for placebo) were also comparable for both groups. Adverse events reported (n = 11 for Echinacin®, n = 7 for placebo) were mainly gastrointestinal upsets, headache, dizziness and tiredness in both groups. In other words, for a period of eight weeks, oral Echinacin® tended to reduce the incidence and severity of the common cold while exhibiting similar tolerability to that of the placebo. No reduction of the CD4/CD8 ratio by Echinacin® was reported.

A more recent randomized, placebo-controlled, double-blind study was carried out on 120 workers at a Swedish factory, who reported to the company physician as soon as they felt the first signs of a cold [31]. They received either Echinacin® lozenges (each containing 88.5 mg aqueous *Echinacea purpurea* extract; n = 60) or placebo (n = 60) initially every 2 h and then three times a day for up to ten days. In the active treatment group, only 24/60 (40%) patients developed a full-blown cold, as opposed to 36/60 (60%) in the placebo group. Moreover, time to improvement was significantly shorter by a median of four days in the Echinacin® as opposed to the placebo group. Tolerability in both treatment groups was comparable. Interestingly, a preparation of the roots of *E. purpurea* has also been reported to shorten the length of the symptoms of the common cold, in a small randomized, single-blind study in 32 subjects, though only by 24 h [32]. Presumably, the active constituents of the preparation are present in different parts of the plant.

The other double-blind, placebo-controlled trial, on file at Madaus in Cologne, was performed on 47 marathon runners, who received either Echinacin® lozenges (each containing 88.5 mg aqueous *Echinacea purpurea* extract; n = 23) or placebo (n = 24) four times a day for a total of 12 weeks. The study was conceived as a pilot study to test in a homogeneous population, closely monitored by sports physicians, whether Echinacin®, as in the Schöneberger [30] study, would decrease the frequency of common colds. The enrolled subjects were non-smoking, long-distance runners of both sexes, aged between 18 and 65 years, who regularly ran between 25 and 120 km per week and who reported that they had had at least three upper airway infections within the six months immediately prior to the start of the study. Exclusion criteria included subjects with recent (one week) infections or with progressive systemic diseases, hypertension, alcohol consumption > 50 g per week, recent (four weeks) immunostimulant therapy, allergy to *Echinacea*, pregnancy and breastfeeding.

Since the marathon runners were extremely fit physically, the original intention of the study was not achievable, all of the subjects being equally insensitive to colds. Several immunological parameters, including leukocyte differential counts, T ($CD3^+$) cells, T helper ($CD4^+$) cells, T suppressor/cytotoxic ($CD8^+$) cells, B ($CD19^+$) cells, natural killer ($CD16^+$) cells, CD4/CD8 ratio, as well as blood levels of IgA, IgM, IgE, C-reactive protein, complement factors C3 and C4 and total neopterin, were measured at three weekly intervals. No differences between the treatment groups were observed (see Tab. 2 for leucocyte counts) and in none of the patients were adverse events reported (in patients' daily diaries or at three weekly examinations) which could be related to treatment. In other words, even given for a period of 12 weeks to healthy subjects, no adverse events on either well-being or immune responses could be observed with Echinacin®. Although no significant changes were observed in this study, the fact that changes in urinary sIL-2 receptor and in serum IL-6 could be observed in triathletes [21], as described earlier, indicates that when immunosuppression does arise during extreme exercise, pretreatment with *E. purpurea* can be effective in stimulating some immune parameters. Once again, in the triathlete study, no adverse events were reported.

Open studies

Another study in marathon runners on file at Madaus AG, this time an open, general practice study was carried out in 1991. The intention was to assess the efficacy and safety of Echinacin® lozenges (qid) given for 6 weeks in the prophylaxis of respiratory or urinary tract infections, in comparison to untreated marathon runners. A total of 79 subjects (19–58 years old) were included, 38 receiving Echinacin® (27 male, 11 female) and 41 untreated (37 male, three female). Nine of the subjects in the Echinacin® group and 3 in the control group considered themselves at risk of infection, when questioned. On the basis of the subjects' training book entries, 20 subjects (52.6%) on Echinacin® and 15 untreated subjects (36.6%) reported the occurrence of infections during the treatment period, which lasted a mean (± SD) of 42 ± 2 days. The subjects were also asked to grade their feelings of well-being on waking each morning, but this highly subjective assessment provided no evaluable data on either efficacy or safety. No adverse events which could be related to the treatment with Echinacin® were reported, however, and complaints such as various muscle aches and joint pain, gastrointestinal complaints (e.g. diarrhoea, nausea, gastric discomfort) and headache were recorded equally by only 1-3 subjects per group. Thus, while these subjects were also extremely fit and healthy and probably less at

Table 2 - Changes in leucocyte counts during treatment of marathon runners with Echinacin® lozenges or placebo for 12 weeks. Values are medians with ranges. (Data from study on file at Madaus AG, Cologne)

Duration of treatment (days)	**Echinacin® (n = 23)**	**Placebo (n = 24)**
Granulocytes (%)		
1	56.1 (36.7–68.5)	54.6 (41.2–77.8)
22	54.6 (39.3–76.1)	57.4 (40.9–78.3)
50	55.7 (43.2–67.9)	54.9 (39.9–73.7)
84	60.1 (41.4–78.6)	56.1 (41.3–73.6)
Monocytes (%)		
1	5.0 (1.0–9.8)	4.6 (1.8–10.2)
22	4.5 (1.0–9.7)	4.9 (2.2–12.9)
50	6.7 (2.3–13.3)	5.7 (1.6–13.4)
84	9.0 (3.4–14.4)	8.6 (5.1–15.3)
Lymphocytes (%)		
1	38.1 (24.9–58.1)	38.7 (18.9–53.9)
22	38.5 (20.2–55.0)	37.3 (24.2–51.8)
50	37.0 (26.8–55.6)	36.6 (21.2–48.9)
84	29.6 (15.7–50.8)	33.8 (17.8–48.6)
CD4/CD8 ratio		
1	1.5 (0.8–2.9)	1.45 (1.0–3.6)
22	1.6 (0.9–2.8)	1.5 (1.0–4.1)
50	1.2 (0.8–3.5)	1.3 (0.8–2.7)
84	1.4 (0.8–2.4)	1.4 (0.9–3.3)

risk of infection than less well-trained subjects, Echinacin® was well-tolerated over the six week treatment period.

Gynaecological infections

Early studies on parenteral treatment

In 1950 Röseler reported on the results of the treatment of 183 women with mixed periuteral infections with Echinacin® 0.2 ml i.v. for 8–9 days. He claimed a 55–70% recovery and reported the characteristic response to Echinacin® as shivering within 30–90 min of injection, followed by fever, accompanied by lymphopenia, which disappeared within 24–48 h at which time a slight leukocytosis was detectable [33]. Similar results were reported two years later [34], by which time Röseler had treated a total of 226 women with periuteral infections. The fact that the lymphopenia in these patients (5–8% lymphocytes 45–120 min after injection, as opposed to 15% lymphocytes before injection) occurred together with the period of maximum fever, would appear to support the proposal, made above, that transient lymphopenia in response to Echinacin® (p.o. or i.v.) is due to redistribution of activated T cells.

In response to Röseler's initial report, Moell treated 120 women with periuteral infections, administering daily i.v. injections of Echinacin® (starting with 0.1 ml and increasing to 1.2 ml, depending on the intensity of the response) over the course of 8–10 days [35]. The response rate of 50–85% was similar to that of Röseler [33, 34]. Moell also reported the same sequence of response to Echinacin®, namely, shivering within 30–90 min, followed by transient lymphopenia and a longer-lasting leukocytosis. In addition, Moell reported the occurrence of subjective complaints (headache, dizziness, tiredness, occasional nausea) and in 10% of cases, abdominal pain [35]. Whether such adverse events were related to the infection or the treatment is unclear.

Priese subsequently reported on the treatment of 60 women with postpartal mastitis with Echinacin® i.v. [36]. The symptomatic response to Echinacin® (shivering, fever) was the same as that observed by Röseler [33, 34] and Moell [35], though in Priese's study, the response rate was over 90%. An important aspect raised by Priese was that the dose used was 0.1–1.0 ml for an average of six days, but that higher doses were not used because above 1 ml i.v. "an inhibition of defence reactions occurred". This would appear to concur with the later *in vitro* data of others that very high concentrations of *E. purpurea* extract are inhibitory to lymphocyte proliferation [37].

Treatment of relapsing candidiasis by different routes

The most recent report on the use of Echinacin® in gynaecological disorders, is as adjuvant therapy to local econazole in the treatment of relapsing vaginal candidiasis [23]. A total of 203 patients were diagnosed as suffering from relapsing candidiasis on the basis of recurrence at least three times after application of at least two antimycotics and recurrence within four weeks of cessation of antimycotic therapy. All patients received an initial six days local econazole therapy. Subsequently, 20 patients received Echinacin® s.c. (0.5 ml increasing to 2 ml), 60 received 2 ml Echinacin® i.m. and 20 received Echinacin® i.v. (0.5 ml increasing to 2 ml) each twice weekly for ten weeks. A further 60 patients were treated orally with 30 drops Echinacin® Liquidum three times daily 1 h before meals for ten weeks. While the recurrence rate within six months was 60.5% with econazole alone, the four groups treated with Echinacin® had recurrence rates of 15% (s.c.), 5% (i.m.), 15% (i.v.)

and 17% (p.o.), respectively. It must be emphasized that this was an open, general practice study and the allocation of the patients to therapy was neither blind nor randomized so the patients were not matched. The immunostimulatory effect of Echinacin, was documented for each group, though, by the use of a multi-antigen skin test for cell-mediated immunity. All patients with relapsing candidiasis exhibited hyposensitivity to antigen testing and sensitivity was enhanced 2–3-fold in each group by ten weeks treatment with Echinacin,, irrespective of the route.

Adverse events were specified as local and mild to moderate (in 8–10% of cases on s.c. or i.m. treatment, but none on i.v. treatment) or general and mild (in 3–5% of cases on s.c., i.m. or i.v. treatment). No adverse events at all were observed in the 60 subjects treated with Echinacin® orally. In other words, oral Echinacin® administered daily for a period of ten weeks produced similar responses to those achieved with parenteral treatment for the same period, but was totally without adverse events.

Safety implications for long-term oral use

Safety in general practice

The German medical literature contains a large number of general practice reports and case studies on the use of Echinacin®, not only for infections, but for other indications as well. For instance, in a recent report on the use of Echinacin® for the treatment of rheumatoid arthritis Reuß states: “In over 3 decades of general practice I have not observed a single case of drug-induced injury, although I have administered Echinacin® to a large extent, not only in primary chronic polyarthritis” [38].

This safety in practice is born out by the results of an unpublished general practice study performed recently by Madaus AG. In a multicentre study, a total of 1,231 patients with relapsing respiratory and urinary infections (median, six infections per annum) were treated for 4–6 weeks with Echinacin® lozenges, one lozenge three times daily. In the documentation forms, to be completed on inclusion in the study and at four further weekly examinations, the presence of a total of eleven clinical symptoms was to be evaluated (together with a baseline assessment of previous infections, previous treatment and concurrent medication). In addition, adverse events were to be specifically recorded. Over 90% of the patients took the medication as planned, 36 patients actually taking 4–6 lozenges per day. In 85.8% of patients, a reduction of the symptoms was recorded, and 80.8% of the attending physicians evaluated the tolerability as very good. Table 3 lists the most frequently cited adverse events. Of these, the unpleasant taste is the only event which can be clearly distinguished from possible infectious symptomology, supporting further the good tolerability of Echinacin® on long-term administration.

Table 3 - Most frequently cited adverse events in 1231 patients with relapsing respiratory and urinary infections treated for 4–6 weeks with Echinacin® lozenges t.i.d. (Data from study on file at Madaus AG, Cologne)

	No. of patients	**% of total**
Patients with adverse events	62	(5.04%)
Unpleasant taste	21	(1.70%)
Nausea/vomiting	6	(0.48%)
Recurrent infection	5	(0.41%)
Sore throat	3	(0.24%)
Abdominal pain	3	(0.24%)
Diarrhoea	3	(0.24%)
Difficulty in swallowing	2	(0.16%)
Other single reports	19	(1.54%)

Over the six years from 1989 to 1995, 13 adverse events in patients receiving oral Echinacin® were reported to the BGA in Germany, on the basis of spontaneous reporting by general practitioners. Of these, in only four cases were the adverse events considered to be causally related to the treatment. All four were cases of allergic skin reactions.

Considerable uncertainty was raised in Germany in 1996 by reports in the popular press that several deaths due to anaphylaxis had occurred over the previous six years in patients taking *Echinacea* preparations. However, investigations by the federal health authorities failed to establish causality between the deaths and *Echinacea* in view of the variety of other treatments being administered [39]. While positive IgE antibodies have been reported in up to 5% of patients taking *Echinacea* preparations [40], this must be set against the millions of packages sold annually without reports of serious adverse events.

Lack of immunotoxicity

Although it has been reported that at very high concentrations *in vitro* the squeezed sap of *E. purpurea* inhibits human lymphocyte proliferation to phytohemagglutinin, this was only observed at a concentration 1000-fold higher than the lowest concentration at which beneficial enhancement of proliferation was observed [37]. Up to 500 µg/ml, the isolated neutral fucogalactoxyloglucan (NFA 10) from *E. purpurea* had no mutagenic effect on human lymphocytes, as determined by sister chromatid exchange and chromosome aberration [41]. The acute toxicity (i.p.) in mice of the four main polysaccharides isolated from *E. purpurea* was also very low (LD50 = 2500 mg/kg) [42]. A direct immunotoxic effect of oral Echinacin® is therefore unlikely. Isolated cases of allergic responses to the drug, though, may be expected.

Immunostimulation at sites of infection

The object of the immunotherapy of infections is to achieve stimulation of immunocompetent cells which are in direct local contact with the infectious agent. That this can be achieved on oral administration of an immunostimulant has been demonstrated experimentally using a lysate of several different bacteria (Luivac®). Oral administration of Luivac® 15 mg/kg p.o. for two periods of five days over a three week period to mice resulted in an enhanced localization of lymphocytes in the respiratory tract after cell transfer to untreated syngeneic mice [43] and a marked increase in IgA synthesis in pulmonary lymphocytes in actively treated animals [44]. Clinically, oral administration of another mixed preparation of bacterial lysates has been shown to increase the concentration of IgA in the saliva of children with recurrent respiratory infections [45]. The transient decrease in peripheral blood CD8 T lymphocyte counts associated with leukocytosis observed by several authors [22, 37] in patients receiving parenteral Echinacin® is, therefore, almost certainly to be accounted for by adherence to the endothelium and migration of activated T helper cells to target organs. This would appear to be supported by the fact that, in the study in triathletes, Echinacin®, given prior to a competition, stimulated the production of cytokines probably derived from activated monocytes [21]. Monocyte-derived cytokines would be capable of stimulating endothelial adhesion molecule expression. The implication of these data is that Echinacin® has little effect, stimulatory or adverse, on the normal immune response, but is most effective as an oral immunostimulant in subjects with slightly to moderately compromised cell-mediated immune responses. This suggestion is supported by the finding that oral Echinacin® given for eight weeks produced a discernible reduction in the incidence and duration of respiratory infections in subjects with a low CD4/CD8 ratio in the peripheral blood [30] and reduced the expression and duration of symptoms of the common cold when given promptly at the first signs that a cold was going to develop [31].

On the other hand, there is no evidence that oral administration of Echinacin® can result in an excessive lymphoproliferative response. The study on marathon runners involved oral treatment for 12 weeks, without a discernible adverse effect on lymphocyte counts. Even when given by various routes of administration to patients with relapsing candidiasis for ten weeks, no adverse immunological overstimulation was observed [23]. The lack of mutagenic activity of the isolated polysaccharide from *E. purpurea* further supports the tolerability of the product [41]. In *in vitro* studies, the purified arabinogalactan actually stimulated macrophage-mediated tumor cell toxicity [15]. While recognizing that studies on the effects of Echinacin® on lymphoproliferative conditions *in vivo* are not available, the data that is available indicate that the product not only has no mutagenic potential, but that it appears to be safe for oral administration for periods longer than eight weeks.

Conclusions

Extracts of *E. purpurea* are widely used in the self-medication of mild respiratory infections. The efficacy of this therapy requires further evaluation, but the safety of the squeezed sap of the flowering coneflower (Echinacin®) can be more clearly assessed from the literature. Echinacin® has been shown, in controlled studies and in general practice, to be very well tolerated when given orally and parenterally. This is the case for subjects over a wide range of ages from infants to adults. Effective particularly in patients at an early stage of a respiratory infection or with slight to moderate depression of cell-mediated immune responses, changes observed with Echinacin® in peripheral blood lymphocyte counts appear to reflect its redistribution of activated lymphocytes to sites of infection. The healthy immune response does not appear to be altered by Echinacin® which has not shown any propensity to enhance pathological lympho-proliferation, though specific studies have not been carried out. Administered orally for up to 12 weeks, no adverse reactions other than aversion to the taste have been reported. Allergic skin responses to Echinacin® have been reported to occur only in isolated cases. Echinacin®, therefore, can be considered a safe product for long-term oral immunostimulation.

References

1 Holzer P, Lembeck F (1983) Analgesia up to the twentieth century. In: MJ Parnham, J Bruinvels (eds): *Psycho- and neuro-pharmacology. Discoveries in Pharmacology* Vol. 1. Elsevier, Amsterdam, 357–377

2 Aronson JK (1984) Digitalis. In: MJ Parnham, J Bruinvels (eds): *Haemodynamics, hormones and inflammation. Discoveries in pharmacology* Vol. 2, Elsevier, Amsterdam, 163–184

3 Collier HOJ (1984) The story of aspirin. In: MJ Parnham, J Bruinvels (eds): *Haemodynamics, hormones and inflammation. Discoveries in pharmacology* Vol. 2, Elsevier, Amsterdam, 555–593

4 Anon (1994) *WHO Drug Information* 8: 208–209

5 Foster S (1991) *Echinacea. Nature's immune enhancer.* Healing Arts Press, Rochester, VT

6 Bauer R, Wagner H (1990) *Echinacea. Handbuch für Ärzte, Apotheker und andere Wissenschaftler.* Wissenschaftliche Verlagsgesellschaft, Stuttgart, 1990

7 Bundesgesundheitsamt (1989) Aufbereitungsmonographien für Arzneimittel der phytotherapeutischen Therapierichtung vom 5.1.1989: *Echinacea purpurea herba* (Purpursonnenhutkraut). *Bundesanzeiger* March 2: 1070

8 Heesen W (1964) Unspezifische Behandlungsmöglichkeiten bei tuberkulösen Erkrankungen. *Erfahrungsheilkunde* 13: 210–217

9 Zimmermann 0 (1969) Die Therapie des Keuchhustens mit Myo-Echinacin®. *Hippokrates* 6: 233–235

10 Choné B, Manidakis G (1969) Echinacin-Test zur Leukozyten-provokation bei effektiver Strahlentherapie. *Dtsch Med Wochenschr* 94: 1406–1410.

11 Lorenz E, Meßner H, Mutz I (1972) Leucocytokinetic studies during viral hepatitis. *Z Kinderheilkunde* 113: 171–174

12 Tympner KD (1981) Der immunologische Wirkungsnachweis von Pflanzenextrakten. *Z angew Phytother* 5: 181–184

13 Bauer R, Remiger P, Jurcic K, Wagner H (1989) Beeinflussung der Phagozytenaktivitat durch *Echinacea*-Extrakte. *Z Phytother* 10: 43–48

14 Bauer R (1987) Standardisierung von *Echinacea-purpurea*-Preßsaft auf Cichoriensäure und Alkamide. *Z Phytother* 18: 270–276

15 Stimpel M, Proksch A, Wagner H, Lohmann-Matthes ML (1984) Macrophage activation and induction of macrophage cytotoxicity by purified polysaccharide fractions from the plant *Echinacea purpurea. Infect Immun* 46: 845–849

16 Luettig B, Steinmüller C, Gifford GE, Wagner H, Lohmann-Matthes ML (1989) Macrophage activation by the polysaccharide arabinogalactan isolated from plant cell cultures of *Echinacea purpurea. J Natl Cancer Inst* 81: 669–675

17 Lohmann-Matthes ML, Wagner H (1989) Aktivierung von Makrophagen durch Polysaccharide aus Gewebekulturen von *Echinacea purpurea. Z Phytother* 10: 52–59

18 Roesler J, Emmendörfer A, Steinmüller C, Luettig B, Wagner H, Lohmann-Matthes M-L (1991) Application of purified polysaccharides from cell cultures of the plant *Echinacea purpurea* to test subjects mediates activation of the phagocyte system. *Int J Immunopharmac* 13: 931–941

19 Möse JR (1983) Zur Wirkung von Echinacin® auf Phagozytoseaktivität und Natural Killer Cells. *Med Welt* 34: 1463–1467

20 Jurcic K, Melchart D, Holzmann M, Martin P, Bauer R, Doenicke A, Wagner H (1989) Zwei Probandenstudien zur Stimulierung der Granulozyten-phagozytose durch *Echinacea*-extrakthaltige Präparate. *Z Phytother* 10: 67–70

21 Berg A, Northoff H, König D, Weinstock C, Grathwohl D, Parnham MJ, Stuhlfauth I, Keul J (1998) Pretreatment with *Echinacea purpurea* modulates the effects of exhaustive exercise on immunological variables in triathletes. *Int J Sports Med; in press*

22 Gaisbauer M, Zimmermann W, Schleich T (1986) Die Veränderung immunologischer Parameter beim Menschen durch *Echinacea purpurea* Moench. *Natura Med* 1: 6–10

23 Coeugniet E, Kühnast R (1986) Rezidividierende Candidiasis. Adjuvante Immuntherapie mit verschiedenen Echinacin® Darreichungsformen. *Therapiewoche* 36: 3352–3358
24 Birr C, Nebe CT, Becker G (1994) Site-specific differentiation induction on T cells *in vivo* by synthetic thymic peptides to fight microbial infections and cancer. In: KN Masihi (ed): *Immunotherapy of infections*. Marcel Dekker, New York, 143–151
25 Parnham MJ, Englberger W (1988) Lipid mediators and lymphocyte function. In: MA Bray, J Morley (eds): *The pharmacology of lymphocytes*. Springer-Verlag, Berlin, 385–414
26 Volz G (1957) Zur Keuchhustenbehandlung mit Myo-Echinacin. *Ther Gegenwart* 96: 312–313
27 Baetgen D (1964) Pertussistherapie mit Myo-Echinacin in der Kinderpraxis. *Med Monatschr* 18: 129–131
28 Heesen W and Orzechowski G (1973) Die Fieberbehandlung mit Echinacin® bei Infektionskrankheiten. *Erfahrungsheilkunde* 22: 163–171
29 Baetgen D (1984) Erfolge in der Keuchhustenbehandlung mit Echinacin. *Therapiewoche* 34: 5115–5119
30 Schöneberger D (1992) Einfluß der immunstimulierenden Wirkung von Preßsaft aus Herba *Echinacea purpurea* auf Verlauf und Schweregrad von Erkältungskrankheiten. *Forum Immunol* 8: 1–8
31 Hoheisel O, Sandberg M, Bertram S, Bulitta M, Schäfer M (1997) Echinagard® treatment shortens the course of the common cold: a double-blind, placebo-controlled clinical trial. *Eur J Clin Res* 9: 261–268
32 Scaglione F, Lund B (1995) Efficacy in the treatment of the common cold of a preparation containing an *Echinacea* extract. *Int J Immunother* 11: 163–166
33 Röseler W (1950) Erfahrungen mit Echinacin bei fieberhaften gynäkologischen Erkrankungen. *Der Krankenhausarzt* 23: 38–40
34 Röseler W (1952) Erfahrungen mit der Echinacin-Therapie fieberhafter gynäkologischer Erkrankungen. *Die Medizinische* 3: 93–95
35 Moell OH (1951) Primäre Ergebnisse der Echinacinbehandlung bei entzündlichen Unterleibserkrankungen. *Der Krankenhausarzt* 24: 299–302
36 Priese H-G (1954) Die Frühbehandlung der Mastitis puerperalis mit Echinacin. *Zentralbl Gynäk* 76: 756–768
37 Coeugniet EG, Elek E (1987) Immunmodulation with Viscum album and *Echinacea purpurea* extracts. *Onkologie* 10 (Suppl): 27–33
38 Reuß D (1986) Behandlung der chronischen Polyarthritis mit Echinacin. *Rheuma* 5: 29–32
39 Bauer R, Wagner H (1996) *Echinacea*: Kein Grund zur Panik. *Dt Apoth Z* 136: 1936–1937
40 Mullins RJ (1998) *Echinacea*-associated anaphylaxis. *Med J Aust* 168: 170–171
41 Schimmer O, Abel G, Behninger C (1989) Untersuchungen zur gentoxischen Potenz eines neutralen Polysaccharids aus *Echinacea*-Gewebekulturen in menschlichen Lymphozyten. Z Phytother 10: 39–42

42 Lenk W (1989). Akute Toxizität von verschiedenen Polysacchariden aus *Echinacea purpurea* an der Maus. *Z Phytother* 1989; 10: 49–51

43 Ruedl C, Albini B, Böck G, Wick G, Wolf H (1993) Oral administration of a bacterial immunomodulator enhances murine intestinal lamina propria and Peyer's patch lymphocyte traffic to the lung: possible implications for infectious disease prophylaxis and therapy. *Int Immunol* 5; 29–34

44 Wolf H (1994) Can orally applied immunomodulators improve local defense? In: Masihi KN (ed): *Immunotherapy of infections.* Marcel Dekker, New York, 351–355

45 Van Aubel A, Hofbauer C, Elsasser U, Kämmereit A, Riedl-Seifert RJ (1994) Immunoglobulins in serum and saliva of children with recurrent infections of the respiratory tract during treatment with an oral immunomodulator. In: KN Masihi (ed): *Immunotherapy of infections.* Marcel Dekker, New York, 357–369

Low-molecular weight compounds with complement activity

Luc A.C. Pieters, Tess E. De Bruyne and Arnold J. Vlietinck

Department of Pharmaceutical Sciences, University of Antwerp, Universiteitsplein 1, B-2610 Antwerp, Belgium

Introduction

The complement system

The complement system is one of the major effector pathways in the process of inflammation. Along with the clotting, fibrinolytic and kallikrein-kinin systems, complement represents one of the complex enzyme systems of blood which can be activated in specific cascade reactions upon a triggering stimulation. Activated complement components mediate various biological effects, each with its specific function in the defence reactions against noxious stimulants. These effects, being beneficial to the host under normal conditions, may also cause adverse reactions depending on the site, extent and duration of complement activation. Pharmacological modulation of the complement system could be of potential interest for the treatment and control of immune-pathological reactions linked with complement activation [1].

Two possible activation routes, referred to as the classical and the alternative pathway, converge at complement factor C3, from which activation proceeds through C5 to the lytic pathway. The classical activation pathway is triggered by antibody-antigen complexes or by the Fc portion of aggregated immunoglobulin belonging to the IgM or IgG class (with the exception of subclass IgG4). The alternative route, on the other hand, can be activated by some polysaccharides, lipopolysaccharides, immune-complexes or aggregated immunoglobulins of classes (e.g. IgA) that do not usually activate the classical sequence. Several mechanisms prevent non-specific, as well as excessive continuous activation and overspill to innocent bystander cells. The terminal route is the final phase of the activation of the complement cascade, resulting in the formation of the membrane attack complex (MAC) (Fig. 1).

Immunomodulatory Agents from Plants, edited by H. Wagner

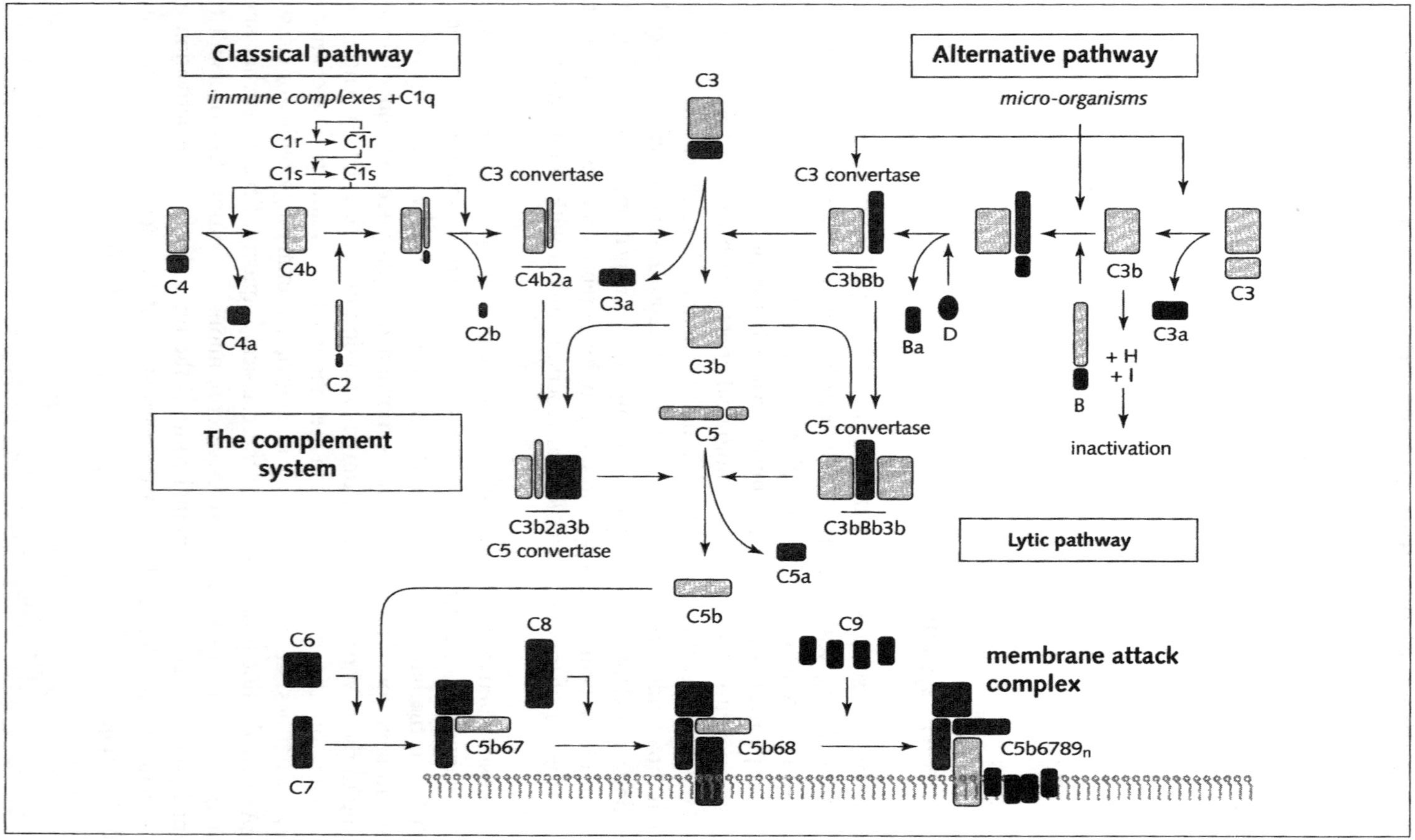

Figure 1 - The complement system

Biological effects of complement

The complement system is a potent mechanism for initiating and amplifying inflammation. The cleavage products C3a and C5a (anaphylatoxins) stimulate chemotaxis and activation of leucocytes. They are chemotactic for neutrophils and trigger degranulation of basophils and mast cells, thus liberating vaso-active substances (e.g. histamine). The net result is an increase in vascular permeability and emigration of neutrophils and monocytes from blood vessels.

Bound C3 and C4 fragments act as opsonins enhancing phagocytosis. Opsonisation involves coating of the target with certain complement proteins. Phagocytic cells carrying receptors for these complement proteins then bind and endocytose the opsonised particles.

By covalent incorporation of C3 into immune complex lattices, it reduces the capacity of the antibody to bind to epitopes on the antigen, thereby limiting the formation of large lattices. The classical pathway of complement is said to inhibit the formation of precipitating immune complexes in plasma, whereas the alternative route can solubilise immune complexes that have already precipitated.

Although a direct lytic effect of the MAC applies only to erythrocytes and not to nucleated cells which can endocytose or exocytose portions of membrane containing MAC, the perturbation of the membrane bilayer can stimulate cells to release and metabolise arachidonic acid, to undertake oxidative metabolism, or to release granules or cytokines. These responses may play an important role in amplifying inflammation following complement activation. The lytic process also interferes with the neutralisation of some Gram-negative bacteria (e.g. *Neisseria* and *Salmonella* species).

Although complement is certainly beneficial, if not essential, for the host's defence against foreign invading organisms as for instance in acute infections by bacteria, fungi or viruses, its activation may contribute to or even evoke pathological reactions in a variety of inflammatory or degenerative diseases. These include immune complex diseases, autoimmune diseases, rheumatoid arthritis, microbial infections, gout and traumatic tissue injury. Drugs that inhibit the complement system could be valuable therapeutics in those cases, while complement-activating drugs could be used in cases of immune-depression or in tumor therapy [2, 3].

HIV shows an intrinsic resistance to complement-mediated virolysis. The role of complement in HIV infection has been largely underestimated in the past. In human plasma, HIV activates the complement system, even in the absence of specific antibodies. If the reactions were allowed to go to completion, complement activation would result in virolysis. This is avoided by complement regulatory molecules, which are either included in the virus membrane upon budding from the infected cells or are secondarily attached to HIV envelope glycoproteins. In this way HIV also takes advantage of human complement activation for enhancement of infectivity, for follicular localisation, and for broadening its target cell range [4].

Complement modulation assay

Screening systems for complement activity are most commonly based on its haemolytic properties, involving a spectrophotometric measurement of the haemoglobin released at $\lambda = 414$ nm. The amount of haemoglobin that is released reflects the degree of lytic action. Complement modulation tests commonly applied are based on the assay models as described by Mayer in 1971 [5] and by Platts-Mills and Ishizaka in 1974 [6] for the classical and the alternative activation pathways, respectively. A haemolytic complement assay on microscale for classical and alternative pathway activation was presented by Klerx et al. in 1983 [7].

In general, sensitised sheep erythrocytes in the presence of Ca^{2+} and Mg^{2+} ions are used for the estimation of classical complement pathway activation and rabbit erythrocytes after addition of Mg^{2+} for alternative pathway activation. For both pathways, the amount of complement needed for the lysis of 50% of the erythrocytes is estimated and denoted by the CH_{50} value (for the classical pathway) and the ACH_{50} value (for the alternative pathway). The inhibitory or activating effect after addition of the test compound is reflected in the shift of the CH_{50} or ACH_{50} value to higher or lower numbers respectively. In the classical pathway assay, several dilutions of the test compound are incubated with human pooled serum, or alternatively Guinea pig serum, as a source for the complement factors, at 37° C. Sheep red blood cells (SRBC), sensibilised with monoclonal anti-SRBC antibodies are added, and after further incubation and subsequent centrifugation, the absorption of the supernatans is read in a multiscan spectrophotometer at $\lambda = 414$ nm. In the alternative pathway assay on the other hand, after incubation of test compound dilutions with serum, rabbit red blood cells are added and the assay is completed as for the classical system.

In 1984 complement-modulating compounds were reviewed by Asghar [8]. The present review will be limited to plant-derived low-molecular weight compounds with complement activity.

Phenolic compounds

Phenolic acids and derivatives

Rosmarinic acid (**1**) was first isolated from *Rosmarinus officinalis* L. (or *Melissa officinalis* L.) (*Labiatae*) [9]. It was found to act as a complement inhibitor, and several investigations were carried out to reveal its mode of action . Rosmarinic acid had effects on both the classical pathway C3-convertase and on the cobra venom factor-induced, alternative pathway convertase. It also exhibited inhibitory activity in a number of *in vivo* models in which complement activation plays a role: Rosmarinic acid (0.316–3.16 mg/kg i.m.) reduced paw oedema induced by cobra venom

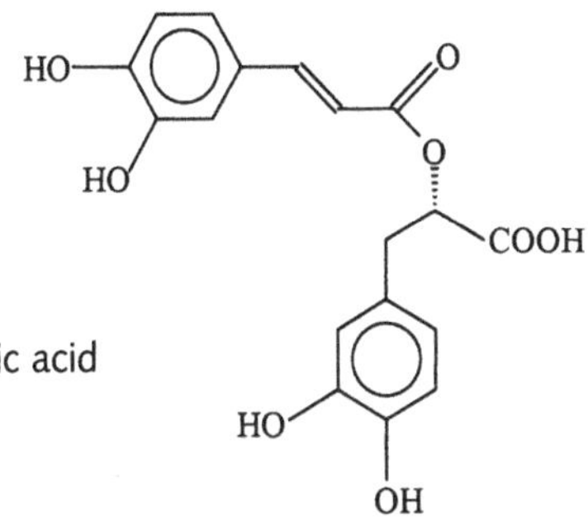

1 Rosmarinic acid

factor in the rat, and at 1–100 mg/kg p.o. it inhibited passive cutaneous anaphylaxis in the rat; at 10 mg/kg i.m. rosmarinic acid impaired *in vivo* activation by heat-killed *Corynebacterium parvum* (i.p.) of mouse macrophages, as measured by the decreased capacity of the activated macrophages to undergo the oxidative burst [10]. Rosmarinic acid (20 mg/kg i.v.) also suppressed endotoxin-induced complement activation in a rabbit model of circulatory shock [11]. Peake et al. reported that the inhibitory effects of rosmarinic acid were principally mediated by inhibition of the C5-convertase [12].

Rosmarinic acid was also identified as one of the complement-inhibiting principles of *Apeiba tibourbou* Aubl. (*Tiliaceae*), interfering with both activation pathways [13]. Its inhibiting properties were more pronounced on the classical than on the alternative pathway (IC_{50} 81 ± 3 mM and 408 ± 53 mM, respectively). A comparative study of the complement-inhibiting properties of rosmarinic acid, a series of phenolic acids, and a series of caffeoyl esters of quinic acid, was carried out by Knaus [14]. Some results are compiled in Table 1 (for the classical pathway) and Table 2 (for the alternative pathway). Results are presented as the reduction of haemolysis (%) at different concentrations of test compound. In the series of the phenolic acids (**2–6**) dihydrocaffeic acid (**6**) was more active as an inhibitor of the classical pathway than caffeic acid (**3**), followed in decreasing order of activity by ferulic acid (**4**), sinapic acid (**5**) and cinnamic acid (**2**). Chlorogenic acid, or 5-caffeoyl quinic acid (**7**), with one caffeoyl moiety, had about the same activity as caffeic acid on the classical pathway, but the dicaffeoyl derivatives of quinic acid, i.e. isochlorogenic acid, a mixture of dicaffeoyl esters of quinic acid (**8**), and cynarin, or 1,3-dicaffeoyl quinic acid (**9**) were more active. These dicaffeoyl derivatives also inhibited the alternative pathway (Tab. 2). However, rosmarinic acid (**1**) was the most potent inhibitor of both the classical and the alternative pathway. It could be concluded that the caffeoyl moieties (with a saturated or an unsaturated side chain, but with two underivatised hydroxyl groups) play an important role in the complement-inhibiting activity, especially on the classical pathway; apparently the quinic acid moiety is not important. Phenolic acid esters of flavonoid glycosides also show complement activity, as discussed in the next section.

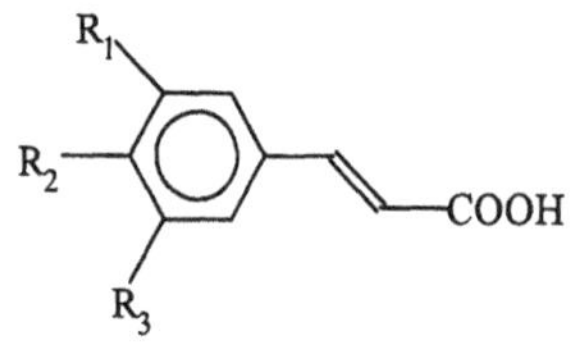

		R_1	R_2	R_3
2	cinnamic acid	H	H	H
3	caffeic acid	OH	OH	H
4	ferulic acid	OCH_3	OH	H
5	sinapic acid	OCH_3	OH	OCH_3

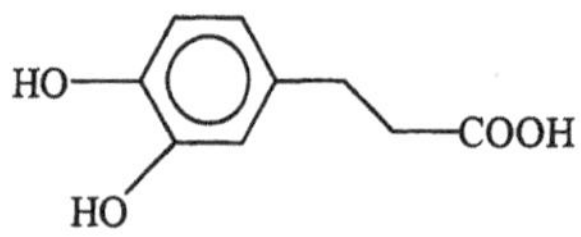

6 Dihydrocaffeic acid

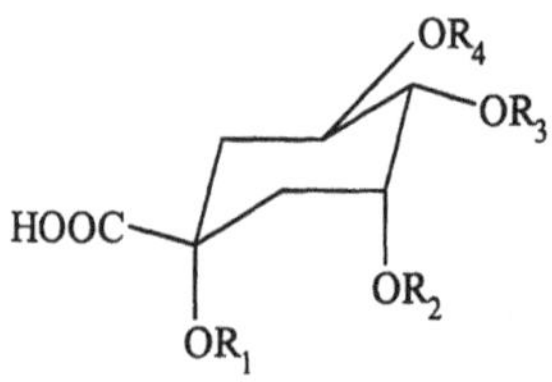

		R_1	R_2	R_3	R_4
7	chlorogenic acid (5-caffeoyl quinic acid)	H	H	H	caf
8	isochlorogenic acid				
	3,4-dicaffeoyl quinic acid	H	caf	caf	H
	3,5-dicaffeoyl quinic acid	H	caf	H	caf
	4,5-dicaffeoyl quinic acid	H	H	caf	caf
9	cynarin (1,3-dicaffeoyl quinic acid)	caf	caf	H	H

(caf = caffeoyl)

Flavonoids and proanthocyanidins

Flavonoids

The flavonoids constitute a large group of naturally occurring compounds that are widely distributed in the plant kingdom. They display a remarkable array of biochemical and pharmacological actions [15]. The influence of 54 flavonoids on both activation pathways of the complement system, using a haemolytic assay, was investigated by Lasure et al. in order to establish a structure-activity relationship [16]. The complement activity was evaluated at a flavonoid concentration of 1 mM. Several compounds exhibited an inhibition on complement-mediated haemolysis in a dose-dependent manner. The most potent inhibitors were quercetin (**10**), quercitrin (**11**), rutin (**12**), hyperoside (**13**), myricetin (**14**), taxifolin (**15**), pelargonidin chlo-

*Table 1 - Inhibition of the classical activation pathway of complement by phenolic compounds and derivatives (**1–9**): Reduction of haemolysis (%) [14].*

		concentration of test compound			
		1000 μM	500 μM	100 μM	50 μM
1	rosmarinic acid	n.d.	94.6 ± 3.5	38.8 ± 5.3	18.7 ± 1.4
2	cinnamic acid	13.2 ± 1.2	–	n.d.	n.d.
3	caffeic acid	67.8 ± 5.8	33.1 ± 7.1	14.7 ± 1.4	n.d.
4	ferulic acid	32.9 ± 2.1	–	n.d.	n.d.
5	sinapic acid	15.4 ± 1.6	–	n.d.	n.d.
6	dihydrocaffeic acid	85.1 ± 1.7	35.7 ± 13.5	–	n.d.
7	chlorogenic acid	65.2 ± 9.5	35.6 ± 9.7	8.8 ± 5.7	n.d.
8	isochlorogenic acid	97.6 ± 3.5	93.3 ± 1.3	32.1 ± 1.2	n.d.
9	cynarin	n.d.	61.4 ± 9.9	25.4 ± 8.3	11.8 ± 2.9

± SD; –, not active; n.d., not determined

*Table 2 - Inhibition of the alternative pathway of complement by phenolic acids and derivatives (**1**, **7**, **8**, **9**): reduction of haemolysis (%) [14].*

		concentration of test compound		
		500 μM	100 μM	50 μM
1	rosmarinic acid	87.6 ± 1.1	50.1 ± 12.1	34.8 ± 7.9
7	chlorogenic acid	42.8	n.d	n.d.
8	isochlorogenic acid	59.7 ± 10.3	8.8	n.d.
9	cynarin	76.9 ± 14.4	27.8	n.d.

± SD; n.d., not determined

ride (**16**) and cyanidin chloride (**17**) for the classical pathway, and hyperoside (**13**), myricetin (**14**), baicalein (**18**) and the anthocyanidins (e.g. pelargonidin chloride (**16**)) for the alternative pathway. Their IC_{50} values are listed in Table 3. Based on the results obtained for this series of 54 flavonoids, the following structure-activity relationship could be proposed for inhibition of the classical pathway [16]:

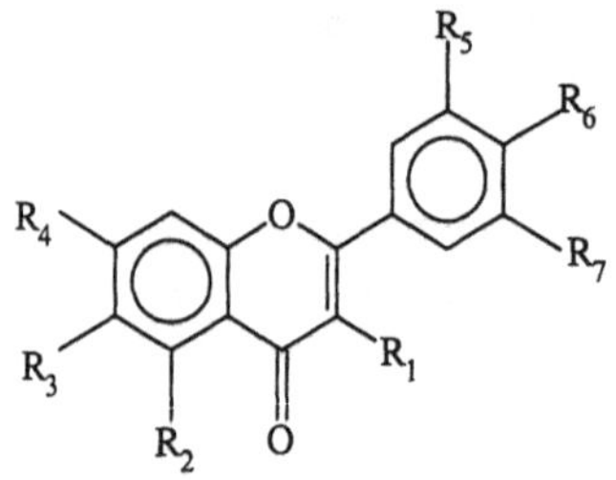

	R_1	R_2	R_3	R_4	R_5	R_6	R_7
10 quercetin	OH	OH	H	OH	OH	OH	H
11 quercitrin	O-rha	OH	H	OH	OH	OH	H
12 rutin	O-rut	OH	H	OH	OH	OH	H
13 hyperoside	O-gal	OH	H	OH	OH	OH	H
14 myricetin	OH	OH	H	OH	OH	OH	OH
18 baicalein	H	OH	OH	OH	H	H	H
19 kaempferol	OH	OH	H	OH	H	OH	H

(rha = rhamnosyl; rut = rutinosyl; gal = galactosyl)

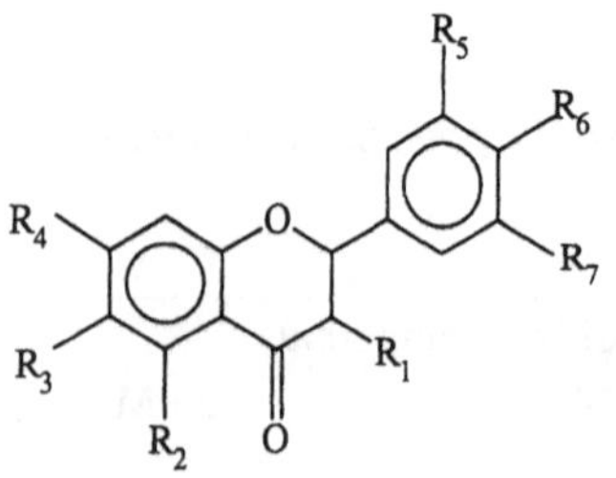

	R_1	R_2	R_3	R_4	R_5	R_6	R_7
15 (±)taxifolin	OH	OH	H	OH	OH	OH	H

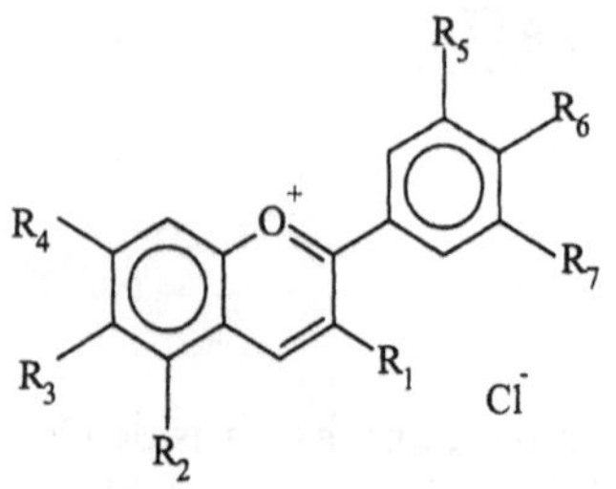

	R_1	R_2	R_3	R_4	R_5	R_6	R_7
16 pelargonidin chloride	OH	OH	H	OH	H	OH	H
17 cynidin chloride	OH	OH	H	OH	OH	OH	H

*Table 3 - IC_{50} values (μM) for flavonoids (**10–18**) on the classical and the alternative pathway of complement [16].*

	CP	AP
10 quercetin	52.6 ± 13.2	n.d.
11 quercitrin	384.1± 8.8	n.d.
12 rutin	357.1 ± 2.9	n.d.
13 hyperoside	n.d.[1]	62.5 ± 5.1
14 myricetin	67.6 ± 1.3	153.8 ± 5.9
15 (±)-taxifolin	402.2 ± 9.2	n.d.
16 pelargonidin Cl	167.2 ± 2.5	120.5 ± 9.4
17 cyanidin Cl	87.7 ± 3.7	n.d.
18 baicalein	n.d.	942.2 ± 11.3

± SD; n.d., not determined;
[1] 41.1 ± 4.6% inhibition at a concentration of 500 μM

- The double bond at C-2 and the carbonyl group at C-4 are not essential;
- Hydroxylation at C-3 increases the inhibitory activity;
- An increasing number of hydroxyl groups in the B-ring (C-1'–C-6') enhances the activity, especially a 3',4',5'-trihydroxyl substitution as in myricetin (**14**);
- Methoxylation decreases the inhibitory effect;
- Glycosylation has an ambiguous effect depending on the nature of the sugar and the aglycone, and on the type of linkage to the aglycone (e.g. C-glycosylation as in vitexin decreases the activity). Also the high inhibitory effect of anthocyanidins is decreased by glycosylation.

This structure-activity relationship is in good agreement with observations made by Knaus for a limited number of flavonoids [14]. In addition a high inhibitory activity was reported for 2",4"-dicoumaroylastragalin (70% inhibition of the classical pathway at a concentration of 50 μM). Astragalin is the 3-O-glucoside of kaempferol (**19**). Tiliroside, or kaempferol 3-O-(6"-coumaroyl)-glucoside, on the other hand, only showed a low activity (4.7 ± 1.5% inhibition at a concentration of 500 μM [16].

For the alternative pathway no clear structure-activity relationship could be established by Lasure et al. However, a few general observations were made [16]:

- Anthocyanidins show a high inhibitory activity;
- The carbonyl group at C-4 is important for a high inhibitory activity;

- Methoxylation in general causes an activation of the alternative pathway, but especially methoxylation at C-4';
- The inhibitory effect increases with the number of hyroxyl groups in ring B.

Lasure et al. also investigated whether the inhibitory activity of the most potent flavonoids on the classical pathway could be explained by chelation of Mg^{2+} or Ca^{2+}. Increasing Ca^{2+} or Mg^{2+} concentrations up to four times the standard concentration did not decrease the inhibition of haemolysis. Thus, inhibition of the classical pathway by flavonoids appeared not to be related to a chelation of essential bivalent cations [16].

The complement-modulating principles of several plants have been identified as flavonoids, e.g. in leaves of *Morinda morindoides* (Baker) Milne Redh. (*Rubiaceae*) [17–19]. It was demonstrated that quercetin, quercitrin and rutin inhibited the classical pathway in a dose-dependent manner, but that the effect on the alternative pathway was not dose-dependent [18]. Morindaoside, a 7-O-rhamnosylsophoroside of kaempferol (kaempferol 7-O-[rhamnosyl-(1-6)]-[glucosyl-(1-2)]-glucoside), showed a dose-dependent inhibition of the classical pathway (40.8 ± 8.6% inhibition at 1 mM), and a dose-dependent activation of the alternative pathway (56.1 ± 4.5% activation at 1 mM). Rosmarinic acid, used as a reference compound, inhibited both the classical and the alternative pathway in a dose-dependent way. Kaempferol (**19**) was about as active as morindaoside as an inhibitor of the classical pathway (33.2 ± 11.5% inhibition at 1 mM), but less active as an activator of the alternative pathway (28.6 ± 3.7% activation at 1 mM) [19].

Flavan-3-ols and proanthocyanidins

The complement-modulating activity of a series of monomeric flavan-3-ols (**20–22**), dimeric (**23–31**) and trimeric (**32**) procyanidins was evaluated by De Bruyne [20]. IC_{50} values for inhibition of the classical and the alternative pathway are listed in Table 4. The results obtained for inhibition of the classical pathway showed clearly that all dimers tested were more active than (+)-catechin (**20**) or (–)-epicatechin (**21**), or than all flavonoids included in Table 3. The only trimer tested, procyanidin C1 (**32**), was even more active. The flavanoid (–)-epigallocatechin (**22**) was an important exception: it was as active as the most potent dimeric procyanidins B6 (**28**) and B8 (**29**). As for myricetin in the flavonoid series, this once again demonstrated the high activity associated with a 3',4',5'-trihydroxyl substitution. This was also confirmed by the high inhibitory activity of gallocatechin-(4'-O-7)-epigallocatechin, a biflavanoid isolated from *Bridelia ferruginea* [20, 21].

With regard to the alternative pathway, no structure-activity relationship could be established, but in Table 4 it is striking that all flavan-3-ols or procyanidins which exhibited an inhibitory activity on the alternative pathway were also potent inhibitors of the classical pathway.

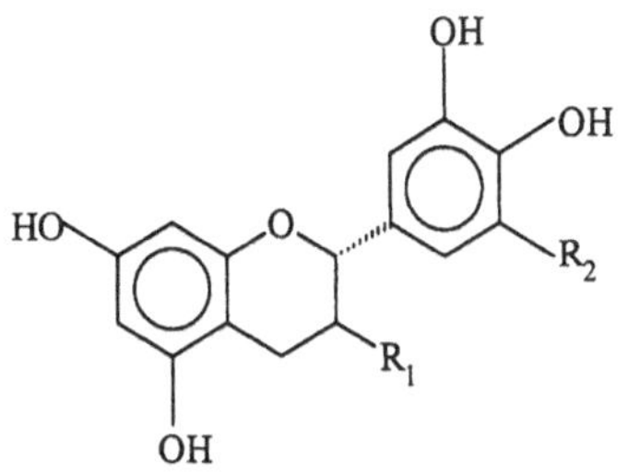

	R_1	R_2
20 (+)-catechin	OH	H
21 (–)-epicatechin	--OH	H
22 (–)-epigallocatechin	--OH	OH

23 procyanidin B1	epicatechin-(4β-8)-catechin
24 procyanidin B2	epicatechin-(4β-8)-epicatechin
25 procyanidin B3	catechin-(4α-8)-catechin
26 procyanidin B4	catechin-(4α-8)-epicatechin
27 procyanidin B5	epicatechin-(4β-6)-epicatechin
28 procyanidin B6	catechin-(4α-6)-catechin
29 procyanidin B8	catechin-(4α-6)-epicatechin
30 proanthocyanidin A1	epicatechin-(4β-8, 2β-O-7)-catechin
31 proanthocyanidin A2	epicatechin-(4β-8, 2β-O-7)-epicatechin
32 procyanidin C1	epicatechin-(4β-8)-epicatechin-(4β-8)-epicatechin
33 gallocatechin-(4′-O-7)-epigallocatechin	

Some flavonoids, such as quercetin (**10**) and rutin (**12**), and proanthocyanidins, such as procyanidin B2 (**24**), B5 (**27**), C1 (**32**) and proanthocyanidin A2 (**31**), were isolated as the complement-inhibiting principles from leaves and fruits of *Crataegus sinaica* Boiss. (*Rosaceae*) [22]. To investigate the mode of action of the anticomplementary activity on the classical pathway, logarithmic dilutions of the ethylacetate extracts of leaves and fruits (containing the phenolic constituents) were tested using different incubation conditions. The inhibitory effect of both extracts was not decreased when preincubation was performed at 4° C, indicating that the interference did not occur at the enzymatic level. A variation in the length of preincubation (0, 15, 30 min) at 37° C had no effect on the inhibition either. Therefore it was concluded that depletion of complement was not the mechanism involved.

Kosasi et al. isolated a high molecular weight proanthocyanidin with catechin or epicatechin as the building unit from latex of *Jathropa multifida* L. (*Euphor-*

*Table 4 - IC_{50} values (μM) for flavan-3-ols and proanthocyanidins (**20–33**) on the classical and the alternative pathway of complement [20].*

	CP	AP
20 catechin	647.2	–
21 epicatechin	655.5	n.d.
22 epigallocatechin	19.6	179.4
23 procyanidin B1	31.3	72.0
24 procyanidin B2	58.0	–
25 procyanidin B3	37.7	–
26 procyanidin B4	45.5	–
27 procyanidin B5	51.7	–
28 procyanidin B6	18.5	–
29 procyanidin B8	19.7	83.7
30 proanthocyanidin A1	57.1	105.0
31 proanthocyanidin A2	11.6	112.8
32 procyanidin C1	6.0	85.5
33 gallocatechin-(4'-O-7)-epigallocatechin	14.6	86.0

–, not active

biaceae), which inhibited complement activation through the classical pathway. The alternative pathway was relatively insensitive to this polymer. This activity was due to the selective depletion of Ca^{2+}, needed for the activation of the classical pathway, but not Mg^{2+}, from the incubation medium [23].

Other phenolic compounds

Guided by the complement activity two phloroglucinol derivatives, multifidol (**34**) (or (2-methylbutyryl)phloroglucinol) and multifidol glucoside (**35**) were isolated from the latex of *Jathropa multifida* L. (*Euphorbiaceae*) [24]. Both compounds inhibited the classical pathway of complement. Multifidol affected a practically complete inhibition at a concentration of 298 μM; multifidol glucoside showed 100% inhibition at a much higher concentration, i.e. 1.3 μM.

The effect of some hydroxycoumarins on complement-mediated haemolysis was evaluated by Ivanovska et al. [25]. Scopoletin (**36**), esculin (**37**) and esculetin (**38**) enhanced complement-mediated haemolysis, while 7-methylesculin (**39**), and the acetylated derivatives of esculin and esculetin significantly inhibited both the classi-

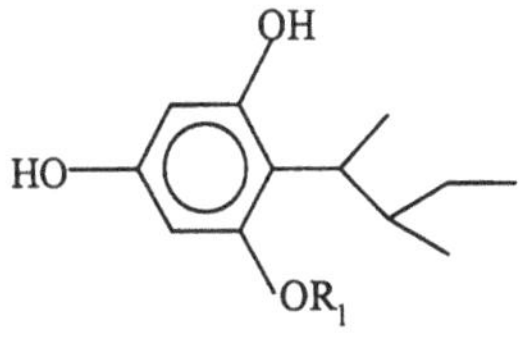

34 multifidol $R_1 = H$
35 multifidol glucoside R_1 = glucosyl

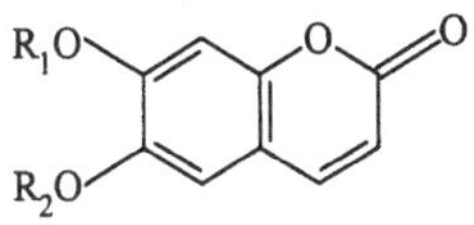

	R_1	R_2
36 scopoletin	H	CH3
37 esculin	H	glc
38 esculetin	H	H
39 7-methylesculin	CH3	glc
40 scoparone	CH3	CH3

(glc = glucosyl)

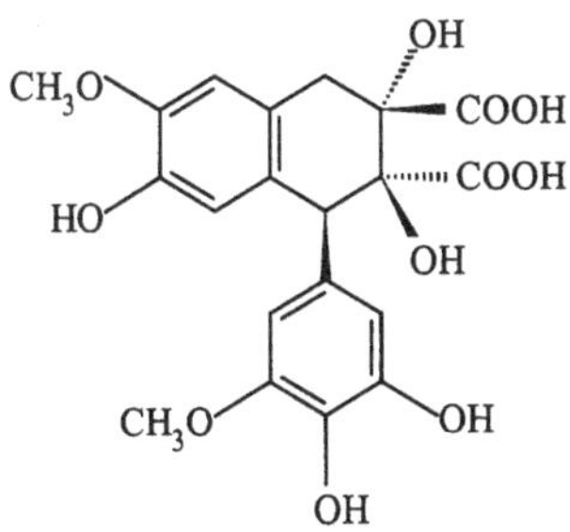

41 plicatic acid

cal and the alternative pathway; compounds were tested at concentrations of 50 μM and 120 μM. Scoparone (**40**) strongly reduced C3 alternative pathway activity. In C1 and C3 functional assays, 7-methylesculin (**39**) had a good effect on reducing total, C1 and C3 haemolysis via both pathways.

Plicatic acid (**41**), a lignan isolated from the heartwood of Western red cedar (*Thuja plicata* D. Don) (*Coniferae*), was found to activate the classical pathway of complement. The mechanism by which this activation occurred was not completely defined at the molecular level, but appeared to involve interference with the control of active C1s in serum by C1-In. By virtue of its ability to interfere with C1-In in its inactivation of active C1, plicatic acid might act as a protector of active C1 [26].

The anticomplementary activity of 19 lignoids obtained from the bark of *Eucommia ulmoides* Oliver (*Eucommiaceae*) was evaluated by Oshima et al. [27]. (+)-Syringaresinol monoglucoside (**42**), (+)-medioresinol monoglucoside (eucommin A) (**43**) and (–)-epipinoresinol (**44**) were active as inhibitors of the classical pathway (inhibition between 25 and 30%) at a concentration of 1.5 mg/ml or about 3 μM.

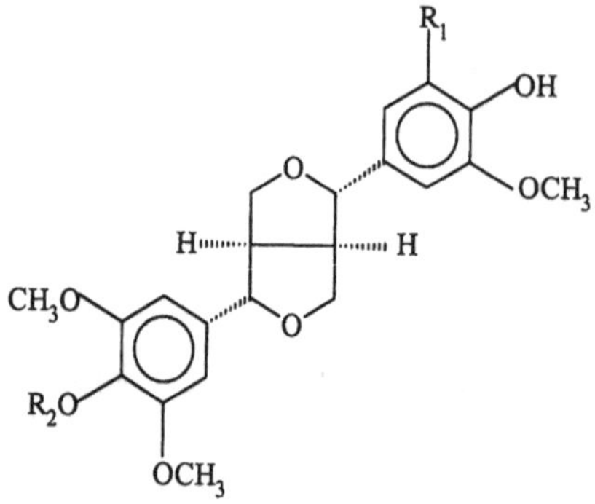

42 (+)-syringaresinol monoglucoside $R_1 = OCH_3$ R_2 = glucosyl
43 (+)-medioresinol monoglucoside $R_1 = H$ R_2 = glucosyl

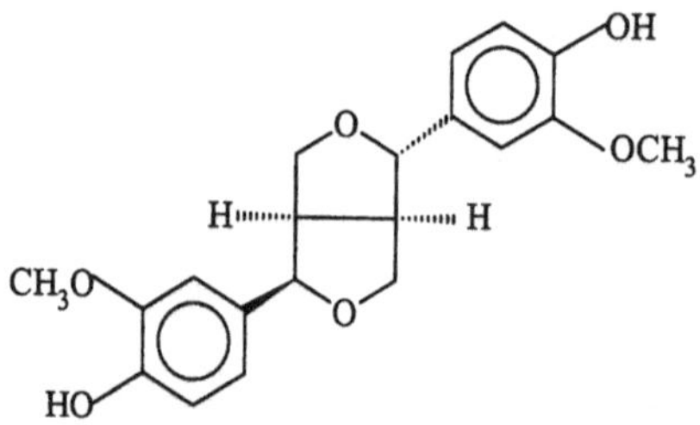

44 (+)-epipinoresinol

Terpenoids

Diterpenes

Glovsky et al. observed an anticomplementary activity for levopimaric acid (**45**), a derivative of abietic acid, and prepared a number of synthetic derivatives such as maleopimaric acid (**46**) and fumaropimaric acid (**47**), being Diels-Alder substitution products of levopimaric acid with maleic anhydride or fumaric acid, respectively [28, 29]. Maleic acid is cis-butenedioic acid, fumaric acid is trans-butenedioic acid. Maleopimaric acid inhibited complement-mediated haemolysis via classical pathway activation (45% inhibition at a concentration of 500 μM). Fumaropimaic acid inhibited *in vivo* complement-dependent systemic Frossman, cutaneous Frossman, and reverse passive Arthus reactions. These pimaric acid derivatives have already been included in earlier reviews on complement-active compounds [8, 30]. The

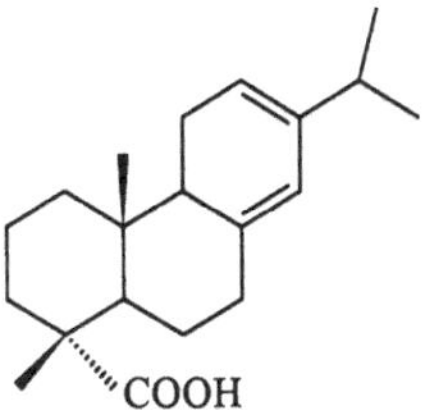

45 levopimaric acid

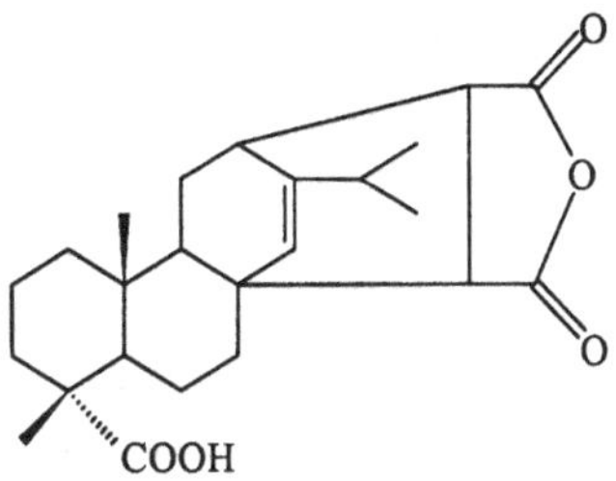

45 levopimaric acid

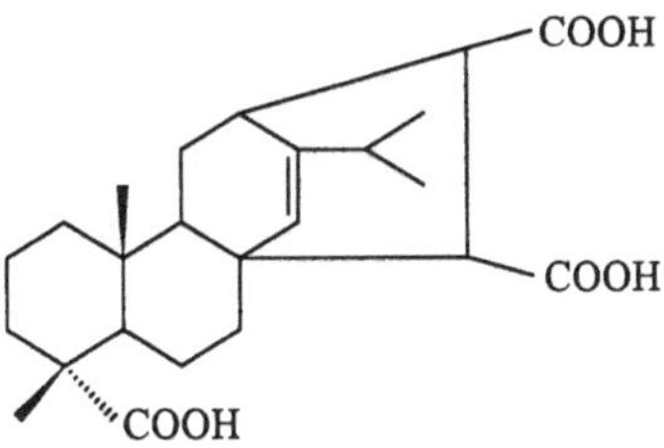

47 fumaropimaric acid

mechanism of action was considered to be inhibition of binding of C1 to sensitised erythrocytes or facilitation of dissociation of the former from the latter, as well as dissociation of the activated trimolecular complex C5b67, destroying its chemotactic activity for PMN (polymorphonuclear neutrophils).

Yagi et al. have isolated a series of diterpenes from the water extract of *Cinnamoni cortex* (*Cinnamonum cassia* Blume) (*Lauraceae*), which showed anticomplement activity; however, no details on the complement-modulating properties of the pure compounds were reported [31].

Triterpenes

An anticomplementary activity was demonstrated by Yamada et al. for some phytosterols, including stigmasterol (being the most potent one), β-sitosterol and campesterol [32]. However, it was suggested that the complement activity of these phytosterols might be due to activation by insoluble particles, as observed for polysaccharides [14]. Knaus and Wagner evaluated the complement-activity of a number of oxygenated triterpenoids such as cucurbitacin I (**48**), glycyrrhetic acid (**49**), oleanolic acid (**50**), quillaic acid (**51**), ursolic acid (**52**), crategolic acid (**53**) and β-boswellic acid (**54**). The latter compound was isolated from the gum resin of *Boswella serrata* Roxb. (*Burseraceae*) [14, 33]. Boswellic acid inhibited immunohaemolysis of the classical pathway in a dose-dependent way. At a concentration of 100 μM, an inhibition of 81 ± 6% was observed using normal human serum as source for complement. Results of a comparative assay with other oxygenated triterpenes and triterpene acids are summarised in Table 5. Boswellic acid (**54**), with a carboxylic group at C-4, ursolic acid (**52**) and crategolic acid (**53**) showed a pronounced anticomplementary activity on the classical pathway. Only boswellic acid demonstrated a pronounced inhibition of the alternative pathway at a concentration of 100 μM (Tab. 5). It was suggested that an inhibition of C3-convertase of the classical pathway was involved in the anticomplementary activty of boswellic acid [34].

Other terpenoids

An iridoid isolated from the bark of *Eucommia ulmoides* Oliv. (*Eucommiaceae*), genipin (**55**), showed a stronger anticomplementary activity (i.e. 75.3 ± 1.8% inhibition of the classical pathway at a concentration of 1.5 mg/ml or 6.6 μM) than

*Table 5 - Inhibition of the classical pathway (CP) and the alternative pathway (AP) of the complement system by triterpenes (**48–54**): reduction of haemolysis (%) [33].*

	concentration of test compound		
	CP		AP
	100 μM	50 μM	100 μM
48 cucurbitacin I	30 ± 2	n.d.	n.d.
49 glycyrrhetic acid	65 ± 9	17 ± 9	14 ± 2
50 oleanolic acid	62 ± 25	25 ± 10	12 ± 1
51 quillaic acid	32 ± 6	n.d.	n.d.
52 ursolic acid	92 ± 8	92 ± 6	16 ± 5
53 crataegolic acid	99 ± 2	91 ± 7	18 ± 8
55 β-boswellic acid	91 ± 5	85 ± 8	90 ± 8

± SD; n.d., not determined

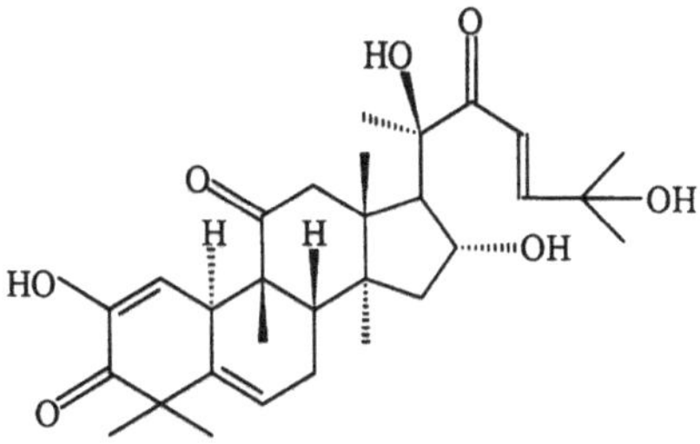

48 cucurbitacin I

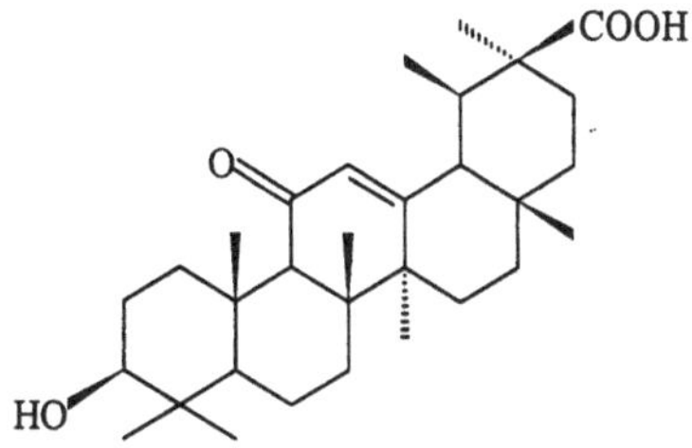

49 glycyrrhetic acid

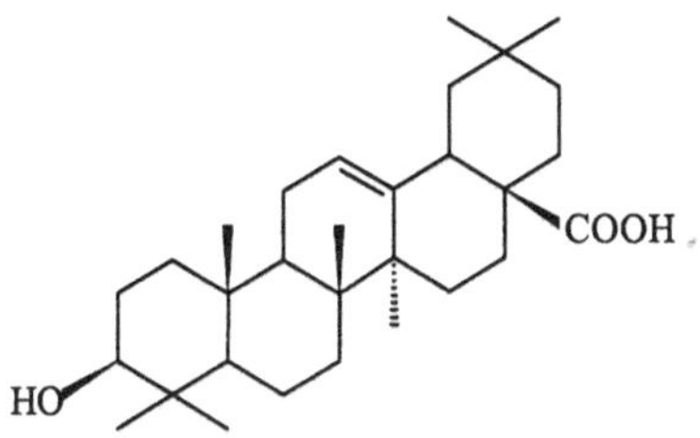

50 oleanolic acid

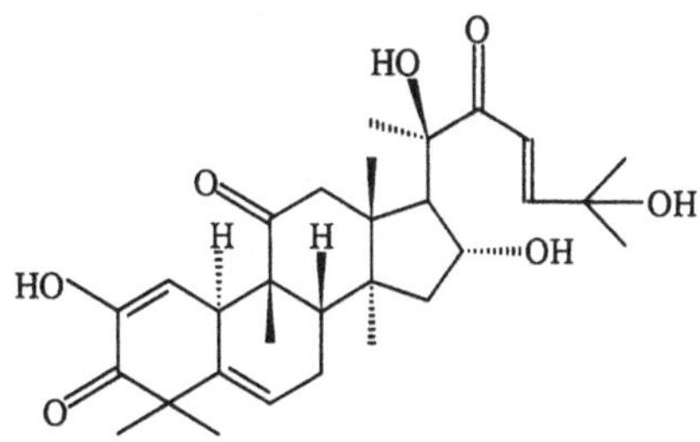

51 quillaic acid

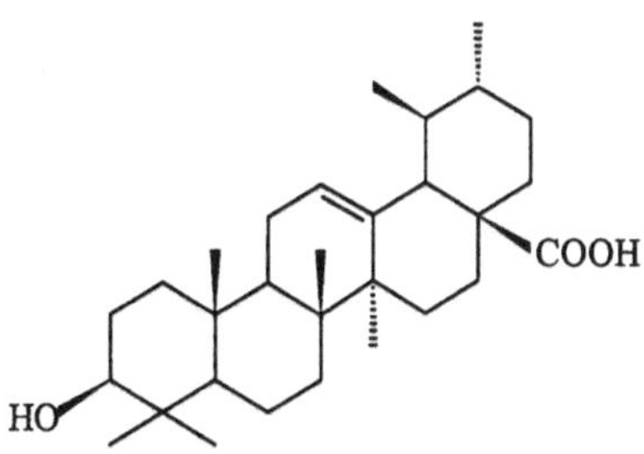

52 ursolic acid

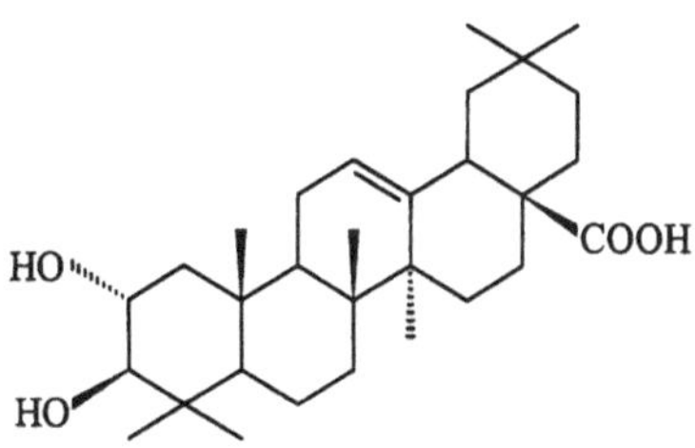

53 crategolic acid

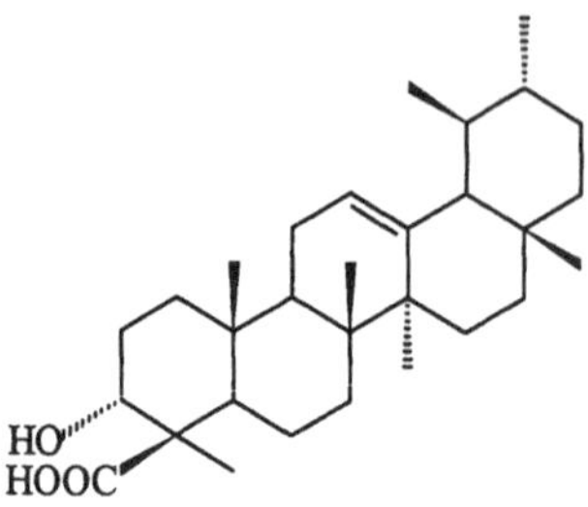

54 β-boswellic acid

some lignoids from the same source (see section "Other phenolic compounds"). Some other iridoids were also active at the same concentration of 1.5 mg/ml, or about 4 μM, e.g. geniposide (**56**), geniposidic acid (**57**), and aucubin (**58**), producing an inhibition of 23.0 ± 8.8%, 14.3 ± 3.0% and 21.7 ± 9.7%, respectively. After enzymatic hydrolysis with a β-glucosidase, however, the inhibition increased up to 87.3 ± 2.3% for geniposidic acid (**57**), and 89.3 ± 0.9% for aucubin (**58**), indicating that the hemiacetal moiety plays an important role in the anticomplementary activity of these iridoids [28].

Another group of iridoids, the valepotriates ocurring in the *Valerianaceae*, exhibited an inhibitory activity on the alternative pathway of the complement system in a dose-dependent manner [35].

Cyclic peptides

In adition to some phenolic compounds with complement-inhibitory activity discussed in previous sections, the latex of *Jathropa multifida* L. (*Euphorbiaceae*) also contained two cyclic peptides with complement activity, labaditin (**59**) (a decapeptide) and biobollein (**60**) (a nonapeptide). These peptides inhibited the classical activation pathway of complement. In mechanistic studies an apparent inactivation of C1 was demonstrated [36]. Curacycline A (**61**), a cyclic octapeptide isolated from the latex of *Jathropa curcas* L. (*Euphorbiaceae*), also displayed an inhibitory activity on the classical pathway, but to a lesser degree than labaditin and biobollein [37].

Alkaloids

Recently a complement-modulatory activity has been reported for a series of alkaloids isolated from *Cryptolepis sanguinolenta* (Lindl.) Schlechter (*Periplocaceae*). The monomeric alkaloids cryptolepine (tested as its hydrochloride) (**62**), quindoline (**63**), and hydroxycryptolepine (**64**) exhibited a dose-dependent inhibitory effect on the classical pathway [38]. The activity (% inhibition) at a concentration of 1 mM

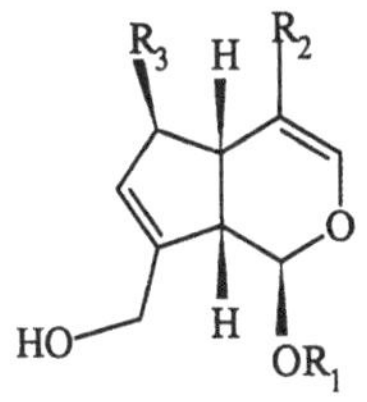

	R_1	R_2	R_3
55 genipin	H	$COOCH_3$	H
56 geniposide	glc	$COOCH_3$	H
57 geniposidic acid	glc	COOH	H
58 aucubin	glc	H	OH

(glc = glucosyl)

is shown in Table 6 for the classical and the alternative pathway. For the alternative pathway only a weak inhibitory or stimulatory effect could be observed.

The dimeric alkaloids biscryptolepine (**65**) and cryptoquindoline (**66**), isolated from the same plant, were more active as inhibitors of the classical pathway: Biscryptolepine showed an IC_{50} of 98 ± 2 µM, and cryptoquindoline an IC_{50} of 38 ± 4 µM. The IC_{50} values on the alternative pathway were 541 ± 4 µM and 726 ± 6 µM, respectively. Cryptoquindoline was more active as an inhibitor of the classical activation pathway of complement than rosmarinic acid (see section "Phenolic acids and derivatives) [39].

Conclusion

This review has been limited, with a few exceptions, to low-molecular weight compounds with complement activity isolated from plants. Naturally occurring complement modulating compounds such as vitamin A, amino acids and derivatives, copper-chlorophyllin, etc., covered in previous reviews, e.g. by Asghar in 1984 [8], have not been included.

It can be concluded from this review that a whole range of low molecular weight compounds exhibits complement-modulating properties. There is little doubt that the use of complement-based assays to guide the isolation of active compounds from plants and plant extracts will add more natural products with a variety of structures to this list.

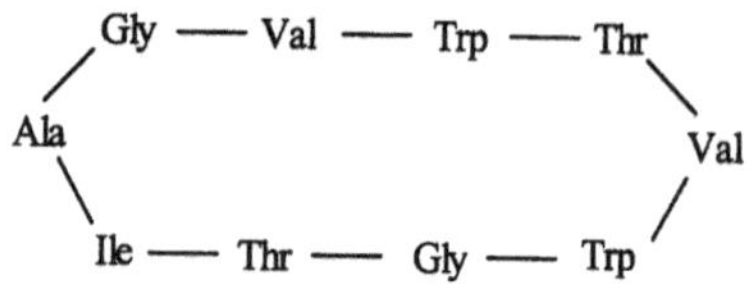

59 labaditin

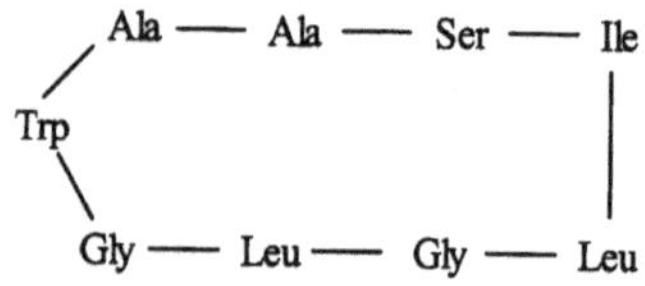

60 biobollein

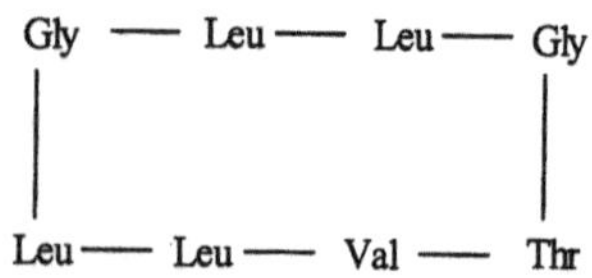

61 curacycline A

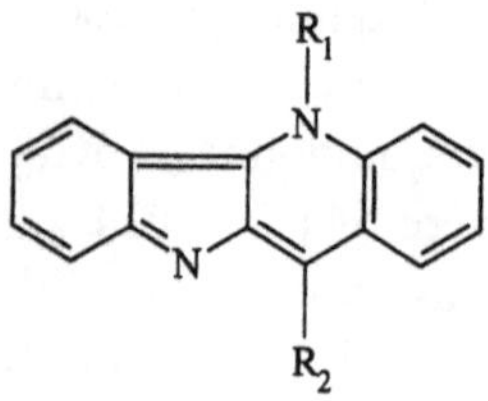

	R_1	R_1
62 cryptolepine	CH_3	H
64 hydroxycryptolepine	CH_3	OH

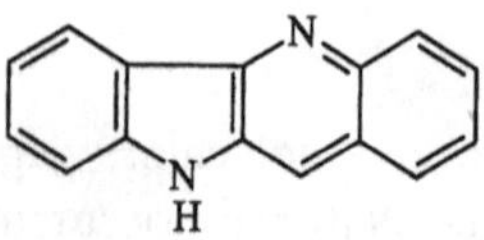

63 quindoline

Acknowledgement

T. De Bruyne is a post-doctoral researcher associated with the Fund for Scientific Research (FWO, Flanders, Belgium).

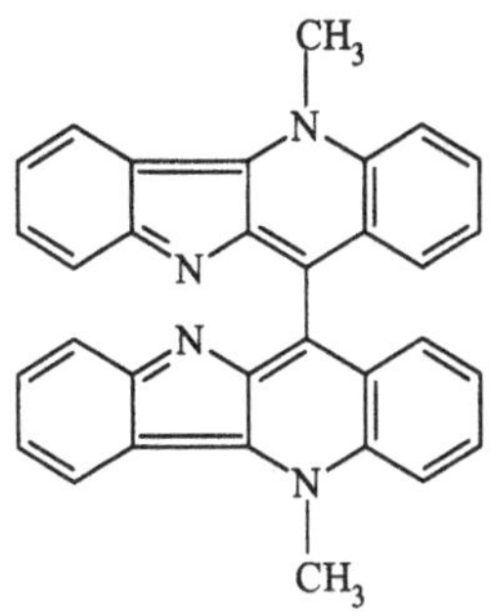

65 biscryptolepine

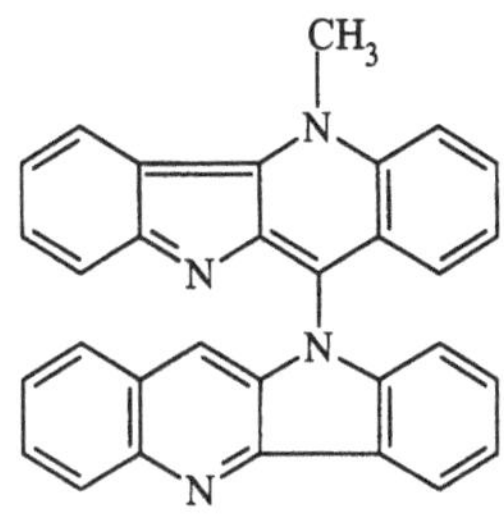

66 cryptoquindoline

*Table 6 - Inhibition of the classical pathway (CP) and the alternative pathway (AP) of the complement system by alkaloids from Cryptolepis sanguinolenta (**62–65**): reduction of haemolysis (%) at a concentration of 1 mM [38].*

	CP	AP
64 cryptolepine (HCl)	57.8 ± 2.7	–27.1 ± 1.2
65 quindoline	41.4 ± 0.9	8.0 ± 0.6
66 hydroxycryptolepine	36.0 ± 1.8	–8.8 ± 1.1

± SD; –, negative sign denotes activation

References

1 Roitt I, Brostoff J, Male D (eds) (1993) *Immunology*. Mosby, London

2 Baumgarten A (1978) Physicochemical and biological features of complement. In: Baumgarten A, Richards FF (eds): *Immunology*. Handbook series in clinical laboratory science, section F. CRC, West Palm Beach (Florida), 89–116

3 Vogt W (1985) Drugs and the complement system. *TIPS* 3: 114–119

4 Stoiber H, Clivio A and Dierich MP (1997) Role of Complement in HIV Infection. *Annu Rev Immunol* 15: 649–674

5 Mayer MM (1971) Complement and complement fixation. In: Kabat EA, Mayer MM (eds): *Experimental immunochemistry*. Thomas, Springfield (Illinois), 133–240

6 Platts-Mills T, Ishizaka K (1974) Activation of the alternate pathway of human complement by rabbit cells. *J Immunol* 113: 348–358

7 Klerx JPAM, Beukelman CJ, Van Dijk H, Willers JMN (1983) Microassay for colorimetric estimation of complement activity in Guinea pig, human and mouse serum. *J Immunol Methods* 63: 215–220

8 Asghar SS (1984) Pharmacological manipulation of complement system. *Pharmacol Rev* 36: 223–244

9 Ellis B, Towers GHN (1970) Biogenesis of rosmarinic acid in *Mentha. Biochem J* 118: 291–297

10 Engleberger W, Hadding U, Etschenberg E, Graf E, Leyck S, Winkelmann J, Parnham MJ (1988) Rosmarinic acid: A new inhibitor of complement C3-convertase with anti-inflammatory activity. *Int J Immunopharmac* 10: 729–737

11 Bult H, Herman AG, Rampart M (1985) Modification of endotoxin-induced haemodynamic and haematological changes in the rabbit by methyl-prednisolone, $F(ab')_2$ fragments and rosmarinic acid. *Br J Pharmacol* 84: 317–327

12 Peake PW, Pussell BA, Martyn P, Timmermans V, Charlesworth JA (1991) The inhibitory effect of rosmarinic acid on complement involves the C5 convertase. *Int J Immunopharmac* 13: 853–857

13 Lasure A, Van Poel B, Pieters L, Claeys M, Gupta M, Vanden Berghe D, Vlietinck A (1994) Complement-inhibiting properties of *Apeiba tibourbou. Planta Med* 60: 276–277

14 Knaus U (1989) *Komplementaktive Verbindungen aus der Grünlippigen Muschel Perna canaliculus (Gmelin) sowie niederen und höheren Pflanzen.* Dissertation, Ludwig-Maximilians-Universität München (Germany)

15 Wagner H, Lacaille-Dubois M-A (1996) Recent pharmacological results on bioflavonoids. In: Antus S, Gábor M, Vetschera K (eds): *Flavonoids and bioflavonoids 1995.* Akadémiai Kiadó, Budapest, 53–72

16 Lasure A, Van Poel B, Cimanga K, Pieters L, Vanden Berghe D, Vlietinck A (1994) Modulation of the complement system by flavonoids. *Pharm Pharmacol Lett* 4: 32–35

17 Cimanga K, De Bruyne T, Lasure A, Li Q, Pieters L, Claeys M, Vanden Berghe D, Kambu K, Tona L, Vlietinck A (1995) Flavonoid O-glycosides from the leaves of *Morinda morindoides. Phytochemistry* 38: 1301–1303

18 Cimanga K, De Bruyne T, Lasure A, Van Poel B, Pieters L, Vanden Berghe D, Vlietinck A (1995) *In vitro* anticomplementary activity of constituents from *Morinda morindoides. J Nat Prod* 58: 372–378

19 Cimanga K, De Bruyne T, Van Poel B, Ma Y, Claeys M., Pieters L, Kambu K, Tona L, Bakana P, Vanden Berghe D, Vlietinck A (1997) Complement-modulating properties of a kaempferol 7-O-rhamnosylsophoroside from the leaves of *Morinda morindoides. Planta Med* 63: 220–223

20 De Bruyne T (1995) *Two-dimensional NMR investigation and biological evaluation of dimeric proanthocyanidins and related polyphenols.* Ph.D. Thesis, Univerity of Antwerp (Belgium)

21 De Bruyne T, Cimanga K, Pieters L, Claeys M, Dommisse R, Vlietinck A (1997) Gallocatechin-(4'-O-7)-epigallocatechin, a new biflavonoid isolated from *Bridelia ferruginea. Nat Prod Lett* 11: 47–52

22 Shahat AA, Hammouda F, Ismail SI, Azzam SA, De Bruyne T, Lasure A, Van Poel B, Pieters L, Vlietinck A (1996) Anticomplementary activity of *Crataegus sinaica. Planta Med* 62: 10–13

23 Kosasi S, 't Hart LA, van Dijk H, Labadie RP (1989) Inhibitory activity of *Jathropa multifida* latex on classical complement pathway activity in human serum mediated by a calcium-binding proanthocyanidin. *J Ethnopharmacol* 27: 81–80

24 Labadie RP, van der Nat JM, Simons JM, Kroes BH, Kosasi S, van den Berg AJJ, 't Hart LA, van der Sluis WG, Abeysekara A, Bamunuarachchi A, De Silva KTD (1989) An ethnopharmacological approach to the search for immunomodulators of plant origin. *Planta Med* 55: 339–348

25 Ivanovska N, Yossifova T, Vassileva E, Kostova I (1994) Effect of some hydroxycoumarins on complement-mediated hemolysis in serum. *Meth Find Exp Clin Pharmacol* 16: 557–562

26 Giclas PC (1982) Effect of plicatic acid on human serum complement includes interference with C1 inhibitor function. *J Immunol* 129: 168–172

27 Oshima Y, Takata S, Hikino H, Deyama T, Kinoshita G (1988) Anticomplementary activity of the constituents of *Eucommia ulmoides* bark. *J Ethnopharmacol* 23: 159–194

28 Glovsky MM, Becker EL, Halbrook NJ (1968) Inhibition of Guinea-pig complement by maleopimaric acid and other derivatives of levopimaric acid. *J Immunol* 100: 979–990

29 Glovsky MM, Ward PA, Becker EL, Halbrook JN (1969) Role of fumaropimaric acid in Guinea-pig complement dependent and non-complement dependent biologic reactions. I. Inhibition of Frossman, reversed passive Arthus, and PCA reactions by fumaropimaric acid. *J Immunol* 102: 1–14

30 Fujii S, Aoyama T (1984) Complement inhibitors. *Drugs of the Future* 9: 849–856

31 Yagi A, Tokubuchi N, Nohara T, Nonaka G, Nishioka I, Koda A (1980) The constituents of Cinnamoni cortex. I. Structures of cinncassiol A and its glucoside. *Chem Pharm Bull* 28: 1432–1436

32 Yamada H, Yoshino M, Matsumoto T, Nagai T, Kiyohara H, Cyong J-C, Nakagawa A, Tanaka H, Omura S (1987) Effects of phytosterols on anticomplementary activity. *Chem Pharm Bull* 35: 4851–4855

33 Knaus U, Wagner H (1996) Effects of boswellic acid of Boswellia serrata and other triterpenic acids on the complement system. *Phytomedicine* 3: 77–81

34 Kapil A, Moza N (1992) Anticomplementary activity of boswellic acids–an inhibitor of C3-convertase of the classical complement pathway. *Int J Immunopharmac* 14: 1139–1143

35 Van Meer JH (1984) Plantaardige stoffen met een effect op het immuunsysteem. *Pharm Weekblad* 119: 836–842

36 Labadie RP (1993) Immunomodulatory compounds. In: Colegate SM, Molyneux RJ (eds): *Bioactive natural products.* CRC Press, Boca Raton, 279–317

37 Van den Berg AJJ, Horsten SFAJ, Kettenes-van den Bosch JJ, Kroes BH, Beukelman CJ, Leeflang BR, Labadie RP (1995) Curcacycline A–a novel cyclic octapeptide isolated from the latex of *Jathropa curcas* L. *FEBS Letters* 358: 215–218

38 Cimanga K, De Bruyne T, Lasure A, Van Poel B, Pieters L, Claeys M, Vanden Berghe D, Kambu K, Tona L, Vlietinck A (1996) *In vitro* biological activities of alkaloids from *Cryptolepis sanguinolenta*. *Planta Med* 62: 22–27

39 Cimanga K, De Bruyne T, Van Poel B, Pieters L, Claeys M, Vanden Berghe D, Vlietinck A (1997) Dimeric alkaloids from *Cryptolepis sanguinolenta* as potent inhibitors of complement pathway activation. *Pharm Pharmacol Lett* 7: 179–180

Complement-activating polysaccharides from medicinal herbs

Haruki Yamada and Hiroaki Kiyohara

Oriental Medicine Research Center, The Kitasato Institute, Minato-ku, Tokyo 108-8642, Japan

Introduction

The complement system consists of over 20 serum proteins including nine complement components (C1 to C9) and their regulators, and is normally present in blood serum in an inactive form. The system is essential for the operation of the innate as well as the adaptive immune defence [1]. The complement proteins can be activated through three cascade pathways: by the classical pathway, by the alternative pathway and by the antibody-independent lectin pathway (Fig. 1). The activation of the classical pathway is initiated by immune complexes containing IgM and IgG antibodies, C1 binds to the Fc region of antibodies through subcomponent C1q, then the complex activates the further complement system by the cascade mechanism. The alternative pathway is directly activated from C3 by microorganisms, protozoa, or some activators such as lipopolysaccharide through an antibody independent mechanism. Recently, an antibody-independent mannan-binding lectin (MBL) pathway has also been established as the third activation pathway of complement systems [2, 3]. This pathway is initiated by the binding of serum MBL (carbohydrate binding component in complement-dependent antibacterial factor, RaRF [4]), which is structurally related to C1q, to the surface carbohydrates and activated through two MBL-associated serine proteases. The MBL pathway is activated by specific carbohydrate structures of microorganisms including bacteria, yeast, parasitic protozoa and viruses, and exhibits antibacterial activity through killing mediated by the terminal, lytic complement components or by promoting phagocytosis [3]. These three pathways activate further common steps (C5–C9) and finally cause cell damage by formation of the terminal complex C5b6789. In general, the alternative and MBL pathways contribute to the early natural defence mechanism of the non-immune host before production of the antibody.

When normal human serum is incubated with some complement regulators, and the remaining complement titer is measured by hemolysis of sensitized sheep ery-

Immunomodulatory Agents from Plants, edited by H. Wagner

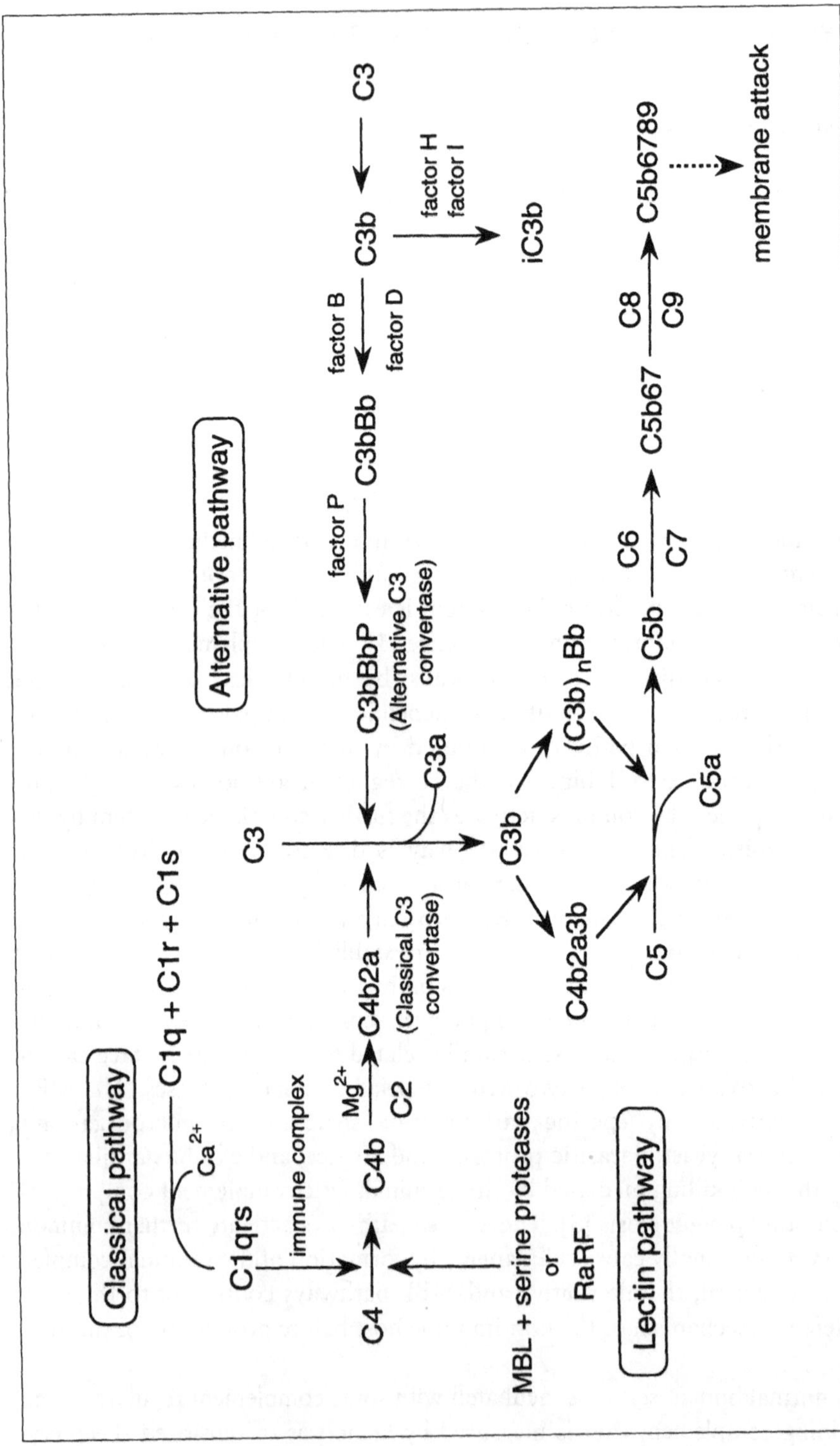

Figure 1
Activation step of the complement system

throcytes as an antigen-antibody complex, the regulating substances for the hemolytic activity of complement are referred to as "anti-complementary substances". Complement activators result in the decrease of hemolysis due to the reduced complement titer by the activation of the complement system, whereas complement inhibitors result in the inhibition of hemolysis due to the inhibition of a certain step in the complement system by the coexistence of the inhibitors in the assay system. Therefore the "anti-complementary activity" seen in the hemolytic assay includes both activation and inhibition of the complement system.

The subsequent proteolytic cleavage of the complement components by the activation of the pathways leads to generation of biologically active complement fragments (mainly the anaphylatoxins C3a and C5a). These released peptide mediators exert many biological activities such as the increment of local vascular permeability, the chemotactic attraction of leukocytes, immune adherence and modulation of antibody production. Therefore, complement activation contributes to inflammatory responses in addition to immunological defence reactions. Activation of complement may become adverse and harmful depending on the site, extent, and duration of complement activation [1]. Enhanced inflammation and resultant tissue damage are the features of various autoimmune and "immune complex diseases" associated with uncontrolled excessive complement consumption [5]. The complement-mediated diseases include systemic lupus erythematosus, certain forms of nephritis and rheumatoid arthritis. Therefore, inhibition of complement activation in inflammation would be a good therapeutic strategy for treating these diseases.

With the activation of the complement system, several kinds of complement fragments, including C3a and C5a, are also formed through the subsequent proteolytic cleavage [1]. These complement fragments are further degraded to generate other fragments (iC3b, C3d, C3g, C3dg etc.) by the actions of complement regulators before and after binding to complement receptors on macrophages and T and B

Table 1 - Immunomodulation associated with activation of the complement system

1	Thymus-dependent antibody response
2	Regulation of specific cyclical antibody production
3	Regulation of IgM-IgG switch
4	Modulation of T and B cell proliferation
5	Induction of supressor or helper T cells
6	Modulation of monokine or lymphokine release

lymphocytes. These primary and secondary complement fragments are also known to activate or supress the functions of macrophages, and T and B cells [1]. Therefore complement activation appears to be intrinsically associated with several immune reactions such as the activation of macrophages and lymphocytes, cellular-co-operation, immunopotentiation and regulation of cyclical antibody production [1, 6], and causes several immunomodulation effects including an anti-inflammatory effect (Tab. 1).

The complement system is also assumed to contribute to the prevention of development of tumors. Host-mediated anti-tumor β-(1→3)-glucans have been indicated to activate the alternative pathway [7]. One such anti-tumor glucan, lentinan, results in the generation of the corresponding complement fragments (C3b, C5a and factor Ba) by the activation of the alternative complement pathway [8]. It has been postulated that the production of these complement fragments leads to activation of macrophages through enhancement of the incorporation of C3b-lentinan complex to macrophages. Hence the anti-tumor effect of lentinan has been suggested to be potentiated by the activation of the complement system.

Several anti-complementary polysaccharides have already been isolated from bacteria, fungi and plants. Examples include LPS [9], a microbial water-insoluble glucan synthesized enzymatically by *Streptococcus mutans* OMZ 176 [10], lentinan, a water-insoluble β-glucan from *Lentinas edodes* (Berk.) sing. [7] and pachyman from *Poria cocos* [7], inulin [11], and a water soluble β-glucan from sugar cane [12]. Inulin is a β-(2→1) fructan, lentinan is a β-(1→3) glucan which has some β-(1→6) glucosidic side chains, and pachyman is a β-(1→3) glucan which has traces of β-(1→6) glucosidic linkages. The streptococcal α-glucan is an α-(1→3) glucan which has some α-(1→6) glucosidic side chains, and are all reported to be insoluble activators of the alternative complement pathway [7]. Zymosan, a yeast cell wall preparation, is also a well-known insoluble activator of the alternative complement pathway [13]. Zymosan is mainly composed of β-(1→3)-glucan and mannan. However, because it also contains a significant amount of lipid and protein, it is not clear whether the polysaccharide moiety is an active principle.

LPS activates complement via the alternative and classical pathways [9]. LPS is composed of lipid A, a core polysaccharide, and O-specific sugar chains. The lipid A portion activates the classical pathway, and the polysaccharide moiety activates the alternative pathway [14]. The lipid A region of LPS can interact directly with complement via an antibody-independent mechanism in which C1 is bound to lipid A [15]. Some anti-complementary polysaccharides also show an anti-inflammatory activity [16].

Several complement activating (anti-complementary) polysaccharides have also been isolated from the hot-water extract of several medicinal herbs (Tab. 2) [16–54], and results have been accumulated during the last ten years. The present review article deals with complement-activating polysaccharides from medicinal herbs.

Table 2 - Anti-complementary and related polysaccharides from medicinal herbs

	Type	MW Da	Biological activity	Plant source	Year	Ref.
polysaccharide I	xyloglucan	35,000	· production of IL-1 and LAF · granulocyte, macrophage stimulating activity	*Echinacea purpurea*, upper part	1984	[87]
polysaccharide II	pectic polysaccharide (rhamnogalacturonan with arabino-3,6-galactan and arabinan)	450,000	· production of IL-1 and LAF · granulocyte, macrophage stimulating activity	*Echinacea purpurea*, upper part	1984	[87]
AGIIa	arabino-β-3,6-galactan		· complement activating activity	*Angelica acutiloba* Kitagawa, roots	1985	[17]
Zizyphus-arabinan	α-2,5-arabinofuranan		· anti-complementary activity	*Zizyphus jujuva*, fruits	1985	[18]
paniculatan	glucuronogalacturono-rhamnan		· anti-complementary activity	*Hydrangea paniculata*, inner barks	1985	[18]
AAFIIb-2	pectin (with arabino-3,6-galactan)	139,000	· anti-complementary activity	*Artemisia princeps* PAMP, leaves	1985-1986	[19–21]
AAFIIb-3	pectin (with arabino-3,6-galactan)	31,000	· anti-complementary activity	*Artemisia princeps* PAMP, leaves	1985-1987	[19–21]
plantago-mucilage A	glucuronoarabinoxylan		· anti-complementary activity	*Plantago asiatica*, seeds	1985	[18, 66]
CS-glucan	amylopectin	> 100,000	· anti-complementary activity	*Coix lacryma-jobi* var. Ma-yuen, seeds	1986	[22]
LR-polysaccharide	acidic heteroglycan	> 500,000	· anti-complementary activity	*Lithospermum euchromum* Royle, roots	1986	[23]
AGIIb-1	pectic arabinogalactan	128,000	· complement activating activity	*Angelica acutiloba* Kitagawa,roots	1986-1989	[24–27]
CA-1	arabinoxylo 3,6-galactan	160,000	· anti-complementary activity	*Coix lacryma-jobi* var. Ma-yuen, seeds	1987	[28]

Table 2 (continued)

	Type	MW Da	Biological activity	Plant source	Year	Ref.
CA-2	arabinoxylo 3,6-galactan	70,000	· anti-complementary activity	*Coix lacryma-jobi* var. Ma-yuen, seeds	1987	[28]
	fucogalactoglucan	25,000	· enhancement of phagocytosis of granulocytes and macrophages	*Echinacea purpurea* plant cell culture	1988	[85, 86]
	acidic arabinogalactan	75,000	· activation of macrophages to cytotoxicity against tumor cells and microorganisms · induction of TNFα, IL-1 interferon-β_2 and oxygen radicals	*Echinacea purpurea* plant cell culture	1988	[85, 86]
RCA-N	arabino-β-3,6-galactan	180,000	· complement activating activity	*Viscum album* L., berries	1988	[29]
RCA-G	arabino-β-3,6-galactan	900,000	· complement activating activity	*Viscum album* L., berries	1988	[29]
BR-5-I	α-3,5-arabinofuranan α-(1→4)glucan complex	18,500	· anti-complementary activity	*Bupleurum falcatum* L., roots	1988	[30]
GL-PI	rhamnogalacturonan with β-galactan	50,000	· anti-complementary activity	*Panax ginseng* C.A. Meyer, leaves	1988 1990	[31] [32]
GL-PII	rhamnogalacturonan with β-galactan	24,000	· anti-complementary activity	*Panax ginseng* C.A. Meyer, leaves	1988 1990	[31] [32]
GL-PIV	rhamnogalacturonan with arabinogalactan	6,000	· anti-complementary activity	*Panax ginseng* C.A. Meyer, leaves	1988 1990	[31] [32]
AR-2IIa	pectin	42,000	· anti-complementary activity	*Angelica acutiloba* Kitagawa, roots	1988–1989	[33, 34]
AR-2IIb	pectin	95,000	· anti-complementary activity	*Angelica acutiloba* Kitagawa, roots	1988–1989	[33, 34]
AR-2IIc	pectin	245,000	· anti-complementary activity	*Angelica acutiloba* Kitagawa, roots	1988–1989	[33, 34]

AR-2IId	pectin	216,000	· anti-complementary activity	*Angelica acutiloba* Kitagawa, roots	1988–1989	[33, 34]
MSL-M	rhamnogalacturonan (with 4-linked galactan)	6,000,000	· anti-complementary activity	*Malva sylvestris* var. *mauritiana*, leaves	1989	[35]
BR-2IIb (bupleuran 2IIb)	pectin (with galactan and arabinogalactan)	36,000	· anti-complementary activity · Fc receptor up-regulation activity	*Bupleurum falcatum* L.,	1989	[36, 92, 93]
CAP-1-IIIa	acidic arabinogalactan	70,000	· anti-complementary activity	*Capsicum anmuem* L., fruits	1989	[37]
CAP-1-IVa	acidic arabinogalactan	195,000	· anti-complementary activity	*Capsicum anmuem* L., fruits	1989	[37]
CAP-1-Va	acidic arabinogalactan	140,000	· anti-complementary activity	*Capsicum anmuem* L., fruits	1989	[37]
PS-III	arabino-β-3,6-galactan	35,000	· phagocytosis enhancing activity	*Calendula officinalis* L., flowers	1989	[89]
Hibiscus mucilage SF	rhamnogalacturonan (with GlcA, 4-linked galacto-oligosaccharide)		· anti-complementary activity	*Hibiscus syriacus* L., flowers	1989	[38]
Hibiscus mucilage ML	rhamnogalacturonan (with GlcA, 4-linked galacto-oligosaccharide)		· anti-complementary activity	*Hibiscus moscheutos* L., leaves	1989	[38]
Hibiscus mucilage SL	rhamnogalacturonan (with GlcA, Gal)		· anti-complementary activity	*Hibiscus syriacus* L., leaves	1989	[38]
Okra-mucilage R	rhamnogalacturonan (with GlcA, 4-linked galacto-oligosaccharide)		· anti-complementary activity	*Abelmoschus esculentus* L., roots	1989	[38]
Hibiscus mucilage MO	rhamnogalacturonan (with GlcA)		· anti-complementary activity	*Hibiscus moscheutos* L., roots	1989	[38]
MVS-I	β-(1→3)glucan with -arabino-β-3,6-galactan	77,000	· anti-complementary activity · hypoglycemic activity	*Malva verticillata*, seeds	1990	[39]
MVS-IIa	arabino-β-3,6-galactan	57,000	· anti-complementary activity	*Malva verticillata*, seeds	1990	[39]
AR-4E-2	pectic arabinogalactan		· anti-tumor activity	*Angelica acutiloba* Kitagawa, roots	1990	[90]
MVS-VI	acidic arabino-β-3,6-galactan	260,000	· anti-complementary activity	*Malva verticillata* L., seeds	1990	[40]

Table 2 (continued)

	Type	MW Da	Biological activity	Plant source	Year	Ref.
MSL-P	rhamnogalacturonan with 4-linked galactan	11,000	· anti-complementary activity	*Malva sylvestris* var. *mauritiana*, leaves	1990	[41]
GL-NIa	arabinogalactan	12,000	· anti-complementary activity	*Panax ginseng* C.A. Meyer, leaves	1991	[42]
GL-NIb	arabinogalactan	5,000	· anti-complementary activity	*Panax ginseng* C.A. Meyer, leaves	1991	[42]
GL-AIa	pectic arabinogalactan	66,000	· anti-complementary activity	Panax ginseng C.A. Meyer, leaves	1991	[42]
GL-AIb	pectic arabinogalactan	5,500	· anti-complementary activity	Panax ginseng C.A. Meyer, leaves	1991	[42]
GR-2IIa	pectic polysaccharides	190,000 –95,000	· anti-complementary activity	*Glycyrrhiza uralensis* Fisch. et DC., roots	1991	[43]
GR-2IIb	pectic polysaccharides	190,000 –160,000	· anti-complementary activity	*Glycyrrhiza uralensis* Fisch. et DC., roots	1991	[43]
GR-2IIc	pectic polysaccharides with β-3,6-galactan	338,000 -160,000	· anti-complementary activity · mitogenic activity	*Glycyrrhiza uralensis* Fisch. et DC., roots	1991	[43,44]
bupleuran 2IIc	pectin	63,000	· anti-complementary activity · anti-ulcer activity · Fc receptor up-regulation activity	*Bupleurum falcatum* L., roots	1991	[45, 71, 95, 98]
A I	arabino-β-3,6-galactan	95,000 ~100,000	· anti-complementary activity · TNF release activity from macrophage	*Arnica montana*, cell culture	1991	[46]
A II	fucogalactoxyloglucan	22,500	· enhancement of carbon clearance	Arnica montana, cell culture	1991	[46]
DWA-2	chondroitin sulfate A and C hybrid.	64,000	· anti-complementary activity	*Cervus nippon* Temminck, pilose antler	1992	[47]
ukonan A	rhamnogalacturonan (with arabino-β-3,6-galactan)		· phagocytosis enhancing activity · anti-complementary activity · B cell mitogenic acitivity	*Curcuma longa* L., rhizomes	1992	[48]

AS-3	pectin	7,600	· anti-complementary activity	*Achyrocline satureioides*, dried aerial parts	1992	[16]
AS-4	pectin	15,000	· anti-complementary activity · anti-inflammatory activity · phagocytosis enhancing activity	*Achyrocline satureioides*, dried aerial parts	1992	[16]
LR-2IId-1a	4-linked GlcA	140,000	· anti-complementary activity	*Lithospermum euchromum*, roots	1993	[49]
LR-2IId-1b	3-linked galactose	92,000	· anti-complementary activity	*Lithospermum euchromum*, roots		
LR-2IId-3a	3-linked fucose	140,000	· anti-complementary activity	*Lithospermum euchromum*, roots		
LR-2IId-5a	4-linked glucose 3-linked mannose	125,000	· anti-complementary activity	*Lithospermum euchromum*, roots		
1A-I	α-3,5-arabinan with β-3,6-galactan and β-3-linked glucose	56,000	· anti-complementary activity	*Artemisia princeps* PAMP, leaves	1994	[50]
1B-I	α-3,5-arabinan with β-6-linked-galactose	56,000 160,000	· anti-complementary activity · anti-complementary activity	*Artemisia princeps* PAMP, leaves	1994	[50]
1C-I	β-(1→4)-glucane with 4-linked mannose	7,000	· anti-complementary activity	*Artemisia princeps* PAMP, leaves	1994	[50]
PR-2	amylopectin	50,000	· enhancement of lymphocyte proliferation · anti-complementary activity	*Urtica dioica*, roots	1994	[51]
PR-3	pectin (rhamnogalacturonan with arabinogalactan)	210,000	· enhancement of lymphocyte proliferation	*Urtica dioica*, roots	1994	[51]
PR-4	pectin (rhamnogalacturonan with arabinogalactan)	18,000	· enhancement of lymphocyte proliferation	*Urtica dioica*, roots	1994	[51]
crude polysaccharide containing PR-2, 3 and 4			· anti-inflammatory activity	*Urtica dioica*, roots	1994	[51]
PMI_{50}	arabino-3,6-galactan	> 130,000	· anti-complementary activity · enhancement of TNFα production from human monocyte	*Plantago major* L., leaves	1995	[52]

Table 2 (continued)

	Type	MW Da	Biological activity	Plant source	Year	Ref.
$PMII_{50}$	pectin	> 520,000	· anti-complementary activity	*Plantago major* L., leaves	1995	[52]
PMII	pectin (with arabino-3,6-galactan)	46,000 ~48,000	· anti-complementary activity	*Plantago major* L., leaves	1996	[53]
DAP-4I-1a	galactoglucan	> 338,000	· anti-complementary activity	*Dipsacus asperoides*, roots	1997	[54]
DAP-4I-1b	galactoglucan (4-linked Gal, 3-linked Glc 6-linked Glc, 4-linked Glc)	137,000	· anti-complementary activity	*Dipsacus asperoides*, roots	1997	[54]
DAP-4I-IIa-1	3,6-galactan with 3-linked Glc	91,000	· anti-complementary activity	*Dipsacus asperoides*, roots	1997	[54]

Classification of anti-complementary polysaccharides from medicinal herbs

Arabinogalactan

Anti-complementary polysaccharide, AGIIa, has been isolated from the hot water extract from the roots of *Angelica acutiloba* as the first complement-activating arabinogalactan in medicinal herbs [17]. AGIIa was a minor constituent and yet possessed the most potent activity among the polysaccharides of an *A. acutiloba* extract. AGIIa was characterized to be arabino β-3,6-galactan by structural analysis, and suggested to contain mainly of a 6-linked galactan backbone with 5-linked α-L-arabinofuranosyl residues and 3-linked galactopyranosyl residues attached at position three of the galactan backbone. AGIIa activates complement via both the alternative and classical pathways. Several other anti-complementary arabino-β-3,6-galactans were also isolated from berries of *Viscum album* (Fig. 2) [29], seeds of *Malva verticillata* [39, 40], leaves of *Panax ginseng* [42], cell culture of *Arnica montana* (Fig. 2) [46], and leaves of *Plantago major* [52].

Glycoproteins containing arabinose and galactose are characteristically associated with cell wall fractions of both higher and lower plants, while the polysaccharides and proteoglycans containing arabinose and galactose are widely distributed in plant tissues and are major components of gum exudates [55]. However, not all extracts of Chinese herbs have anti-complementary activity [56]. The arabinogalactans can be grouped into three major structure types [55]; the arabino-4-galactans are classified as type I by Aspinall, the arabino-3,6-galactans as type II, and polysaccharides with arabinogalactan side chains as another type. Most of the anti-complementary arabinogalactans in medicinal herbs are characterized as type II arabinogalactans. However, type II arabinogalactan from larch wood was found to have no anti-complementary activity.

Some other anti-complementary acidic pectic arabinogalactans including rhamnogalacturonan core and arabinan have also been isolated from medicinal herbs such as the roots of *Angelica acutiloba* (AGIIb-1) [24–27], berries of *Viscum album* (Fig. 2) [29], and the roots of *Urtica dioica* [51]. Their arabinogalactan parts were also characterized as arabino-β-3,6-galactan.

AGIIb-1 was a complex pectic arabinogalactan consisting of four carbohydrate units; one neutral (N-1) and two acidic (A-I and A-II) arabinogalactans and one neutral arabinan (N-II), which are linked to each other by acid-labile linkages (Fig. 3) [26, 27]. A-I and A-II consist of rhamnogalacturonan cores in which 2-linked and/or 2,4-disubstituted rhamnosyl residues alternate with 4-linked galacturonic acid in the sequences, and at least three kinds of high-molecular weight arabinogalactan side chains probably attach to the core. N-I is a high molecular weight neutral arabinogalactan consisting of a β-(1→3) linked galactan backbone with a β-(1→6) linked galactosyl side chain at position six and some arabinofuranosyl side chains attached

A

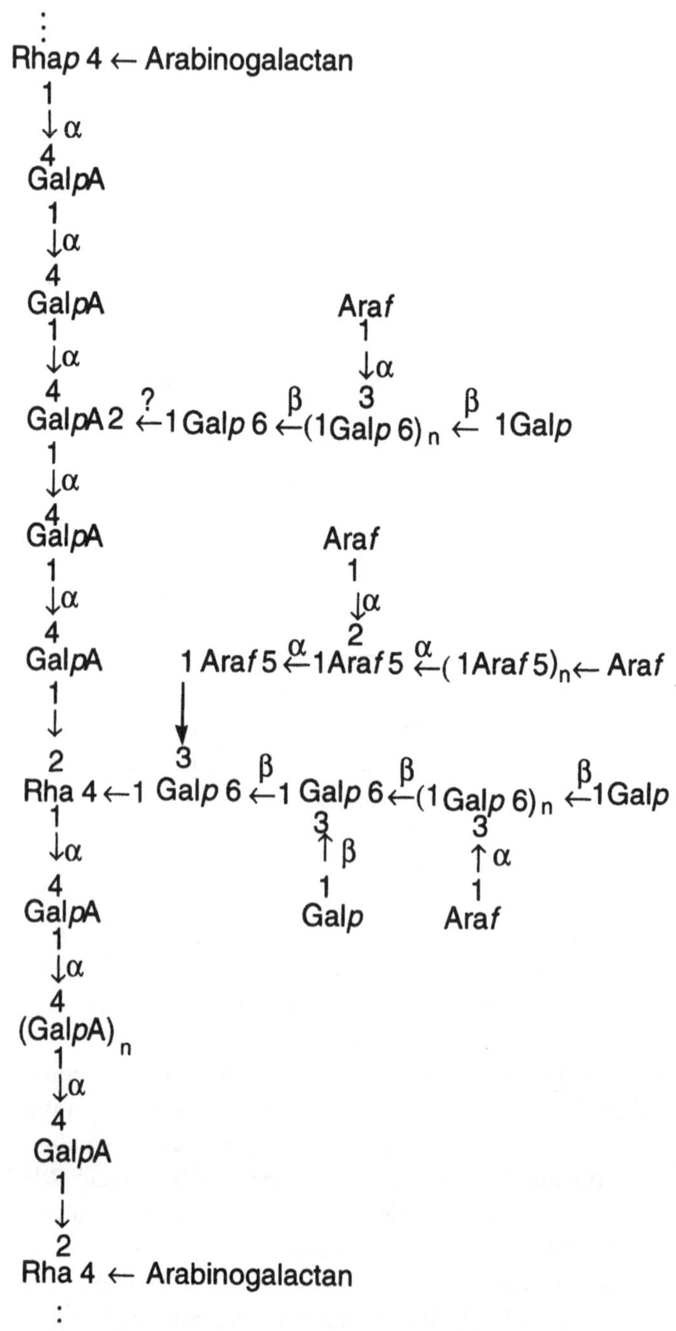
Rhap 4 ← Arabinogalactan
GalpA
GalpA
Araf
GalpA 2 ←1 Galp 6 ←(1Galp 6)n ← 1Galp
GalpA
Araf
GalpA
1 Araf 5 ←1Araf 5 ←(1Araf 5)n← Araf
Rha 4 ←1 Galp 6 ←1 Galp 6←(1 Galp 6)n ←1Galp
GalpA
Galp
Araf
(GalpA)n
GalpA
Rha 4 ← Arabinogalactan

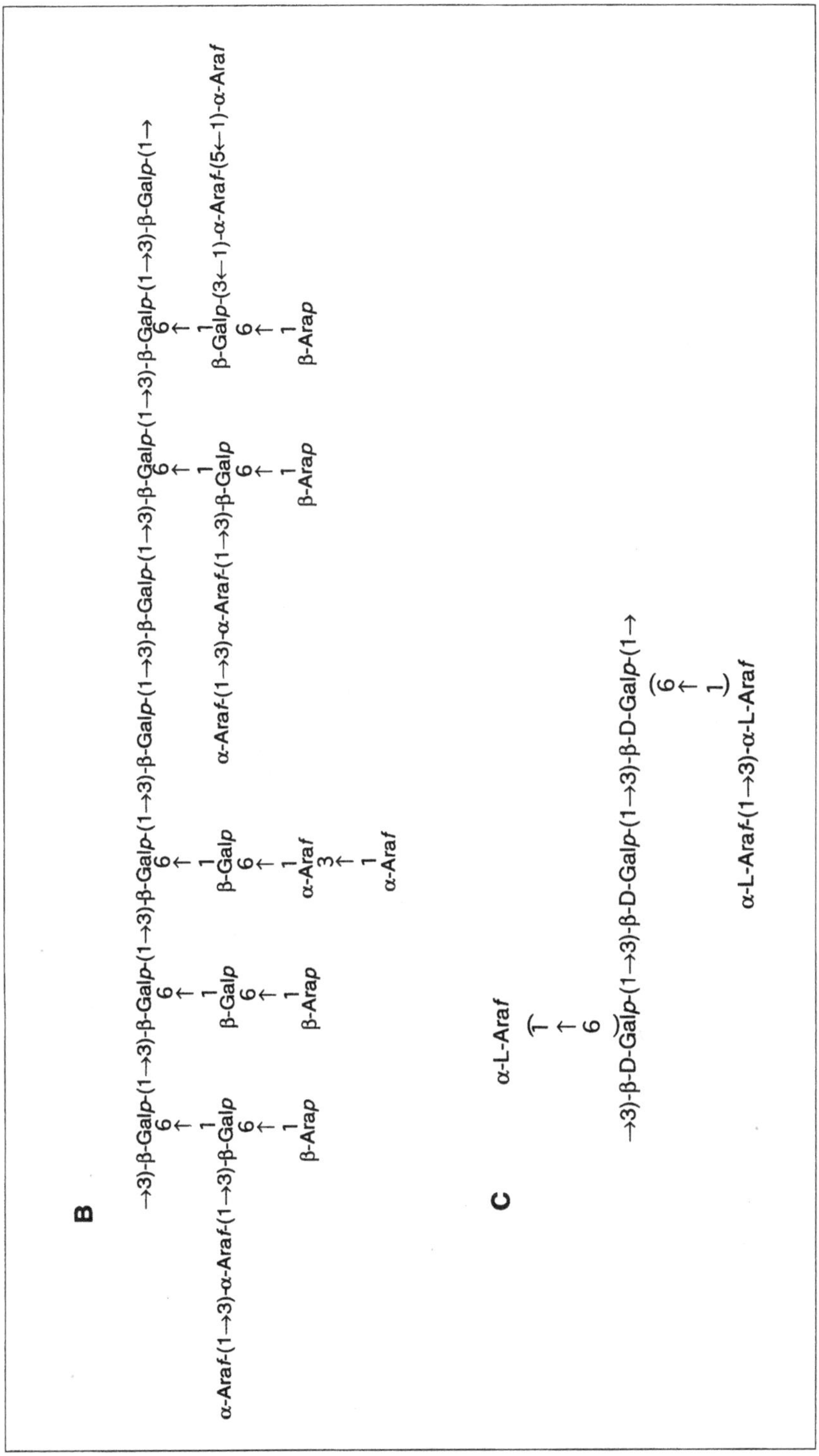

Figure 2
Structures of anti-complementary polysaccharides from Viscum album *[RCA-N and RCA-G (A)] and from* Arnica montana *[A-I (B)] and related polysaccharide from* Calendula officinalis *[PS-III (C)].*

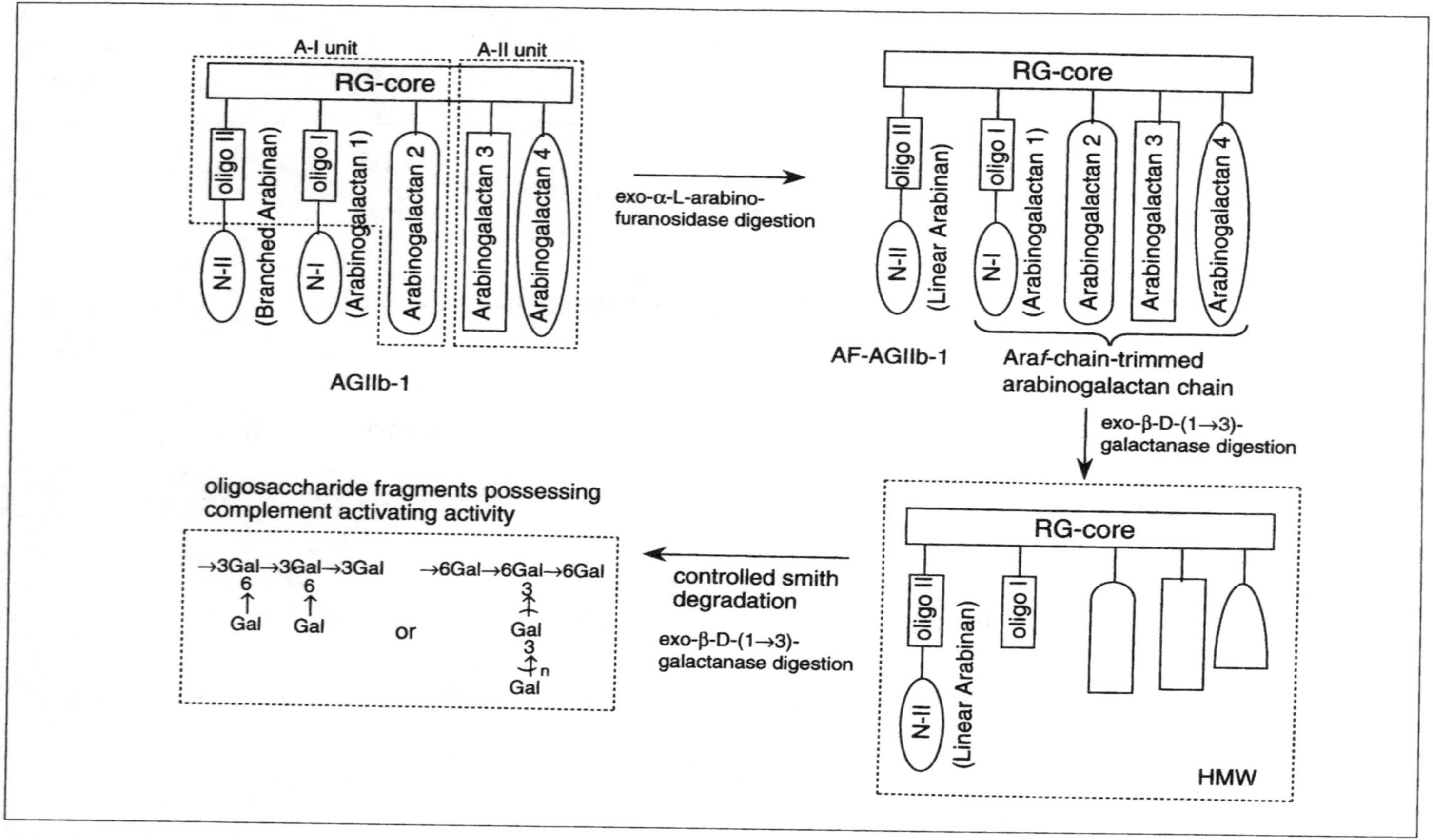

Figure 3
Sequential degradation of AGIIb-1 from roots of Angelica acutiloba *by using enzymic and chemical treatments.*

to position three of the galactosyl side chains. N-II is a highly branched α-L-(1→5)-linked arabinan possessing some arabinofuranosyl side chains at position three. N-I is probably attached to galactosyl chains (oligo I) in A-I through galactosyl residues and N-II to arabinosyl chains (oligo II) in A-I through arabinosyl residues. The structure of AGIIb-1 resembles certain pectins, but it contains either a lesser galacturonan moiety than pectins or no galacturonan moiety at all.

Certain pectins had anti-complementary activity, in which potently active polysaccharides also contained a β-3,6-galactan moiety as neutral sugar side chains [19, 20, 53]. Several heteroglycans having potent anti-complementary activity also contained a (1→3,6)-galactan moiety [28, 39, 42, 44, 50, 54]. Therefore, these facts indicate that (1→3,6)-β-galactan is one of the typical units in the complement-activating polysaccharides from medicinal herbs. Since α-L-arabinofuranosidase digestion enhanced or did not change the anti-complementary activity of arabino-β-3,6-galactan-rich polysaccharides, the β-3,6-galactan part might be essential for the expression of the activity [25, 33, 36, 57].

The β-glucosyl-Yariv antigen (1,3,5-tri-(4-β-D-glucopyranosyloxyphenylazo)-2,4,6-trihydroxybenzene; Fig. 4) is known to react with (1→3,6)-β-galactan to form a red dye. The mechanism of the reaction between the antigen and (1→3,6)-β-galactan is not completely understood [55]. However, the reaction has been extremely useful and (1→3,6)-β-galactan can be quantified by single radial gel diffusion with the β-glucosyl-Yariv antigen [58]. This dye binding assay is also very useful for the analysis of anti-complementary arabino-β-3,6-galactan in the medicinal herbs, and was first applied to the detection of the (1→3,6)-β-galactan moiety in the anti-complementary pectins and pectic arabinogalactan from the roots of *A. acutiloba* [57, 59] and the leaves of *P. ginseng* [42].

Pectin

Anti-complementary pectins have been isolated from several medicinal herbs such as the leaves of *Artemisia princeps* [19], the roots of *Angelica acutiloba* [33, 34], the roots of *Bupleurum falcatum* [36, 45], the leaves of *Panax ginseng* [31, 32], the roots of *Glycyrrhiza uralensis* [44], the dried aerial parts of *Achyrocline satureioides* [16] and the leaves of *Plantago major* [53]. Pectins are generally known to be comprised of a large quantity of an α-(1→4)-linked galacturonan region, and a small "ramified" region which consists of rhamnogalacturonan core substituted with side chains rich in neutral sugars such as arabinogalactan, arabinan, galacto-oligosaccharides and arabino-oligosaccharides [60]. Pharmacologically active pectins also contain a rhamnogalacturonan II (RG-II)-like region containing rarely observed component sugars such as 3-deoxy-D-*manno*-2-octulosonic acid (KDO), 3-deoxy-D-*lyxo*-2-heptulosaric acid (DHA), 2-methylfucose, 2-methylxylose, apiose, and aceric acid [61,62].

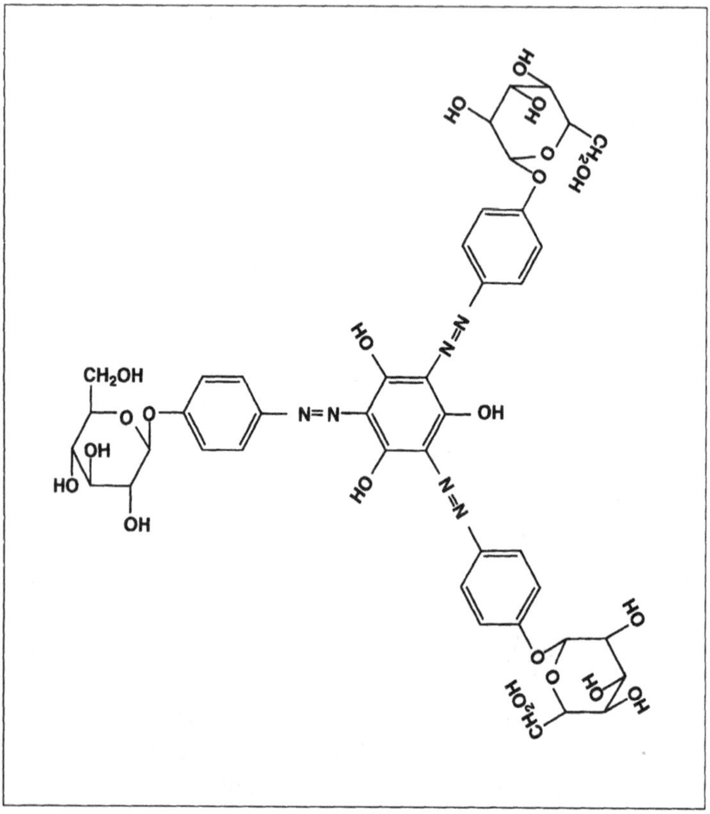

Figure 4
Structure of β-D-glucosyl-Yariv antigen.

Anti-complementary pectins, AR-2IIa, 2IIb, 2IIc and 2IId, which were isolated from *A. acutiloba*, were composed of over 90% of the galacturonan region with a small amount of the "ramified" region [33]. The "ramified" region contained the rhamnogalacturonan core possessing side chains rich in neutral carbohydrate chains which were directly attached to position four of rhamnose [34, 57]. A part of the neutral carbohydrate chains was also suggested to attach to the rhamnose through 4-linked galacturonic acid [34, 57]. Digestion of each pectin with endo-α-(1→4) polygalacturonase after de-esterification gave the "ramified" region (PG-1a, PG-1b, PG-1c and PG-1d from AR-2IIa, 2IIb, 2IIc, and 2IId, respectively) and several α-(1→4) linked oligogalacturonides [33]. The "ramified" region from each pectin had a more potent complement-activating activity than the corresponding original pectins, but the oligogalacturonides had weak or negligible activities. These facts suggest that the complement-activating potency of these pectins are expressed mainly by their "ramified" regions [33]. The results which were observed in complement activating pectins and pectic polysaccharides from roots of *B. falcatum* [36], *A. acutiloba* [27] and *G. uralensis* [44], seeds of *C. lacryma-jobi* [28], leaves of *A. princeps* [20] and *P. ginseng* [31] also supported the theory that their structural units of "ramified" regions are responsible for expression of the activity. Lithium-mediated degradation of the "ramified" regions from the four pectins of *A. acutiloba* gave several neutral oligosaccharides originating from the side chains which were attached to the rhamnogalacturonan core [34, 57]. Since this oligosaccharide mixture had a reduced activity [57], and the pectin from *Zizyphus jujuba*, which brings different side chains from that of *A. acutiloba*, did not show the activity [18], it has been suggested that the potent complement activation by the "ramified" region may be due to a combination of the rhamnogalacturonan core and the neutral sugar chains [57]. Of these neutral carbohydrate chains, a high molecular weight fraction and the oligosaccharides, which appeared in the same elution volume with glucopentaose, showed potent activity. Exo-β-galactosidase-treated "ramified" regions of the active pectins contained β-(1→6) linked galactosyl di- to tetra-saccharides which were suggested to attach to position four of the 2,4-disubstituted rhamnosyl residue in the rhamnogalacturonan cores either directly or through 4-linked galacturonic acid [34, 57]. The "ramified" region of AR-2IIa also contained a large proportion of (1→3,6)-linked, long β-galacto-oligosaccharide chains, whereas the regions of AR-2IIb, -2IIc and -2IId contained only a trace or very few of such a moiety (Fig. 5) [34]. These results indicated that the original "ramified" regions have more long galactosyl side chains and β-3,6-galactan chains. Of these neutral oligosaccharides eliminated by β-elimination, the (1→3,6)-linked long β-galactosyl chain showed potent activity, but the mixture of β-(1→6)-linked galacto-oligosaccharides, having rhamnosyl or galactosyl residues as a reducing terminals, also showed significant activity (Fig. 6) [57]. Therefore the neutral carbohydrate chains containing β-(1→6)-linked galactose attached to the rhamnogalacturonan core might be the minimum essential structure in the active pectins for the expression of complement activating activity. No all pectins have anti-complementary activity although structures of pectins are highly heterogenous, therefore only limited neutral sugar side chains might be responsible for the expression of the activity in the "ramified" region.

Arabinan

Some anti-complementary arabinans such as *Zizyphus arabinan* (α-2,5-arabinofuranan) and BR-5-I (α-3,5-arabinofuranan-α-(1→4)-glucan complex) have been isolated from the fruits of *Zizyphus jujuva* and from the roots of *B. falcatum*, respectively [18, 30]. The α-3,5-arabinofuranan unit (N-II), which was released from AGIIb-1, also showed moderate anti-complementary activity [26].

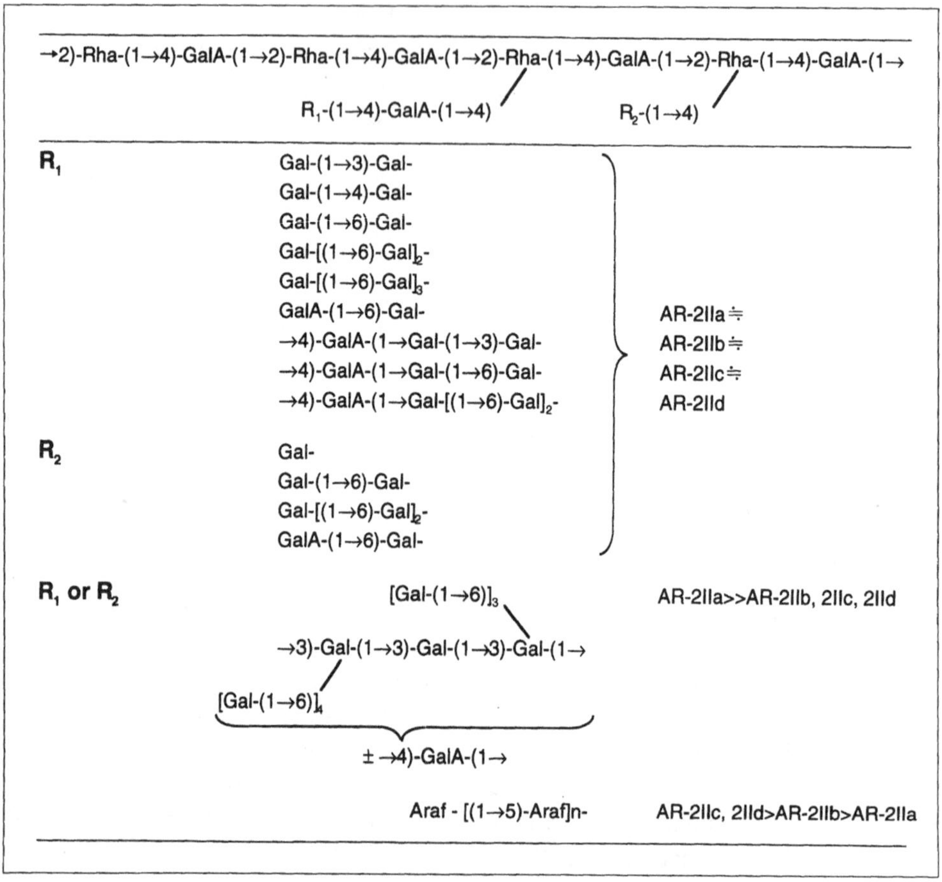

Figure 5
Structure of enzyme-treated "ramified" region of complement activating pectins from Angelica acutiloba.
Modes of substitutions [R_1 and R_2] of the neutral side chains to the rhamnogalacturonan core were suggested from the results of base-catalyzed β-elimination [57].

Other heteroglycans

Some other acidic heteroglycans also showed potent anti-complementary activity. Such active polysaccharides included paniculatan (highly branched, partially O-acetylated, acidic mucous polysaccharide composed of (1→2)-linked-α-L-rhamnose having branches of 4-O-Me-D-GlcA-(1→4)-β-D-Gal at position four and of (1→4)-linked-α-D-GalA and β-D-GlcA at position three) which was isolated from the inner bark of *Hydrangea paniculata* [18, 63], and plantago-mucilage A (highly branched,

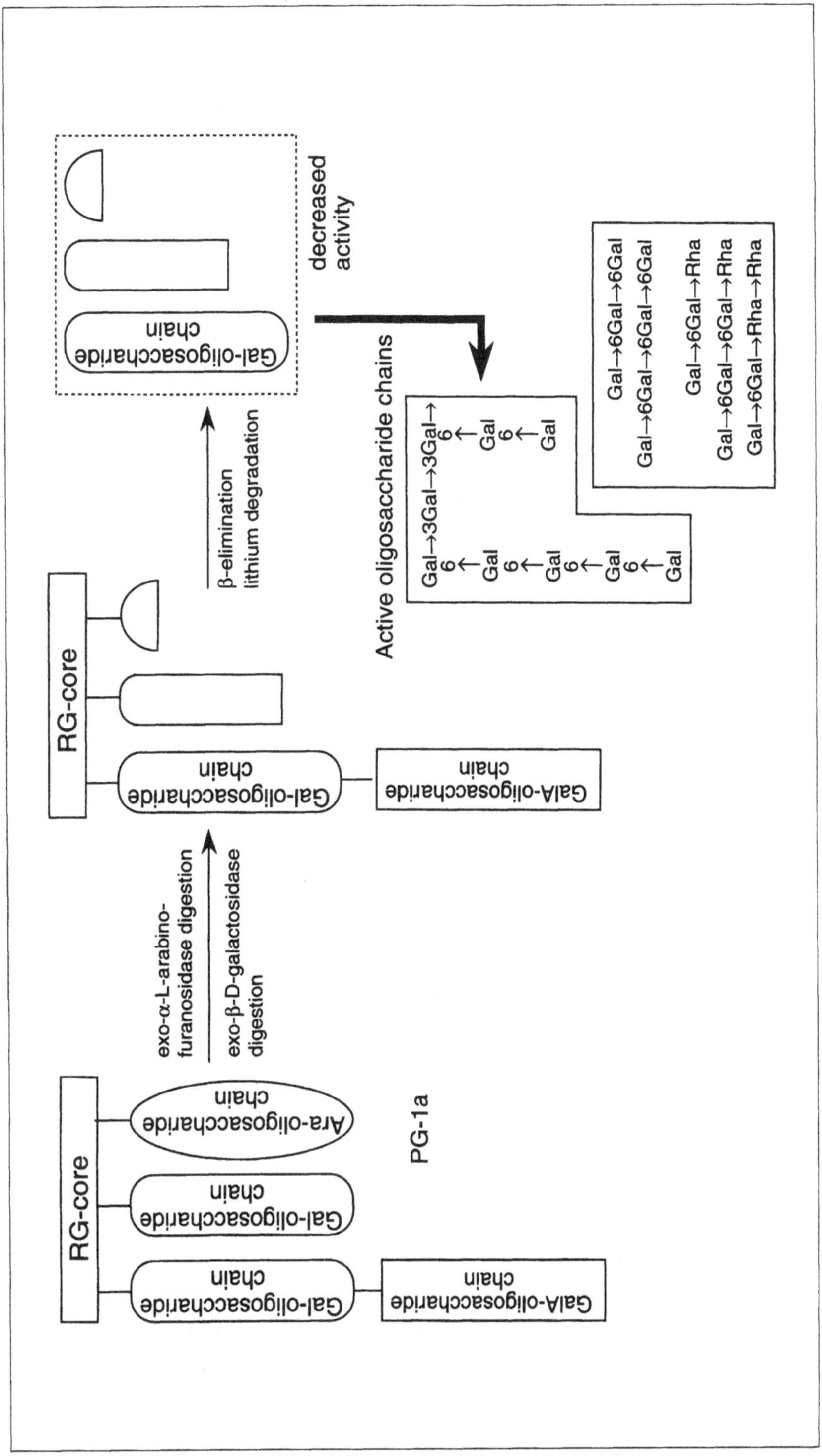

Figure 6
Sequential degradation of the "ramified" region (PG-1a) of AR-2IIa from roots of Angelica acutiloba by using enzymic and chemical treatments.

partially O-acetylated, acidic mucous polysaccharide with a main chain of (1→4)-β-D-xylan having branches consisting of other β-D-Xyl and α-D-Glc-(1→3)-α-L-Araf at position three) from the seed of *Plantago asiatica* [18, 64]. However, glucomannans from the several plant species did not show any significant anti-complementary activity [18]. Extremely potent anti-complementary polysaccharides (LR-2IId-1a, -1b, -3a and 5a) were isolated from the roots of *Lithospermum euchromum* [49]. These polysaccharides were highly heterogenous and mainly composed of 4-linked glucose, in addition to 3-linked galactose, 3-linked fucose, 4-linked glucuronic acid and 3-linked mannose. Another anti-complementary heteroglycan, DAP-4I-1b, from the roots of *Dipsacus asperoides*, also contained 4-linked glucose in addition to 3-linked glucose and 6-linked glucose [54].

Mode of action

The mode of anti-complementary activities has been studied for pectic polysaccharides from *A. acutiloba* (AGIIa, AGIIb-1, AR-2IIa, AR-2IIb, AR-2IIc and AR-2IId) [17, 33, 59], *A. princeps* (AAF-IIb-2 and IIb-3) [65] and *Z. jujuba* (*Zyziphus* arabinan), glucuronoarabinoxylan (Plantago-mucilage A) from *P. asiatica*, acidic polysaccharide (paniculatan) from *H. paniculata* [18, 66], inulin from Dahlias [11], and sulfated fucans from brown seaweed [67].

Modes of actions for the anti-complementary activities of water soluble pectic polysaccharides have been estimated by measurements of anti-complementary activity in the presence or absence of Ca^{2+} ion, which is required for the activation of the classical complement pathway, the hemolytic activity of the alternative complement pathway using rabbit erythrocytes, functional assay of C4 (C4 titration), and crossed immunoelectrophoresis using anti-C3 antibody [5, 17, 23, 33, 59, 65]. All the active pectic polysaccharides activate both the classical and alternative complement pathways. Other acidic polysaccharides such as Plantago-mucilage A and paniculatan also activate both pathways [18,66]. Six-branched β-D-(1→3)glucans such as lentinan from *Lentinas edodes* and inulin are reported to be insoluble activators of the alternative pathway [7,11]. Inulin activates late-acting complement components (C3-C9) but not the early-acting component (C2) [11]. β-D-(1→3)-glucan also activates C3 but not C1 [7].

In the alternative pathway, the initial complement component C3 is activated to C3b on the target surface, combined with factor B (C3bB), and is then converted into the catalytically active C3 convertase (C3bBbP) through the activation with factors D and P (Fig. 1). C3bBbP can activate other C3 molecule to C3b, resulting in the activation of the alternative pathway. The alternative pathway also contains other regulatory components, factors H and I as inhibitory components, and C3b is converted to inactive C3 convertase (iC3b) by the actions of the inhibitory components in the absence of the activating substances (Fig. 1). C3b is attached to complement-activating polysaccharides such as inulin and dextran in the alternative pathway through transesterification of the thioester of C3b with hydroxy groups on the polysaccharides [68]. The resulting C3b-polysaccharide conjugates (C3b-CHO) decrease its affinity for factor H in comparison with C3b, and inactivation rate of C3b-CHO is slower in the presence of factor H and I than in that of C3b (Fig. 7) [69].

The initial complement component, C1 of the classical pathway is activated by immune complexes, and catalyzes the assembly of classical C3 convertase (C4b2a) (Fig. 1). This raises the question as to how the active polysaccharides can activate complement through the classical pathway. The effect of the serum component on the active pectic polysaccharides (AAF-IIb-2 and IIb-3) from *A. priceps* has been studied [65]. When asialofetuin-conjugated-Sepharose-passed serum was used for the assay, no change in the anti-complementary activity of the polysaccharides was observed. However, when protein A-coupled-Sepharose-passed serum was used for the same assay, the anti-complementary activity decreased significantly, and the activity was restored to the original level by the addition of the protein A-Sepharose-bound fraction (Fig. 8). When protein A-Sepharose passed serum was absorbed with anti-human IgG antibody, no more reduction of the activity was observed. The presence of natural antibody of IgM and IgG classes, which can recognize the complement activating pectic polysaccharides from *A. acutiloba*, *B. falcatum*, *G. uralensis*, and *A. princeps* has been detected in normal human serum by enzyme-linked immunosorbent assay (ELISA), however, inactive polysaccharide could not be reacted with these antibodies (H. Kiyohara and H. Yamada, unpublished data). When the presence of the polysaccharide-recognizing antibody was tested for in the sera from eight healthy adults, all sera were found to contain the antibodies of IgM and IgG classes (H. Kiyohara and H. Yamada, unpublished data). These results indicate that natural antibody-dependent mechanisms are likely to be involved in activation of the classical complement pathway by the active pectic polysaccharides (Fig. 7).

Some of the complement activating activity of AAF-IIb2 and IIb-3 still remained even when protein A-Sepharose-passed serum was used for the assay (Fig. 7) [65]. Therefore it is suggested that other mechanisms may also be involved in expression of the complement activating activity of pectic polysaccharides in addition to the classical and alternative pathways. The MBL lectin pathway also has a possibility to be involved in activation of complement by the active pectic polysaccharides (Fig. 1), however, further studies are required.

Sulfated fucan from brown seaweed shows anti-complementary activity by inhibition of the complement system [67]. The polysaccharide has been found to inhibit C4 cleavage which results in the formation of the classical C3 convertase (C4b2a), and to inhibit formation and function of alternative C3 convertase (C3bBb) by interfering with the binding of factor B to C3b and accelerating the decay of factor P-stabilized sites on the alternative C3 convertase (Fig. 7) [67].

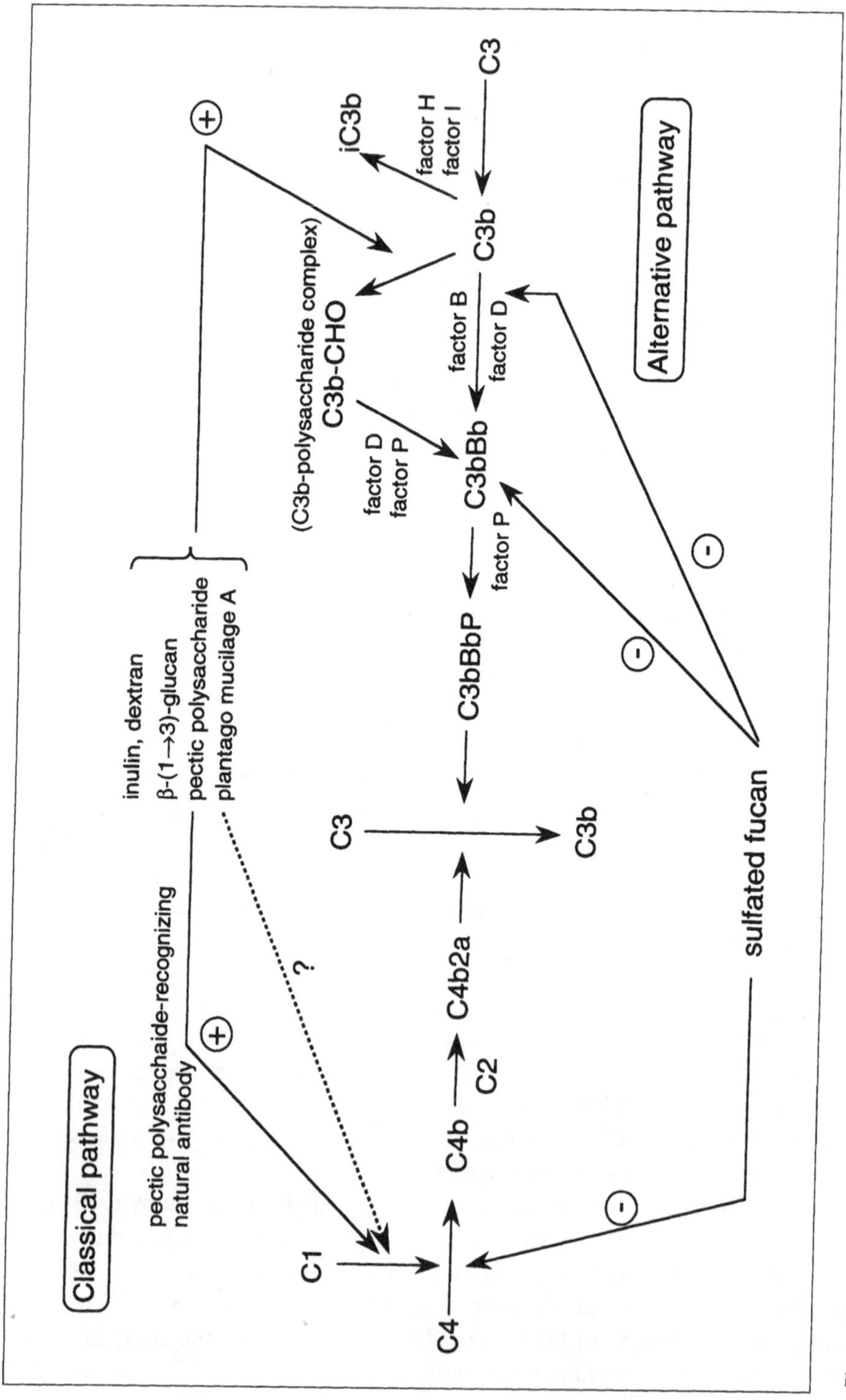

Figure 7
Modes of action of anti-complementary polysaccharides.

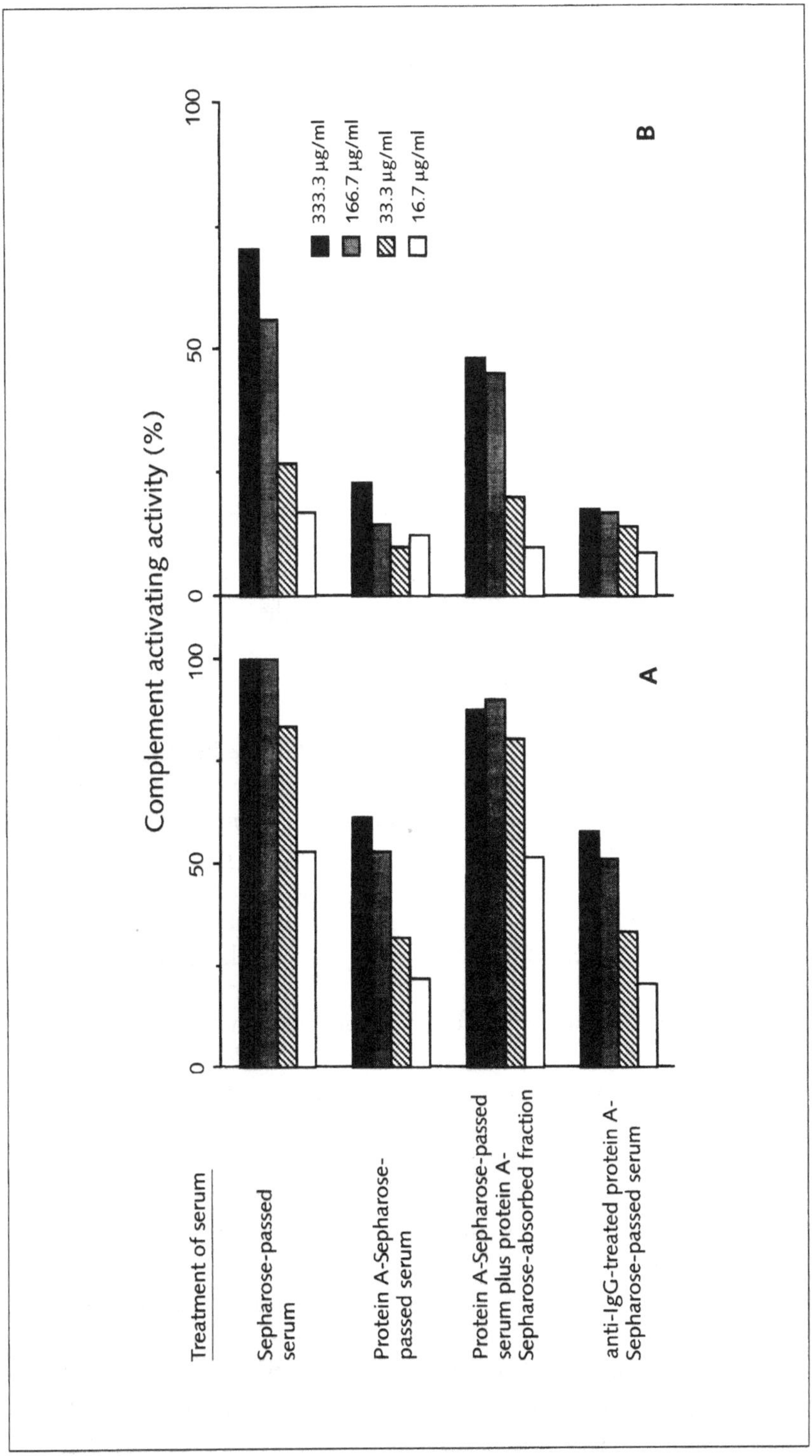

Figure 8
Effects of Protein A-Sepharose and anti-IgG treatments of the serum on anti-complementary activity of AAF-IIb-2 (A) or AAF-IIb-3 (B) from Artemisia princeps.

Structure-activity relationship

The "ramified" regions of complement activating pectins (AR-2IIa, IIb, IIc and IId), purified from the roots of *A. acutiloba*, were proposed to be active sites for expression of the complement-activating activity [33]. All the "ramified" regions of AR-2IIa, IIb, IIc and IId activated both alternative and classical pathways of the complement system whereas the original pectins, AR-2IIa, IIb and IIc activated only the classical pathway but AR-2IId activated both pathways. This fact suggests that the galacturonan regions in the pectins regulate the activities of the "ramified" regions through the alternative pathway [33].

Analysis of the distribution of methyl-esters proposed that partially methyl-esterified oligogalacturonide blocks were linked each other through unesterified oligogalacturonide blocks in the galacturonan regions of the active pectins. Comparison of the frequency of methyl-ester suggests that AR-2IIa, IIb, IIc and IId have the structural difference on chain-length of unesterified oligogalacturonide blocks in their galacturonan regions [70]. Methyl-esterfication of the galacturonan region is known to actually affect the formation of the "egg-box" structure on the three-dimensional network of pectins [60]. These postulate that the three-dimensional difference of the galacturonan region modulates the complement activating activities of the "ramified" regions in the pectins through the alternative pathway.

Some pectic polysaccharides have been found to have side chains in the galacturonan region [32,71]. Three pectic polysaccharides (GL-PI, PII and PIV) from leaves of *P. ginseng* showed potent anti-complementary activity but one other polysaccharide form *P. ginseng* (GL-PIII) did not (Tab. 3) [31]. Comparison of structural features in these polysaccharides indicated that the inactive polysaccharide, GL-PIII, possessed a higher proportion of branched galacturonan sequences than the active polysaccharides (Tab. 3) [32]. Therefore it is postulated that the branching frequency in the galacturonan region also affects the anti-complementary activity of pectic polysaccharides.

The carbohydrate chains responsible for the complement-activating activity of AGIIb-1 have been studied by using enzymic and chemical degradations (Fig. 3) [59]. Removal of arabinofuranosyl side chains from branched arabinan and arabinogalactan chains in AGIIb-1 increased the potency of its complement-activating activity through alternative complement pathway, suggesting that arabinofuranosyl side chains inhibit the activity of AGIIb-1 through the alternative pathway [25, 72]. When arabinofuranosidase-digested AGIIb-1 was digested with exo-β-D-(1→3)-galactanase, which is able to cleave the β-(1→3)-galactan backbone with or without side chains by exo-fashion [73], outer chains of arabinogalactan side chains were hydrolyzed and gave remarkable amounts of galactosyl oligosaccharide chains [72]. However, rhamnogalacturonan core possessing side chains (HMW), which were resistant to the galactanase digestion, still showed almost the same complement activating activity as AGIIb-1, suggesting that the activity of AF-AGIIb-1 is expressed

Table 3 - Structural feature and complement-activating activity of polysaccharides (GL-PI, PII, PIII and PIV) isolated from leaves of P. ginseng

Proposed structure	$\left[2)\text{-Rha-}(1\rightarrow 4)\text{-GalA-}(1\right]_m$ (4 ↓ SC)	$\left[2)\text{-Rha-}(1\rightarrow 4)\text{-GalA-}(1\right]_n$	$\left[4)\text{-GalA-}(1\right]_x$	$\left[4)\text{-GalA-}(1\right]_y$ (2 or 3 ↓ SC)
	Ratio of structural sequence			
	GL-PI	GL-PII	GL-PIII	GL-PIV
m	1.0	1.0	1.0	1 0
n	4.2	2.6	3.3	0.6
x	1.3	0	34	39
y	0.7	0.3	4.7	1.4
Degree of complement-activating activity	+++	+++	+	+++

SC: side chains consisting of β-D-galactan (GL-PI and PII) or arabinogalactan (GL-PIII and PIV)

by carbohydrate chains present in the inner portion of the polysaccharide but not by the chains present in the outer portion of AGIIb-1. Studies using controlled Smith degradation and exo-β-D-(1→3)-galactanase digestion indicated that the carbohydrate chains of the inner portion of AGIIb-1 consisted of weak but notable complement-activating galactosyl oligosaccharide chains, and that the active chains mainly comprised of terminal, 3- and 3,6-linked galactosyl residues (Fig. 3). These results suggest that the β-(1→3)-galactan chain possessing the sequences of the active galactosyl chains in the inner portion contributes to expression of the activity of AGIIb-1 (Fig. 3) [72].

Because many anti-complementary pectic polysaccharides consists of arabino-3,6-galactan chains, it is postulated that these carbohydrate chains are also responsible for expression of the activity in the active polysaccharides [17, 20, 25, 26, 28]. However, typical arabino-3,6-galactan from Larch wood and β-(1→3)-galactan did not show the anti-complementary activity [17] (H. Kiyohara and H. Yamada, unpublished data), therefore a certain particular structure may be necessary for expression of the activity. Complement-activating and typical arabino-3,6-galactan (N-I unit) has been released from the active pectic arabinogalactan (AGIIb-1) of *A. acutiloba* by mild acid hydrolysis [26]. When arabinofuranosidase-digested N-I unit (AF-N-I unit) was digested with exo-β-D-(1→3)-galactanase, the complement-activating activity of the AF-N-I unit slightly decreased, and the digested products still had the activity [74]. Gel filtration of the products gave long (GN-1A amd GN-1B), intermediate-size and shorter oligosaccharide chains which were derived from side chains in the AF-N-I unit, and GN-1A, GN-1B and intermediate-sized oligosaccharides had marked complement-activating activity. These active side chains consisted mainly of a 6-linked galactosyl residue. These results suggest that the side chains composed mainly of 6-linked galactosyl residues in the N-I unit are responsible for expression of the complement activating activity of the N-I unit, and that the attachment of the active side chains to the β-D-(1→3)-galactan backbone is necessary to express the potent activity [74].

A pectin (GR-2IIc) from *G. uralensis* showed not only complement activating activity but also mitogenic activity against spleen B lymphocytes [44, 75, 76]. The "ramified" region of GR-2IIc also acted as an active site for expression of both activities [44]. Degradation of the rhamnogalacturonan core of the "ramified" region significantly reduced the activities. However, acidic tetrasaccharide possessing a similar partial structure as rhamnogalacturonan core did not show the activities. Some neutral oligosaccharide-alditols derived from the "ramified" region by lithium-degradation expressed potent complement-activating activity, and all of the fractions containing the oligosaccharide-alditols also had weak but statistically active mitogenic activity (Fig. 9) [75, 76]. Commercially available glucosyloligosaccharides and glucosyloligosaccharide-alditols had no complement activating and mitogenic activities, suggesting that certain neutral oligosaccharide side chains in the "ramified" region of GR-2IIc are responsible for expression of both activities [75,76]. Although the potencies of complement-activating activity and mitogenic activity of the oligosaccharide-alditols were not correlated (Fig. 9), it is not known whether different oligosaccharides are involved in the expressions of both activities of the "ramified" region in GR-2IIc. It has been reported that heparin showed anti-complementary activity due to inhibition of the alternative complement pathway in addition to anti-coagulant activity [77, 78], and that the pentasaccharide unit in heparin is required as the minimum carbohydrate sequence for its affinity to anti-thrombin III. Maillet et al. have found that the minimally critical oligosaccharide structure, which is required for anti-thrombin III binding, is different from that required for anti-complementary activity [79].

Yamada et al. [66] have studied the structure-activity relationship of Plantago-mucilage A from seeds of *Plantago asiatica*. Deacetylation of Plantago-mucilage A enhanced the activation of complement through only the classical pathway whereas its polyalcohol, which was derived from the polysaccharide by periodate oxidation followed by reduction, enhanced the activation of complement through only the alternative pathway. Therefore these observations suggest that O-acetyl groups on the polysaccharide prevent the activation of the classical pathway, and that polyhydroxyl groups are important for the activation of complement through the alternative pathway. Carboxyl-reduction of uronic acids in the polysaccharide significantly reduced the activation of complement through only the classical pathway, therefore it is proposed that carboxyl groups of uronic acids are also essential for the activation of complement through the classical pathway.

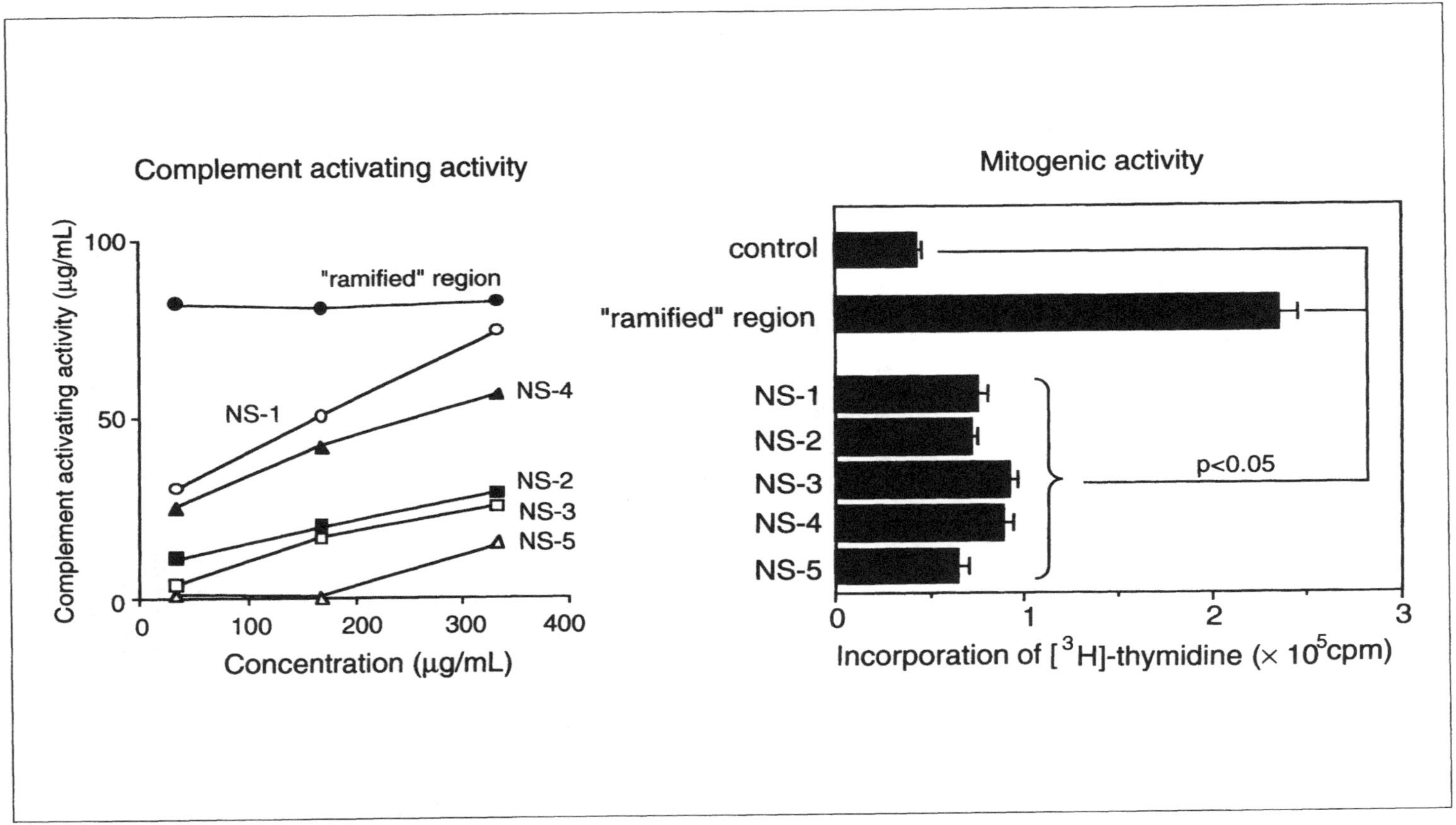

Figure 9
Comparison of complement activating and mitogenic activities of neutral oligosaccharide side chains derived from the "ramified" region of the active pectin (GR-2IIc) in roots of Glycyrrhiza uralensis.

The complement-activating pectic arabinogalactan (AGIIb-1) from *A. acutiloba* has been found to form self-aggregates by analysis of its elution behavior on gel filtration in various concentrations of salt solution [24]. AGIIb-1 was eluted as the aggregate having the highest molecular weight on gel filtration in water. The aggregate was dissociated with an increasing concentration of sodium chloride, and AGIIb-1 gave the lowest molecular weight in 0.2 M sodium chloride solution. AGIIb-1 showed the most potent complement-activating activity when AGIIb-1 was dissolved in water in the assay. However, the activity was reduced with increasing of sodium chloride concentration, and AGIIb-1 did not have the activity in 0.2 M sodium chloride solution although the solvent control had no effect on the activity. These results propose that self-aggregation of AGIIb-1 is involved in the expression of the complement-activating activity.

Particulate inulin from Dahlias activates the alternative complement pathway [80]. Inulin is known to have various forms termed "the polymorphic solubility forms" of its particle (alpha, beta and gamma form) [81]. Gamma inulin potently activated complement through the alternative pathway whereas alpha and beta inulins showed weak activity [80]. Solubilization of inulin completely decreased the activity, but the particle size of the inulin molecule in each solubility form had no effect on the complement activating activity. However, among the three solubility forms, gamma inulin had the highest molecular weight. These results suggest that the particulate formation of polysaccharides is also involved in the expression of the complement-activating activity through the alternative pathway [80].

From the studies on structure-activity relationship, typical structures and structural requirements of polysaccharides can be summarized for expression of complement-activating activity as shown in Figure 10 and Table 4. The active polysaccharides are grouped into four kinds of typical structures. In the case of pectins (Type I and II), 6-linked galacto-oligosaccharides and/or heteroglycosyl oligosaccharides contribute to expression of the activity, and the attachment of these oligosaccharide side chains to the rhamnnogalacturonan core is necessary to express the potent complement-activating activity through the alternative and classical pathways. Galacturonan regions in the active pectins are suggested to modulate the complement-activating activity of the "ramified" region, and methyl-ester distribution (type I) and branching frequency (type II) in the galacturonan regions inhibit the activity of the "ramified" region.

In the case of complement activating polysaccharides consisting of an arabinogalactan chain (type III), (1→6)-linked galacto-oligosaccharides, which are attached to the β-D-(1→3)-galactan backbone, instead of the rhamnogalacturonan core, are suggested to be another minimum carbohydrate chain needed for expression of complement-activating activity through the classical and alternative pathways. It is also indicated that the addition of arabinofuranose to the side chains of the galactan disturbs the potency of the activity through the classical pathway. In the case of plantago-mucilage A (type IV), it is assumed that attachment of side chains such as

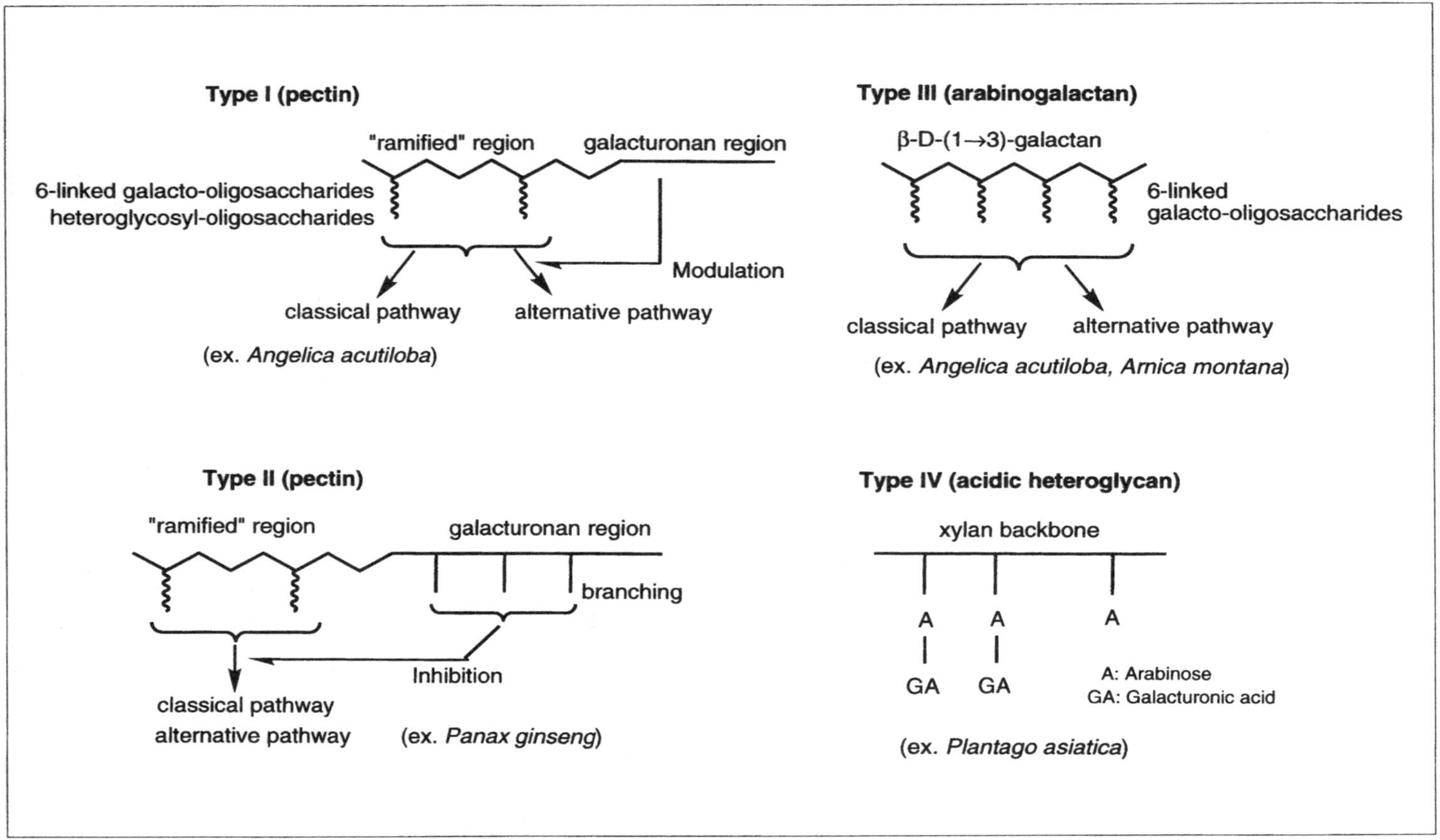

Figure 10
Typical structures of polysaccharides for complement activation.

Table 4 - Structural requirement for expression and modulation of complement-activating activity of polysaccharides of plant origin

	Activation or modulation factor		Other factor
Activation	(1→6)-linked galacto-oligosaccharides heteroglycosyl oligosaccharides		attachment of the oligosaccharides to rhamnogalacturonan core for expression of the potent activity
	(1→6)-linked galacto-oligosaccharides (1→6)- or (1→3)-linked galacto-oligosaccharides branched at position 3 or 6 of the backbone		attachement of the oligosaccharides to β-D-(1→3)-galactan backbone for expression of the potent activity
Modulation	acceleration	polyalcoholization of polysaccharide (alternative pathway) carboxyl group of uronic acids (classical pathway) aggregate formation particulate formation (alternative pathway)	
	inhibition	arabinofuranosyl side chains (classical pathway) acetyl group (classical pathway) methyl-ester distribution in galacturonan region (alternative pathway) branching frequency in galacturonan region	

β-D-xyl, α-D-GalA-(1→3)-α-L-Araf, and α-D-GlcA-(1→3)-α-L-Araf to the β-D-(1→4)-xylan backbone, instead of the rhamnogalacturonan core, may also be responsible for expression of the activity. In all the types, it seems that the structure of the side chains is important for the activity. Complement-activating acidic polysaccharide, paniculatan, also consists of an acidic backbone possessing side chains such as 4-O-Me-α-D-GlcA-(1→4)-β-D-Gal and the side chain may be responsible for the activity [18, 63].

With regard to other modulation factors for complement activation by the polysaccharides, acetyl groups on the polysaccharide molecules inhibited the anti-complementary activity of plantago-mucilage A through the classical pathway, however, polyalcoholization of the side chains in plantago-mucilage A enhanced its activity through the alternative pathway (Tab. 4) [66]. Although the carboxyl groups of uronic acids are suggested to stimulate the activity through the classical pathway of plantago-mucilage A [66] and the active pectins from *A. acutiloba* [33], it is not known whether the same mechanisms contribute or not because the tertiary structures of the pectins are strongly dependent on the carboxyl group of the galacturonan region [60]. The three dimensional structure is also suggested to affect the activities of arabinogalactan, pectin and inulin. β-D-(1→3)-glucan and amylopectin-type polysaccharide were found to be complement-activating polysaccharides [7, 22].

Honda et al. have reported that chain length having over 20 as the degree of polymeization (DP) is responsible for the activity of β-D-(1→3)-glucan through the alternative pathway, however, that induction of the carboxyl methyl group decreases the activity of β-D-(1→3)-glucan [82]. It has been clarified that β-D-(1→3)-glucan having over DP 20 takes the ordered conformation. It is also indicated that amylopectin-type polysaccharide, which can bind with iodine, is able to activate the complement system [22]. Therefore these observations propose that the three dimensional conformation is another factor for expression of complement activation by anti-complementary polysaccharides.

Effects of anti-complementary polysaccharides on complement level *in vivo*

When the anti-complementary polysaccharide, LR-polysaccharide, purified from the roots of *Lithospermum euchromum* was injected intraperitoneally into guinea pigs (20 mg/kg or 100 mg/kg), the complement level in the blood was reduced about 30–40% in comparison with that of the control 2–12 h after the injection [23]. Visual reduction of the complement level was observed in the injected animals with the dose of 20mg/kg of the polysaccharide. This result suggests that anti-complementary polysaccharides also activate the complement system *in vivo*.

Other biological activities

Several pharmacological activities have been reported in the polysaccharides isolated from medicinal herbs (Tab. 5) [83, 84]. Anti-complementary polysaccharides also have a variety of other immunopharmacological activities.

The roots of *Echinacea purpurea* or *E. angustifolia* have been used by the Indians of North America for wound healing and treatment of infections [85]. Extracts of both plants are claimed to have immunostimulating activity and are used prophylactically and therapeutically as adjuvants for the management of infectious diseases and in particular for the treatment of chronic bronchitis, sinusitis and influenza [85]. Both a xyloglucan and an acidic arabinogalactan (polysaccharide II) containing the arabino β-3,6-galactan part from the upper part of *E. purpurea* stimulated granulocytes and macrophages and induced the production of monokines (IL-1, LAF) in stimulated marrow macrophages and revealed high toxicity against tumor target cells as measured by a ^{51}Cr-release assay [85–87]. The acidic arabino β-3,6-galactan from plant cell cultures of *E. purpurea* was also effective in activating macrophages for cytotoxicity against tumor cells [85–87] and *in vitro* as well as *in vivo* against microorganisms such as *Leishmania enriiettii* and *Candida albicans* [85]. This acidic arabinogalactan also induced macrophages to

Table 5 - Pharmacological activity of polysaccharides isolated from plants

Immune system	Complemet activating activity Anti-tumor activity Mitogenic activity Stimulation of macrophage phagocytosis Stimulation of tumor-cytotoxicity by macrophage Induction of cytokines (IL-1, LAF, TNFα, INF-β2) and oxigen radical Enhancing activity of NK cell cytotoxicity Anti-inflammatory activity Anti-metastasis activity
Coagulation system	Anti-coagulant activity
Digestive system	Anti-emetic activity Anti-ulcer activity
Others	Hypoglycemic activity Anti-glaucoma activity Anti-nephritis activity and anti-nephrosis activity Cholesterol decreasing effect

produce tumor necrosis factor (TNFα), interleukin-1 (IL-1), interferon-β2 and oxygen radicals [88]. Although acidic arabinogalactan from mistletoe (*Viscum album*), having a similar chemical composition to that from *E. purpurea*, did not enhance TNFα from macrophages, it strongly activated complement [29]. Arabino β-3,6-galactan from the flower of *Calendula officinalis* (Fig. 2) enhanced phagocytosis of granulocytes *in vitro* [89].

Anti-complementary pectins (AS-3 and AS-4) from the aerial parts of *Achyrocline saturoioides*, which strongly enhanced phagocytosis of granulocytes and macrophages, showed a moderate effect on TNFα induction [16]. It is likely that the anti-complementary activity is responsible for the antiphlogistic activities of both polysaccharides as measured in the rat paw edema model [16]. In comparison to indomethacin (10 mg/kg), both polysaccharides exhibited the same activity (25–30% edema reduction in 8 h) at concentrations of 3 mg/kg by intravenous administration. The same correlation between the *in vitro* anti-complementary activity and the antiphlogistic activity in experimental animals has also been found for a polysaccharide mixture from *Urtica dioica* [51] (see also H. Wagner et al., this volume).

Pectic polysaccharide, AR-4E-2, isolated from the roots of *A. acutiloba*, showed a potent anti-tumor activity against the ascitic form of sarcoma-180, IMC carcinoma, and Meth A fibrosarcoma as well as the solid form of MM-46 tumor [90]. AR-4E-2 contained a rhamnogalacturonan core, and highly branched 3,5-arabinan and

(1→4)-linked-galactan attached to the rhamnogalacturonan core. It is known that most of the anti-tumor polysaccharides have anti-complementary activity [7], however, the anti-tumor polysaccharide fraction from *A. acutiloba*, containing AR-4E-2, showed weak anti-complementary activity. This result suggests that the structure of neutral carbohydrate side chains in AR-4E-2 might be important for the expression of anti-tumor activity but not for that of anti-complementary activity.

When excessive quantities of immune complex are formed, immune complex are deposited at several tissues, in which case the complement system is activated, resulting in anaphylatoxin formation and then severe inflammation occurs. A primary function of mononuclear phagocytic cells is to bind immune complexes through the Fc and complement receptors, followed by subsequent endocytosis and degradation of the complexes. Therefore the binding of immune complexes to these cells is an important functional parameter for immune complex clearance, and the enhancing substance for this binding has a possibility of being able to treat such inflammations. A photometric microassay was developed for measurement of immune complex (IC) binding to macrophages in a homologous system using glucose oxidase-anti-glucose oxidase complexes (GAG) as a model for IC clearance *in vitro* [91], and applied to the extracts of medicinal herbs. Anti-complementary pectins, bupleuran 2IIb and 2IIc, from the roots of *B. falcatum* L., remarkably enhanced the GAG binding activity of the macrophages through Fc receptors (FcR), and bupleuran 2IIb showed higher activity than bupleuran 2IIc [92]. When bupleuran 2IIb was administrated to mice, immune complex was cleared from the circulating blood stream more rapidly in a dose-dependent manner when compared with control mice [93]. However, bupleuran 2IIb did not affect carbon clearance. These results suggest that bupleuran 2IIb specifically enhances the clearance potency of immune complex through the FcR. Among the structural parts of bupleuran 2IIb, only its "ramified" region showed a potent activity, suggesting that the "ramified" region is important for expression of this enhancing activity as similar as anti-complementary activity [36, 92]. The result of a Scatchard analysis of GAG binding to macrophages indicated that bupleuran 2IIb enhanced Fc receptor expression on the cell surface. Fc receptors of macrophages have a variety of biological activities concerning immune complex clearance, antibody-dependent cell-mediated cytotoxicity, release of arachidonic acid metabolites, release of lysozomal enzymes, release of active oxygens and release of IL-1. Therefore, bupleuran 2IIb and 2IIc may regulate these activities. Bupleuran 2IIb induced the up-regulation of FcR on macrophages due to enhancement of transcription of both FcγRI and FcγRII genes by a mechanism dependent on an increase in intracellular Ca^{2+} followed by activation of the calmodulin, but not by a protein kinase C or protein kinase A, pathway [92, 94]. Excess amounts of immune complex may bind to the newly formed FcR and then may be degraded by the macrophages.

Oral administration of bupleuran 2IIb and 2IIc also showed the potent anti-ulcer activity against HCl-ethanol induced ulcerogenesis in mice [95]. Bupleuran 2IIc showed higher activity than a clinically-used anti-ulcer drug, sucralfate, at the same dose, and the activity of bupleuran 2IIb was a little weaker than bupleuran 2IIc. Although the oral administration of a pectin fraction, BR-2 (mainly contained bupleuran 2IIb and 2IIc), at doses of 50 to 200 mg/kg dose-dependently prevented the formation of gastric lesions induced by HCl-ethanol, the intraperitoneal and the subcutaneous administrations of BR-2 also dose-dependently reduced this gastric lesion [95]. Therefore BR-2 was suggested to exert not only a local action, but also a systemic action, for the stomach. BR-2 inhibited the ulcerogenesis of a variety of acute experimental ulcer models and a chronic ulcer model by oral administration [96]. The results on the mechanism of action suggest that the major mechanism of mucosal protection by BR-2 may be due to its anti-secretory activity on gastric acid and pepsin, its increased protective coating, and its radical scavenging effects, but not involved in the action of endogenous prostaglandins and mucus synthesis [96, 97]. Although the anti-ulcer activity of BR-2 decreased after endo-polygalacturonase digestion, the activity of apple pectin, which contained over 95% galacturonic acid, showed no significant activity [95]. These results indicate that not only the galacturonan moiety but also other minor parts such as "ramified" region and rhamnogalacturonan II-like region, and the branched galacturonan part may be important for the expression of the anti-ulcer activity of bupleuran 2IIb and 2IIc [95, 98].

Some other polysaccharides having anti-complementary activity such as MVS-I from *Malva verticillata* also showed hypoglycemic activity [39].

Concluding remarks

Anti-complementary polysaccharides have been classified into typical structural types such as arabino-β-3,6-galactan and rhamnogalacturonan with several neutral sugar side chains ("ramified" region of pectins). Both typical anti-complementary polysaccharides also reveal other pharmacological activities, and their immunopotentiating activities may somehow relate to the anti-complementary activity.

Although these pectic polysaccharides have been considered to be essential for the expression of the clinical effects of some medicinal herbs, the relationship between anti-complementary activity and other biological activities have not been fully elucidated. In order to clarify their detailed mode of action, receptor proteins on the immune cells and/or binding proteins in the serum have to be clarified. Pharmacokinetics (absorption from digestive organs, tissue distribution, metabolism and excretion) of the pectic polysaccharides also have not yet been established, because no specific reagent for the detection and quantification of pharmacologically active pectic polysaccharides is available. For this purpose, an antibody against pharmacologically active pectic polysaccharide would be a useful tool for investigating the contribution of the antigenic epitopes for the activity, and for the tissue distribution of the administered polysaccharides. Since herbal medicines are generally given orally to patients, it is necessary to analyze the pharmacokinetics after oral administration of the polysaccharides. Anti-polysaccharide antibody is also useful for the quality control of herbal medicines. When the crude polysaccharide fraction (BR-2), containing mainly bupleuran 2IIb and 2IIc from *B. falcatum*, was administrated orally to the mice, the polysaccharides were detected in the liver and Peyer's patch by using specific antibody against the "ramified" region of the anti-complementary polysaccharides [99]. Although we could detect bupleuran 2IIc in the liver when it was administrated to the mice orally, it is not yet clear whether bupleuran 2IIc was modified in the body by the action of endogenous enzymes and other factors, but a certain molecular size should be retained in order to be recognized by the antigenic epitope of the antibody. These observations suggest that at least a part of the pharmacologically active pectic polysaccharides may be absorbed from digestive organs and metabolize in the liver. Other parts of active polysaccharides may stimulate immune cells in systemic and/or intestinal immune systems through receptor-polysaccharide interaction. Anti-idiotypic antibody against anti-polysaccharide antibody would also give important information on the receptor proteins against the active polysaccharides [100].

References

1 Law SKA, Reid KBM (eds) (1995) *Complement,* 2nd ed. IRL Press, New York, Oxford

2 Thiel S, Vorup-Jensen T, Stover CM, Schwaeble W, Laursen SB, Paulsen K, Willis AC, Eggleton P, Hamsen S, Holmskov U et al (1997) A second serine protease associated with mannan-binding lectin that activates complement. *Nature* 386: 506–510

3 Turner WT (1996) Mannose-binding lectin: the pluripotent molecule of the innate immune system. *Immunol Today* 17: 532–540

4 Matsushita M, Takahashi A, Hatsuse H, Kawakami M, Fujita T (1992) Human mannose-binding protein is identical to a component of Ra-reactive factor. *Biochem Biophys Res Commun* 183: 645–651

5 Wagner H, Jurcic K (1991) Assays for immunomodulation and effects on mediators of inflammation. *Methods in Plant Biochemistry* 6: 195–217

6 Egivang TG, Befus AD (1984) The role of complement in the induction and regulation of immune responses. *Immunology* 51: 207–224

7 Okuda T, Yoshioka Y, Ikekawa T, Chihara G, Nishioka K (1972) Anti-complementary activity of anti-tumor polysaccharides. *Nature* (London) 238: 59–60

8 Hamuro J, Hadding U, Bitter-Suermann (1978) Solid phase activation of alternative pathway of complement by β-1,3-glucans and its possible role for tumor regressing activity. *Immunol* 34: 695–705

9 Morrison DC, Ulevitch RJ (1978) The effects of bacterial endotoxins on host mediation systems. *Am J Path* 93: 526–617

10 Inai S, Nagai K, Ebisu S, Kato K, Kotani S, Misaki A (1976) Activation of the alternative complement pathway by water insoluble glucans of Streptococus mutans: The relation between their chemical structures and activating potencies. *J Immunol* 117: 1256–1260
11 Götze O, Müller-Eberhard HJ (1971) The C3-activation system: An alternate pathway of complement activation. *J Exp Med* 134: 905–1085
12 Li XY, Nolte R, Vogt W (1983) Natural antibodies against a polysaccharide (B0) from sugar cane mediate its complement -activating effect. *Immunobiology* 164: 110–117
13 Pillemer L, Blum L, Lepow IH, Ross OA, Todd EW, Wardlaw AC (1954) The properdin system and immunity I. Demonstration and isolation of new serum protein, properdin and its role in immune phenomenon. *Science* 120: 279–285
14 Morrison DC, Kline LF (1977) Activation of the classical and properdin pathways of complement by bacterial lipopolysaccharides (LPS). *J Immunol* 118: 362–368
15 Wilson ME, Morrison DC (1982) Evidence for different requirements in physical state for the interaction of lipopolysaccharides with the classical and alternative pathway of complement. *Eur J Biochem* 128: 137–141
16 Puhlmann J, Knams U, Tubaro L, Schaefer W, Wagner H (1992) Immunologically active metallic ion-containing polysaccharides of *Achyrocline satureioides*. *Phytochem* 31: 2617–2621
17 Yamada H, Kiyohara H, Cyong JC, Otsuka Y (1985) Studies on polysaccharides from *Angelica acutiloba* IV. Characterization of anti-complementary arabinogalactan from *Angelica acutiloba* Kitagawa. *Molec Immunol* 22: 295–304
18 Yamada H, Nagai T, Cyong JC, Otsuka Y, Tomoda M, Shimizu N, Shimada K (1985) Relationship between chemical structure and anti-complementary activity of plant polysaccharides. *Carbohydr Res* 144: 101–111
19 Yamada H, Ohtani K, Kiyohara H, Cyong JC, Otsuka Y, Ueno Y, Omura S (1985) Purification and chemical properties of anti-complementary polysaccharide from the leaves of *Artemisia princeps*. *Planta Medica* 51: 121–125
20 Yamada H, Otsuka Y, Omura S (1986) Structural characterization of anti-complementary polysaccharides from the leaves of *Artemisia princeps* PAMP. *Planta Medica* 52: 311–314
21 Yamada H, Kiyohara H, Otsuka Y (1987) Further structural studies of an anti-complementary acidic heteroglycan from the leaves of *Artemisia princeps*. *Carbohydr Res* 170: 181–191
22 Yamada H, Yanahira S, Kiyohara H, Cyong JC, Otsuka Y (1986) Water soluble glucans from the seed of *Coix lacryma-jobi var. ma-yuen*. *Phytochem* 25: 129–132
23 Yamada H, Cyong JC, Otsuka Y (1986) Purification and chracterization of complement activating-acidic polysaccharide form the root of *Lithospermum euchromum* Royle. *Int J Immunopharmacol* 8: 71–82
24 Kiyohara H, Yamada H, Cyong JC, Otsuka Y (1986) Molecular aggregation and anti-complementary activity of arabinogalactan from *Angelica acutiloba*. (Studies on polysaccharides from *Angelica acutiloba*, part V). *J Pharmacobio-Dyn* 9: 339–346

25 Yamada H, Kiyohara H, Cyong JC, Otsuka Y (1987) Structural characterization of an anti-complementary arabinogalactan form the roots of *Angelica acutiloba* Kitagawa. (Studies on polysaccharides from *Angelica acutiloba*, part VI). *Carbohydr Res* 159: 275–291

26 Kiyohara H, Yamada H, Otsuka Y (1987) Unit structure of anti-complementary arabinogalactan form *Angelica acutiloba* Kitagawa. (Studies on polysaccharides from *Angelica acutiloba*, part VII). *Carbohydr Res* 167: 221–237

27 Kiyohara H, Yamada H (1989) Structure of an anti-complementary arabinogalactan form the root of *Angelica acutiloba* Kitagawa. (Studies on polysaccharides from *Angelica acutiloba*, Part X). *Carbohydr Res* 193: 173–192

28 Yamada H, Yanahira S, Kiyohara H, Cyong JC, Otsuka Y (1987) Characterization of anti-complementary acidic heteroglycans from the seed of *Coix lacryma-jobi var. Ma-Yuen*. *Phytochem* 26: 3269–3275

29 Wagner H, Jordan E (1988) An immunologically active arabinogalactan from *Viscus album*. *Phytochem* 27: 2511–2517

30 Yamada H, Ra K-S, Kiyohara H, Cyong JC, Yang HC, Otsuka Y (1988) Characterization of anti-complementary neutral polysaccharide from the roots of *Bupleurum falcatum* L. *Phytochem* 27: 3163–3168

31 Gao QP, Kiyohara H, Cyong JC, Yamada H (1988) Characterization of anti-complementary acidic heteroglycans from the leaves of *Panax ginseng* C. A. Meyer. *Carbohydr Res* 181: 175–187

32 Gao QP, Kiyohara H, Yamada H (1990) Further structural studies of anti-complementary acidic heteroglycans from the leaves of *Panax ginseng* C. A. Meyer. *Carbohydr Res* 196: 111–125

33 Kiyohara H, Cyong JC, Yamada H (1988) Structure and anti-complementary activity of pectic polysaccharides isolated form the roots of *Angelica acutiloba* Kitagawa. (Studies on polysaccharides from *Angelica acutiloba*, Part VIII). *Carbohydr Res* 182: 259–275

34 Kiyohara H, Yamada H (1989) Structure of neutral carbohydrate side chains in anti-complementary acidic polysaccharides from the roots of *Angelica acutiloba* Kitagawa. (Studies on polysaccharides from *Angelica acutiloba*, Part IX). *Carbohydr Res* 187: 255–265

35 Tomoda M, Gonda R, Shimizu N, Yamada H, (1989) Plant Mucilages. XLII. An anti-complementary mucilages form the leaves of *Malva sylvetris var. mauritana*. *Chem Pharm Bull* 37: 3029–3032

36 Yamada H, Ra KS, Kiyohara H, Cyong JC, Otsuka Y (1989) Structural characterization of an anti-complementary pectic polysaccharide from the roots of *Bupleurum falcatum* L. *Carbohydr Res* 189: 209–226

37 Ra KS, Yamada H, Sung HJ, Cyong JC, Yang H-C (1989) Purification and chemical properties of anti-complementary polysaccharide from *Capsici Fructus*. *J Kor Agr Chem Soc* 32: 378–385

38 Tomoda M, Shimizu N, Gonda R, Kanari M, Yamada H, Hikino H (1989) Anti-com-

plementary and hypoglycemic activities of okra- and hibiscus mucilages. *Carbohydr Res* 190: 323–328
39 Tomoda M, Shimizu N, Gonda R, Kanari M, Yamada H, Hikino H (1990) Anti-complementary and hypoglycemic activities of the glycans from the seed of *Malva verticillata*. *Planta Medica* 56: 168–170
40 Gonda R, Tomoda M, Kanari M, Shimizu N, Yamada H (1990) Constituents of the seed of *Malva verticillata* VI. Characterization and immunological activities of a novel acidic polysaccharide. *Chem Pharm Bull* 38: 2771–2774
41 Gonda R, Tomoda M, Shimizu N, Yamada H (1990) Structure and anti-complementary activity of an acidic polysaccharide from the leaves of *Malva sylvestris var. mauritiana*. *Carbohydr Res* 198: 323–329
42 Gao QP, Kiyohara H, Cyong JC, Yamada H (1991) Chemical properties and anti-complementary activity of heteroglycans from the leaves of *Panax ginseng* C. A. Meyer. *Planta Medica* 57: 132–136
43 Zhao JF, Kiyohara H, Sun XB, Matsumto T, Cyong JC, Yamada H, Takemoto N, Kawamura H (1991)In vitro immunostimulating polysaccharide fractions from roots of *Glycyrrhiza uralensis* Fisch. et DC. *Phytother Res* 5: 206–210
44 Zhao JF, Kiyohara H, Yamada H, Takemoto N, Kawamura H (1991) Heterogeneity and characterization of mitogenic and anti-complementary pectic polysaccharides from the roots of *Glycyrrhiza uralensis* Fisch. et DC. *Carbohydr Res* 219: 149–172
45 Hirano M, Matsumoto T, Kiyohara H, Yamada H (1994) Lipopolysaccharide-independent limulus amebocyte lysate activating, mitogenic and anti-complementary activities of pectic polysaccharides from Chinese herbs. *Planta Medica* 60: 248–252
46 Puhlmann J, Zenk M, Wagner H (1991) Immunologically active polysaccharides of *Arnica montana* cell cultures. *Phytochem* 30: 1141–1145
47 Zhao Q-C, Kiyohara H, Nagai T, Yamada H (1992) Structure of the complement activating proteoglycan from pilose antler of *Cervus nippon* Temminck. *Carbohydr Res* 230: 361–372
48 Gonda R, Tomoda M, Takada K, Ohara N, Shimizu N (1992) The core structure of ukonan A, a phagocytosis-activating polysaccharide from the rhizome of *Curcuma longa*, and immunological activities of degradation products. *Chem Pharm Bull* 40: 990–993
49 Zhao JF, Kiyohara H, Matsumoto T, Yamada H (1993) Characterisations of anti-complementary acidic polysaccharides from the roots of *Lithospermum euchromum* Loyle. *Phytochem* 34: 719–724
50 Zhao QC, Kiyohara H, Yamada H (1994) Purification and characterisation of anti-complementary neutral polysaccharides from the leaves of *Artemisia princeps* PAMP. *Phytochem* 35: 73–77
51 Wagner H, Willer F, Samtleben R, Boos G (1994) Search for antiprostatic principle of stinging nettle (*Urtica dioica*) roots. *Phytomedicine* 1: 213–224
52 Samuelsen AB, Paulsen BS, Wold JK, Otsuka H, Yamada H, Espevik T (1995) Isolation

and partial characterization of biologically active polysaccharides from *Plantago major* L. *Phytotherapy Res* 9: 211–218

53 Samuelsen AB, Paulsen BS, Wold JK, Otsuka H, Kiyohara H, Yamada H, Knutsen SH (1996) Characterization of a biological active pectin from *Plantago major* L. *Carbohydr Polymers* 30: 37–44

54 Zhang YW, Kiyohara H, Matsumoto T, Yamada H (1997) Fractionation and chemical properties of immunomodulating polysaccharides from roots of *Dipsacus asperoides*. *Plant Medica* 63: 393–399

55 Clarke AE, Anderson RL, Stone BA (1979) Form and function of arabinogalactans and arabinogalactan-proteins. *Phytochem* 18: 521–540

56 Yamada H, Kiyohara H, Takemoto N, Zhao JF, Kawamura H, Komatsu Y, Cyong JC, Aburada M, Hosoya E (1992) Mitogenic and complement activating activities of the herbal components of Juzen-Taiho-To. *Planta Medica* 58: 166–170

57 Kiyohara H, Cyong JC, Yamada H (1989) Relationship between structure and activity of the "ramified" region in anti-complementary pectic polysaccharides from *Angelica acutiloba* Kitagawa. (Studies on polysaccharides from *Angelica acutiloba*, Part XII).*Carbohydr Res* 193: 201–214

58 Holst GJ, Clarke AE (1985) Quantification of arabinogalactan-protein plant extracts by single radial gel diffusion. *Anal Biochem* 148: 446–450

59 Kiyohara H, Cyong JC, Yamada H (1989) Relationship between structure and activity of an anti-complementary arabinogalactan from the roots of *Angelica acutiloba* Kitagawa. (Studies on polysaccharides from *Angelica acutiloba*, Part XI). *Carbohydr Res* 193: 193–200

60 Dey PM, Brinson K (1987) Plant cell-walls. *Adv Carbohydr Chem Biochem* 42: 265–382

61 Hirano M, Kiyohara H, Yamada H (1994) Existence of rhamnogalacturonan II-like region in bioactive pectins from medicinal herbs. *Planta Medica* 60: 450–454

62 Albersheim P, An J, Freshour G, Fuller MS, Guillen R, Ham KS, Hahn MG, Huang J, O'Neill M, Whitcombe A et al. (1994) Structure and function studies of plant cell wall polysaccharides. *Biochem Soc Trans* 22: 374–378

63 Tomoda M, Satoh N (1977) Plant mucilage XVII. Partial hydrolysis and a possible structure of paniculatan. *Chem Pharm Bull* 25: 2910–2916

64 Tomoda M, Shimizu N, Shimada K, Gonda R, Sakabe H (1984) Plant mucilages XXXIV. The location of O-acetyl groups and the structural features of plantago-mucilage A, the mucous polysaccharide from the seeds of *Plantago asiatica*. *Chem Pharm Bull* 32: 2182–2186

65 Yamada H, Nagai T, Cyong JC, Otsuka Y (1991) Mode of complement activation by acidic heteroglycans from the leaves of *Artemisia princeps* PAMP. *Chem Pharm Bull* 39: 2077–2081

66 Yamada H, Nagai T, Cyong JC, Otsuka Y, Tomoda M, Shimizu N, Gonda R (1986) Relationship between chemical structure and activating potencies of complement by an

acidic polysaccharide, Plantago-mucilage A, from the seed of *Plantago asiatica. Carbohydr Res* 156: 137–145

67 Blondin C, Fischer E, Boisson-Vidal C, Kazatchkine MD, Jozefonvicz J (1994) Inhibition of complement activation by natural sulfated polysaccharide (fucans) from brown seaweed. *Molec Immunol* 31: 247–253

68 Law S K, Lichtenberg NA, Levine RP (1979) Evidence for an ester linkage between the labile binding site of C3b and receptive surfaces. *J Immunomol* 123: 1388–1394

69 Pangburn MK (1989) Analysis of the mechanism of recognition in the complement alternative pathway using C3b-bound low molecular weight polysaccharides. *J Immunomol* 142: 2759–2765

70 Kiyohara H, Yamada H (1994) Characterisation of methyl-ester distributions in galacturonan regions of complement activating pectins from the roots of *Angelica acutiloba* Kitagawa. *Carbohydr Polymers* 25: 117–122

71 Yamada H, Hirano M, Kiyohara H (1991) Partial structure of an anti-ulcer pectic polysaccharide from the roots of *Bupleurum falcatum* L.*Carbohydr Res* 219: 173–192

72 Zhang YW, Kiyohara H, Sakurai M, Yamada H (1996) Complement activating galactan chains in a pectic arabinogalactan (AGIIb-1) from the roots of *Angelica acutiloba* Kitagawa. *Carbohydr Polymers* 31: 149–156.

73 Tsumuraya Y, Mochizuki N, Hashimoto Y, Kovác P (1990) Purification of an exo-β-(1→3)-galactanase of *Irpex lacteus* (*Polyporus tulipiferae*) and its action on arabinogalactan-proteins. *J Biol Chem* 265: 7207–7215

74 Kiyohara H, Zhang YW, Yamada H (1997) Effect of exo-β-D-(1→3) galactanase digestion on complement activating activity of neutral arabinogalactan unit in a pectic arabinogalactan from roots of *Angelica acutiloba* Kitagawa. *Carbohydr Polymers* 32: 249–253

75 Kiyohara H, Takemoto N, Zhao JF, Kawamura H, Yamada H (1996) Pectic polysaccharide from roots of Glycyrrhiza uralensis: Possible contribution of neutral oligosaccharide in the galacturonase-resistant region to anti-complementary and mitogenic activities. In: Visser J, Voragen AGJ (eds): *Pectin and pectinase. Progress in biotechnology*, Vol. 4. Elsevier, Amsterdam, 673–678

76 Kiyohara H, Takemoto N, Zhao JF, Kawamura H, Yamada H (1996) Pectic polysaccharide from roots of *Glycyrrhiza uralensis*: Possible contribution of neutral oligosaccharide in the galacturonase-resistant region to anti-complementary and mitogenic activities. *Planta Medica* 62: 14–19

77 Rosenberg RD (1977) Chemistry of the hemostatic mechanism and its relationship to the action of heparin. *Fed Proc* 36: 10–18

78 Maillet F, Kazatchkine MD, Glotz D, Fischer E, Row M (1983) Heparin prevents formation of the human C3 amplification convertase by inhibiting the binding site for B on C3b. *Molec Immunol* 20: 1401–1404

79 Maillet F, Petitou M, Choay J, Kazatchkine MD (1988) Structure-function relationships in the inhibitory effect of heparin on complement activation: In dependency of the anti-

coagulant and anti-complementary sites on the heparin molecule. *Molec Immunol* 25: 917–923
80 Cooper PD, Carter M (1986) Anti-complementary action of polymorphic "solubility forms" of particulate inulin. *Molec Immunol* 23: 895–901
81 McDonald EJ (1946) The polyfructosans and difructose anhydrides. *Adv Carbohydr Chem* 2: 253–277
82 Honda S, Sugino H, Asano T, Kakinuma A (1986) Activation of the alternative pathway of complement by an anti-tumor (1→3)-β-D-glucan from *Alcaligenes faecalis* var. myxogenes IFO 13140 and its lower molecular weight and carboxymethylated derivatives. *Immunopharmacol* 11: 29–37
83 Yamada H (1994) Pectic polysaccharides from Chinese herbs: Structure and biological activity. *Carbohydr Polymers* 25: 269–276
84 Yamada H (1996) Contribution of pectins on health care. In: Visser J, Voragen AGJ (eds): *Pectin and pectinase. Progress in biotechnology.* Vol. 4, Elsevier, Amsterdam, 173–190
85 Wagner H (1990) Search for plant derived natural products with immunostimulatory activity (recent advances). *Pure & Appl Chem* 62: 1217–1222
86 Wagner H, Stuppner H, Schafer W, Zenk M (1988) Immunologically active polysaccharides of *Echinacea purpurea* cell cultures. *Phytochem* 27: 119–126
87 Stimple M, Proksch A, Wagner H, Lohmann-Matthes ML (1984) Macrophage activation and induction of macrophage cytotoxicity by purified polysaccharide fractions from the plant *Echinacea purpurea. Infection and Immunity* 46: 845–849
88 Luettg B, Steinmüller C, Gifford GE, Wagner H, Lohmann-Matthes ML (1989) Macrophage activation by the polysaccharide arabinogalactan isolated from plant cell cultures of *Echinacea purpurea. J Natl Canc Inst* 81: 669–675
89 Varljen J, Liptak A, Wagner H (1989) Structural analysis of a rhamnoarabinogalactan and arabinogalactans with immuno-stimulating activity from *Calendula officinalis. Phytochem* 28: 2379–2383
90 Yamada H, Komiyama K, Kiyohara H, Cyong JC, Hirakawa Y, Otsuka Y (1990) Structural characterization and antitumor activity of a pectic polysaccharide from the roots of Angelica acutiloba. (Studies on polysaccharides form *Angelica acutiloba,* Part XIII). *Planta Medica* 56: 182–186
91 Matsumoto T, Tanaka M, Yamada H, Cyong JC (1990) A new photometric microassay for quantitation of macrophage Fc receptor function: *in vitro* enzyme-containing immune complex clearance (EIC) assay. *J Immunol Methods* 129: 283–290
92 Matsumoto T, Cyong JC, Kiyohara H, Matsui H, Abe A, Hirano M, Danbara H, Yamada H (1993) The pectic polysaccharides from *Bupleurum falcatum* L. enhances immune-complexes binding to peritoneal macrophages through Fc receptor expression. *Int J Immunopharmacol* 15: 683–693
93 Matsumoto T, Yamada H (1996) The pectic polysaccharide from *Bupleurum falcatum* enhances immune complexes clearance in mice. *Phytotherapy Res* 10: 585–588
94 Matsumoto T, Yamada H (1995) Regulation of immune-complex binding of

macrophages by pectic polysaccharide from *Bupleurum falcatum* L.: Pharmacological evidence for the requirement of intracellular calcium/calmodulin on Fc receptor up-regulation by bupleuran 2IIb. *J Pharmacy Pharmacol* 47: 152–156

95 Yamada H, Sun XB, Matsumoto T, Ra KS, Hirano M, Kiyohara H (1991) Purification of anti-ulcer polysaccharides from the roots of *Bupleurum falcatum* L.*Planta Medica* 57: 555–559.

96 Sun XB, Matsumoto T, Yamada H (1991) Effects of a polysaccharide fraction from the roots of *Bupleurum falcatum* L. on experimental gastric ulcer models in rats and mice. *J Pharmacy Pharmacol* 43: 699–704

97 Matsumoto T, Moriguchi R, Yamada H (1993) Role of polymorphonuclear leukocytes and oxygen-derived free radicals in the formation of gastric lesions induced by HCl/ethenol, and a possible mechanism of protection by anti-ulcer polysaccharide. *J Pharmacy Pharmacol* 45: 535–539

98 Hirano M, Kiyohara H, Matsumoto T, Yamada H (1994) Structural studies of endo-polygalacturonase-resistant fragments in anti-ulcer pectin from the roots of *Bupleurum falcatum* L. *Carbohydr Res* 251: 145–162

99 Sakurai MH, Matsumoto T, Kiyohara H, Yamada H (1996) Detection and tissue distribution of anti-ulcer polysaccharides from *Bupleurum falcatum* L. by polyclonal antibody. *Planta Medica* 62: 341–346

100 Czop JK, Gurish MF, Kadish JL (1990) Production and isolation of rabbit anti-idiotypic antibodies directed against the human monocyte receptor for yeast β-glucans. *J Immunol* 145: 995–1001

Lentinan and other antitumoral polysaccharides

Yukiko Y. Maeda[1] *and Goro Chihara*[2]

[1]Dept. of Laboratory Animal Science, The Tokyo Metropolitan Institute of Medical Science, 3-18-22 Honkomagome, Bunkyo-ku, Tokyo 113-8613, Japan; [2]Ajinomoto Co. Ltd, 49-15 Tanacho, Aoba-ku, Yokohama 227-0064, Japan

Despite a great deal of effort made by many researchers throughout the world, chemotherapeutic agents that attack cancer cells directly do not seem to have the expected effects except on some leukaemias. Besides, these agents show strong toxicity to the host, and reduce the host defense against infections, especially destroying lymphocytes and bone marrow cells. To find a new cancer drug that can activate or restore host defense mechanisms, we examined fungi, which had traditionally been said to be effective against cancer in Japan and other Asian countries, such as *Ganoderma applanatum* (Pers.) Pat. and *Coriolus versicolor* (Fr.) Quél., and several kinds of Japanese edible mushrooms. Test substances were administered intraperitoneally and screened for their ability to inhibit the growth of sarcoma 180 cells subcutaneously transplanted into swiss or ICR mice. This method, reported by Nakahara et al. [1], has been proven to be simple and suitable for screening of host-mediated anticancer drugs. Table 1 shows various antitumoral polysaccharides including lentinan that were isolated from fungi, basidiomysetes and yeast. Lentinan, a (1→3)-β-D-glucan with (1→6)-β-D-glucopyranoside branches isolated from an edible mushroom, *Lentinus edodes* (Berk.) Sing., exhibits a marked antitumor effect against sarcoma 180 cells transplanted subcutaneously at a dose of 1 mg/kg/day for ten days (Fig. 1) [2–4]. Its chemical and physical characteristics are listed in Table 2. In this report, we mainly review various studies on lentinan, since it is a purified and well characterized antitumoral polysaccharide, and because much data on the biological activities of lentinan and the relationship between its structure and biological activities have been accumulated and genetic research and clinical studies on lentinan have been carried out. Lentinan used here was obtained from Ajinomoto Central Laboratories (Kawasaki, Japan), and was isolated by the method described by Chihara et al. [2, 3]. For the basic study, lentinan at a concentration of 1–5 mg/ml of distilled water was autoclaved at 121° C for 20 min for both solubilization and sterilization. LENTINAN ‹Ajinomoto› (Hoechst Marion Roussel, Tokyo, Japan), which includes 1 mg of lentinan, 2 mg of Dextran 40 and 100 mg of D-mannitol, was dissolved in 2 ml of physiological saline solution and used clinically.

Immunomodulatory Agents from Plants, edited by H. Wagner

Table 1 - Antitumoral activity of some polysaccharides against subcutaneously implanted sarcoma180 cells in mice

Polysaccharide	Source	Linkage	Dose (mg/kg x 10)	Inhibition ratio (%)	References
Lentinan	*Lentinus edodes*	(1→6)-, (1→3)-β-D-glucan	1	100	[2,3,4]
LC11	*Lentinus edodes*	(1→4)-, β-(1→6)-β-D-glucan	5	93.6	[3]
Schizophyllan	*Schizophyllum commune*	(1→6)-, (1→3)-β-D-glucan	5	89	[39]
Pachymaran	*Poria cocos*	(1→3)-β-glucan	5	96	[31]
Scleroglucan	*Sclerotium glucanicum*	(1→6)-, (1→3)-β-D-glucan	0.5	91.6	[42]
Pustulan	*Gyrophera esculenta*	(1→6)-β-D-glucan	150	85.5	[42]
Lichenan	*Cetraria islandica*	(1→3)-, (1→4)-β-D-glucan	100	99.7	[42]
Isolichenan	*Cetraria islandica*	(1→3)-, (1→4)-α-D-glucan	150	98.9	[42]
D-glucan (DP_n)540	*Alcaligenes faecalis*	(1→3)-β-D-glucan	5	99.7	[41]
Yeast glucan	*Saccharomyces cerevisiae*	(1→6)-, (1→3)-β-D-glucan	150	88.6	[42]
Yeast mannan	*Saccharomyces cerevisiae*	(1→6)-, (1→2)-α-D-mannan	100	100	[42]
Hemicellulose B	*Wheat straw*	Xyl 70%, Ara 17%, Glc 7.5%, Gal 3% and uronic acid 2%	100	99.5	[1]

Polysaccharides were administered i.p. daily for 10 days, starting 24 h after tumor transplantation and the inhibition ratios of tumor-growth were calculated after 5 weeks.

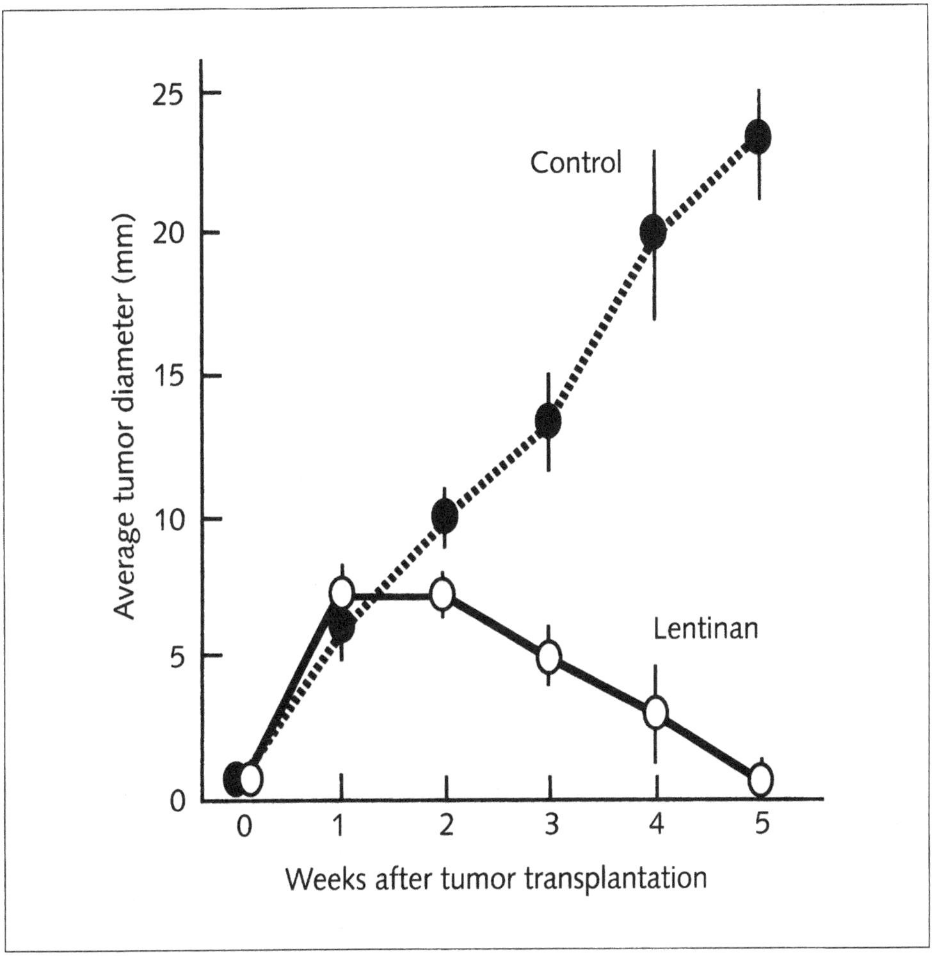

Figure 1
Antitumoral activity of lentinan against sarcoma 180 cells. Lentinan (1 mg/kg) was intraperitoneally injected once a day for ten days in ICR mice 24 h after subcutaneous transplantation of 6 × 10⁶ tumor cells.

Antitumor activity of lentinan

Lentinan exerts prominent antitumor effects on various syngeneic and autochthonous tumors induced by 3-methylcholanthrene as well as on allogeneic tumors, as shown in Table 3 [5–8]. Carcinogenesis induced by 3-methylcholanthrene in SWM/Ms and DBA/2 mice is also suppressed by lentinan from 83% to 33%, and

Table 2 - Chemical and physical characteristics of lentinan

1. Primary structure:	(1→6)-, (1→3)-β-D-glucan

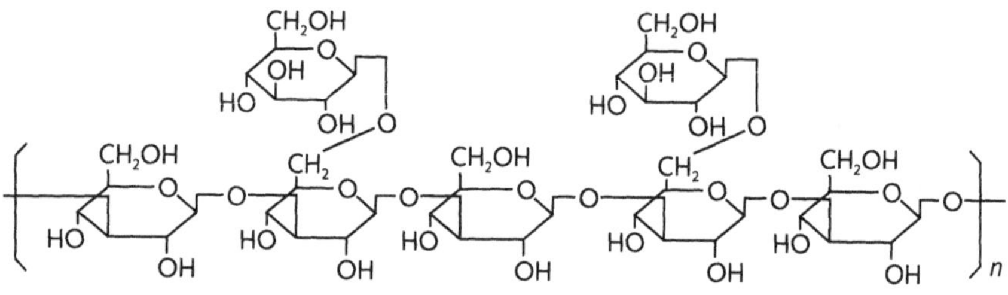

2. Three-dimensional structure:	Right-handed triple helical structure (X-ray analysis)
3. Molecular formula:	$(C_6H_{12}O_5)n$ (elementary analysis)
	Measured: C: 44.16%, H: 6.27%, N, P and S: negative
	Estimated: C: 44.44%, H: 6.22%
4. Molecular weight:	in the range of 4×10^5 to 8×10^5 Da
	(gel permeation chromatography and Laser Raman light scattering)
5. Sugar component:	glucose only (gas chromatography)
6. Physical constants	$[\alpha]_D^{20}$: 13.5–14.5° (2% NaOH), 19.5–21.5 (10% NaOH)
	UV: No absorption
	I.R. spectrum: 890 cm^{-1} (β-glucose)
	Solubility: slightly soluble in water (0.1%)
	Ultracentrifugation and high-voltage glass fiber electrophoresis: one peak

from 78% to 37%, respectively [9]. Lentinan markedly inhibited spontaneous pulmonary metastases of DBA/2.MC.CS-T fibrosarcomas in DBA/2 mice, of Lewis lung carcinomas in C57BL/6 mice, and of B16-BL6 melanomas in C57BL/6 mice that were considered as metastasis models (Fig. 2) [10]. Regarding the mechanism of antitumoral action, interesting characteristics are; (1) Lentinan does not exhibit any direct cytotoxicity against tumor cells and its action is host-mediated. (2) Toxicity towards the host is not observed (LD50 > 100 mg/kg, i.p. in mice). (3) Lentinan administered at a high dose (80 mg/kg/day × 5) does not exhibit any antitumor activity. This phenomenon of an optimal dose suggests that lentinan molecules interact with certain substances, either cellular or humoral, in the host (Tab. 3).

Table 3. Antitumor activity of lentinan and its suppressive effect on carcinogenesis

Tumor	mice	Dose mg/kg x day	Inhibition ratio (%)	References
Sarcoma 180	ICR	0.2 × 10 (i.p.)	78.1	[2, 3, 5,]
		1 × 10 (i.p.)	100	
		25 × 10 (i.p.)	88.2	
		80 × 5 (i.p.)	–8.5	
A/Ph, MC, SI sarcoma	A/Ph	1 × 10 (i.p.)	100	[6]
DBA/2.MC.CS-1 fibrosarcoma	DBA/2	1 × 10 (i.p.)	76.5	[9]
P-815 mastocytoma	DBA/2	5 × 4 (i.v.)	82	[7]
L-5178Y lymphoma	DBA/2	10 × 3 (i.v.)	89	[7]
MM-46 carcinoma	C3H/HeN	5 × 2 (i.v.)	100	[7]
MM-102 carcinoma	C3H/HeN	10 × 1 (i.v.)	60	[8]
EL-4 lymphoma	C57BL/6	10 × 1 (i.v.)	72	[8]
Lewis lung cancer	C57BL/6	1 × 6 (i.p.)	59.3	[8]
MC-induced primary tumor	DBA/2	1 × 10 (i.p.)	80.5	[9]
			Tumor occurrence (%)	
MC-induced carcinogenesis	SWM/Ms	Control	83	[9]
		1 × 10 (i.p.)	33	
MC-induced carcinogenesis	DBA/2	Control	78	
		1 × 10 (i.p.)	37	

Tumor cells were transplanted subcutaneously into mice.

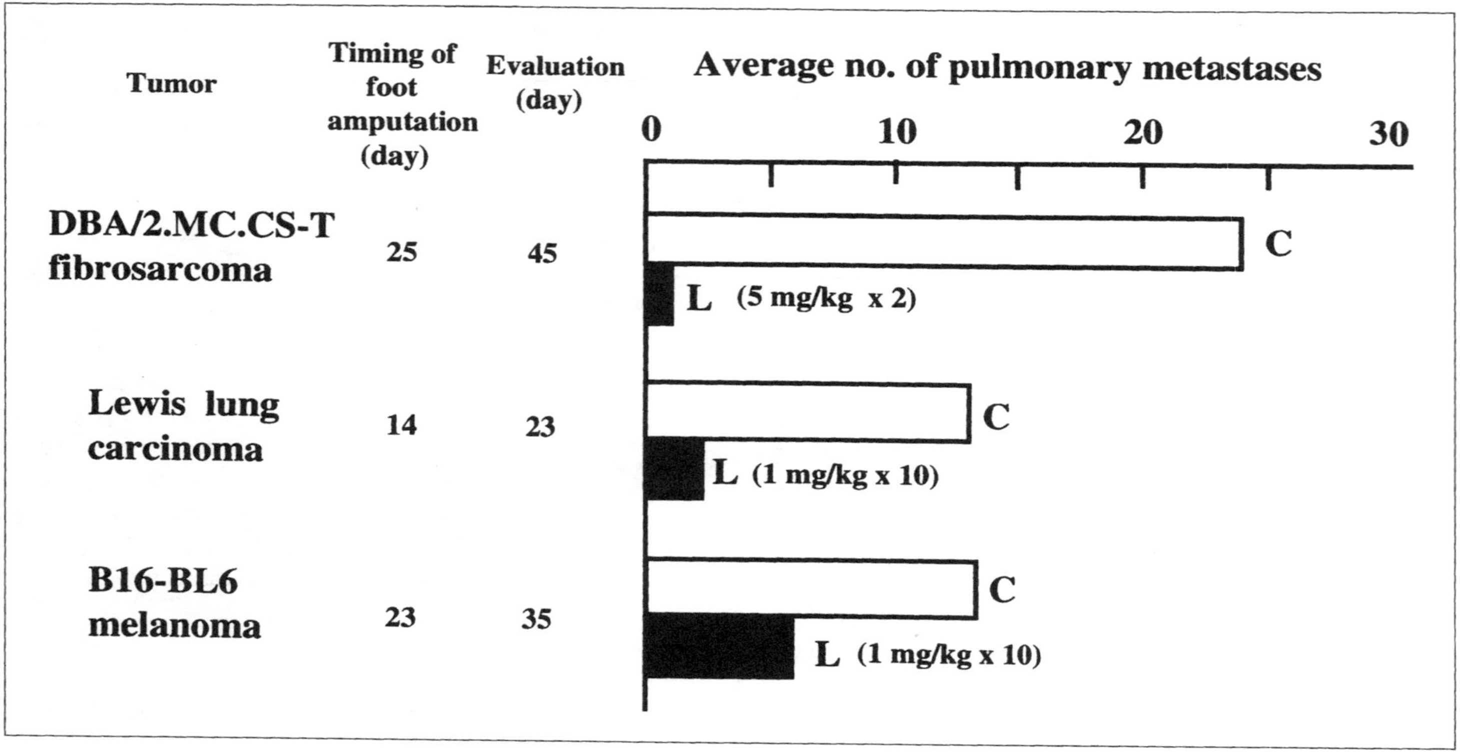

Figure 2

Suppressive effect of lentinan on spontaneous pulmonary metastasis of tumors.
DBA/2.MC.CS-T fibrosarcoma (2×10^6 cells/mouse), Lewis lung carcinoma (1×10^6 cells/mouse) and B16-BL6 melanoma cells (2.5×10^5 cells/mouse) were transplanted subcutaneously into the right side of the footpad of DBA/2, C57BL/6N and C57BL/6N mice, respectively. After the mice were intravenously injected with lentinan and footpad amputation was carried out, the mice were sacrificed and the numbers of pulmonary metastasizing tumors were counted [10].

Effect of lentinan on various immune and inflammatory responses

Various biological responses to lentinan are listed in Table 4. One of the distinct characteristics of lentinan is its capacity to act as a T cell immune adjuvant. The antitumoral activity of lentinan is absent in neonatally thymectomized mice or nude mice, and is decreased by the administration of antilymphocyte serum, suggesting that participatipation of T cells is neccessary for the exhibition of this activity [5, 11]. In particular, lentinan appears to restore or potentiate helper T cell functions, but not to stimulate B cells or T suppressor cells. Lentinan markedly enhances γG responses to sheep erythrocytes (SRBC) in CBA/J mice with the 'sham' treatment (T^+ mice), whereas adjuvant activity cannot be seen in CBA/J mice with grossly reduced populations of T cells (T mice) [12]. Dennart et al. found that lentinan stimulates the trinitrophenyl (TNP) response markedly when hapten-carrier (TNP-SRBC) conjugates were used as antigens [13]. T cell secretion of cytokines such as IL-3, IFNγ, CSF and MIF is also stimulated by lentinan [14, 15]. Hamuro et al. [16] and Akiyama et al. [7] found that lentinan increases the generation of cytotoxic T lymphocytes and NK cells in the presence of IL-2. When thymocytes or splenocytes obtained from lentinan-treated mice were cultured in the presence of IL-2, cytotoxic activities of these cells against EL-4 lymphoma cells or YAC-1 cells markedly increased, respectively. Recent immunology revealed that helper T cell clones can be classified into subsets that produce different sets of cytokines upon activation. T helper type 1 (Th1) cells produce IL-2, IFNγ and TNFβ, thereby activating macrophages and inducing delayed-type hypersensitivity responses. T helper type 2 (Th2) cells produce IL-3, IL-4, IL-5, IL-6, IL-10 and IL-13, stimulating production of mast cells, eosinophils, and immunoglobulin G1 and E antibodies and possibly suppressing cell-mediated immunity. Considering these various results on lentinan, its antitumoral activity appears to be mediated by Th1, but not Th2. Th1 activation by lentinan is consistent with the fact that lentinan stimulates delayed type hypersensitivity (DTH) against tumor-associated antigens *in vivo* [13]. In addition to the antitumoral activity and DTH, lentinan can markedly induce two *in vivo* responses, delayed-type acute phase responses (DT-APR) [17] and vascular dilation and hemorrhage (VDH) [18] (Fig. 3). DT-APR is characterized by a slow increase (four to seven days after administration) in the amount of acute phase proteins (APPs) such as haptoglobin, ceruloplasmin and hemopexin, as compared with lipopolysaccharide (LPS) showing a rapid increase (several hours to one day) in the production of APPs. DT-APR is a non-T cell-mediated response, since this response is observed in nude mice as well as in normal mice. VDH is a T cell-mediated response observed in highly localized areas such as the ears, feet and tails of mice, two to four days after lentinan administration. VDH induction as well as the antitumoral activity and DTH may be mediated by Th1 cells. DT-APR appears to have activation pathways distinct from those of the above responses. Extrathymic T cells expressing $CD3^+$ and $NK1.1^+$ might concern the expression of

Table 4 - Various immunological and inflammatory responses activated by lentinan

1. *In vivo* responses		**References**
Neonatal thymectomy	Decreased antitumoral activity	[5, 11]
Antilymphocyte serum	Decreased antitumoral activity	[5, 11]
Helper T cell function	Restoration or potentiation	[12, 13]
Generation of cytotoxic T cells	Augmentation in the presence of IL-2	[7, 16]
Suppressor T-cell function	No effect	[7]
NK-cell activity	Augmentation in the presence of IL-2	[7]
Treatment with antimacrophage agents	Decreased antitumoral activity, VDH, and DT-APR	[18, 19]
Phagocytosis	Weak	[5]
Secretion of cytokines	Augmentation of IL-1, CSF, MIF, IL-3, IL-6 and IFNγ	[7, 14, 15, 22]
Generation of cytotoxic macrophages	Activation	[7, 20]
Antibodies against SRBC, BSA	Augmentation	[12, 13]
Delayed-type hypersensitivity	Potentiation	[14]
Granuloma formation	Increase around schistosoma	[43]
Local cellularreaction	Stimulation around tumor	[44]
Delayed type acute phase response (DT-APR)	Induction	[17]
Vascular dilation and hemorrhage (VDH)	Induction	[18]
2. *In vitro* responses		**References**
Alternative C3 pathway	Activation	[25]
α Helix of bovine serum albumin	Increased its content	[27]

DT-APR. Macrophages are considered to be the first cells which lentinan comes into contact with and activates in the host. Simultaneous administration of anti-macrophage agents such as silica and carrageenan suppressed the induction of the antitumoral activity, VDH and DT-APR by lentinan [18, 19]. Lentinan induces non-specific cytotoxicity in macrophages [7, 20] and stimulates IL-1, IL-6, TNFα and prostaglandin E2 secretion [7, 21, 22]. For both basic and clinical studies, it is a notable characteristic that antiboides against lentinan are extremely difficult to prepare. Preparation of such antibodies was achieved by immunization with lentinan conjugated with BSA [23]. Monoclonal antibody against lentinan revealed that lentinan binds to monocytes, but not to neutrophils or lymphocytes, via CR1 or CR3 [24]. Lentinan activates the C3 alternative pathways *in vitro*, resulting in

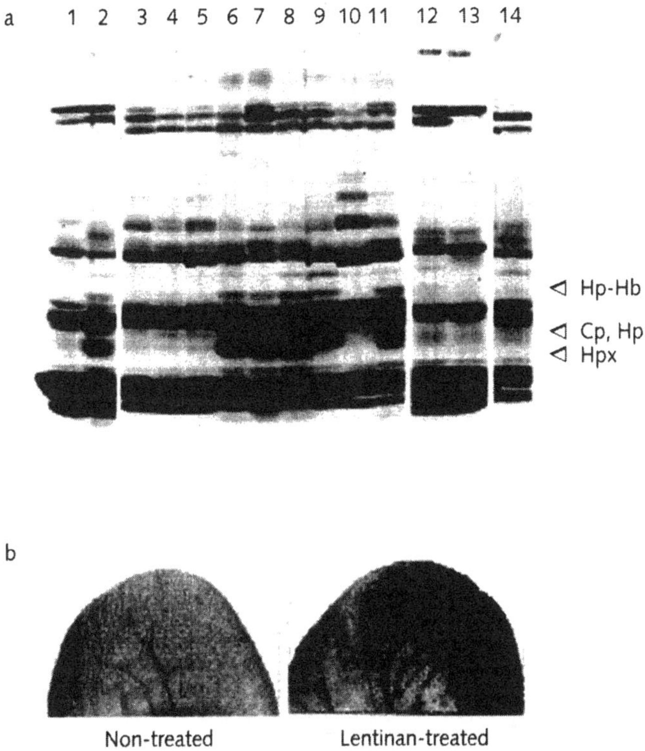

Figure 3
(a) DT-APR: change in the levels of acute phase proteins in the sera from several strains of mice obtained seven days after an intraperitoneal injection of lentinan (10 mg/kg). Five microliters of serum was applied to a 4–30% gradient polyacrylamide gel. Lanes: (1) AKR/J (non-treated), (2) C57BL10SnSlc (3) A/J, (4) BALB/cAnN, (5) C3H/HeN, (6) C58/J, (7) DBA/2J, (8) RIIIS/J, (9) SJL/J, (10) SM/J, (11) SWR/J, (12) C57BL/6ByJ, (13) AKR/J, and (14) MA/MyJ. Hp haptoglobin; Hb hemoglobin; Cp ceruloplasmin; Hpx hemopexin. (b) VDH induced in ears of ICR mice three days after lentinan administration [17, 18].

the splitting of C3 into C3a and C3b [25]. Lentinan opsonized with C3b is considered to bind to CR1 or CR3 on monocytes. Lentinan may also bind monocytes through β-glucan receptors as reported by Czop and Austen [26]. Antitumoral polysaccharides change the amount of helixes in bovine serum albumin *in vitro*, suggesting that these polysaccharides bind to certain proteins such as albumin in a host [27]. Possible pathways activated by lentinan in the immune and inflammatory systems are shown in Figure 4.

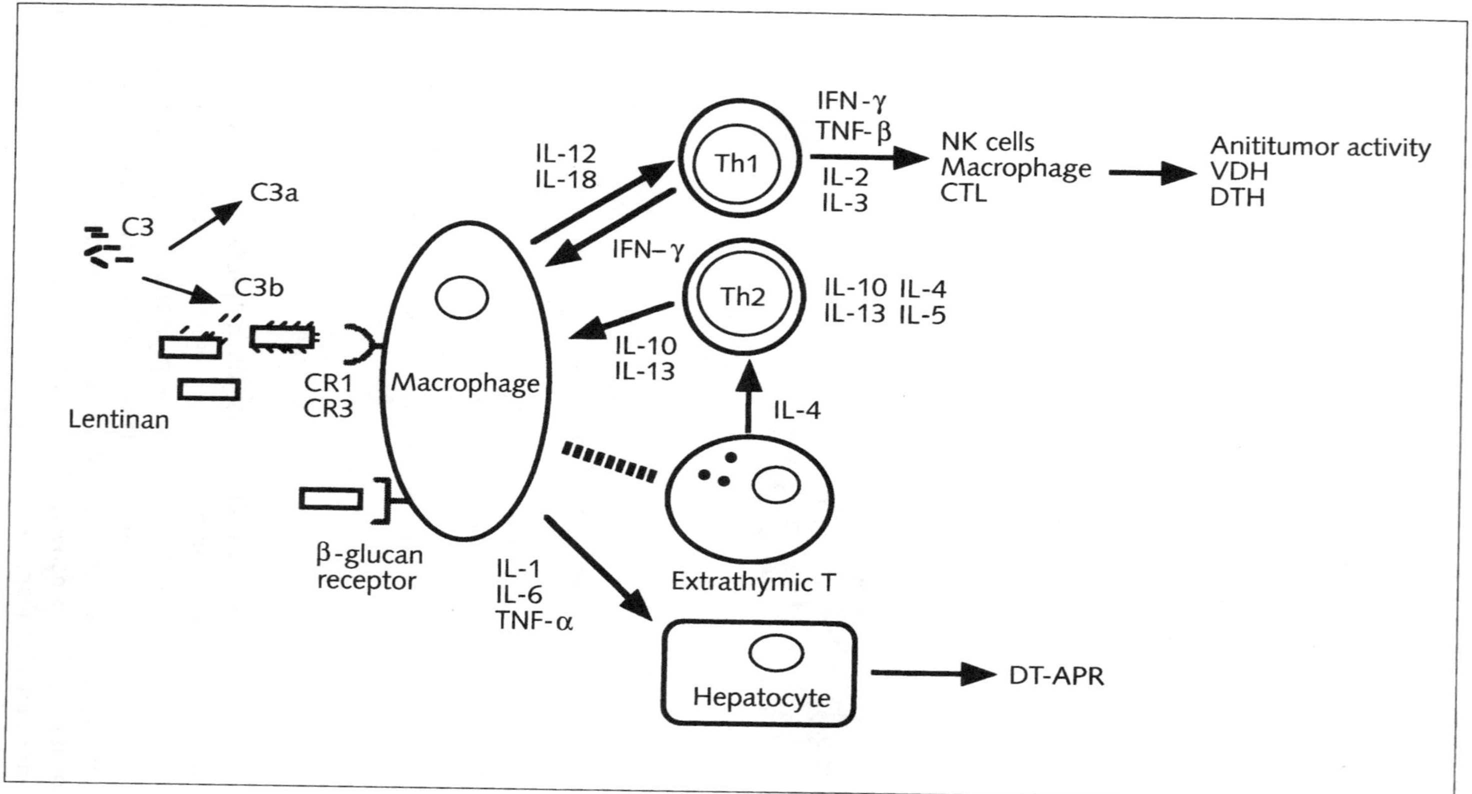

Figure 4

Possible mode of action of lentinan.

VDH, vascular dilation and hemorrhage; DTH, delayed-type hypersensitivity; DT-APR, delayed-type acute phase response; Th1and Th2, T helper type 1 and 2 cells; NK, natural killer ; IL, interleukin; TNF, tumor necrosis factor; INF, interferon.

Increase in the resistance of the host to infections

Lentinan and yeast glucan can enhance the resistance of a host to bacterial, fungal, viral or parasitic infections (Tab. 5) [28–30], which is a marked advantage for cancer patients, since infections caused by microorganisms often cause serious problems in tumor-bearing or AIDS patients whose immune responsiveness has deteriorated.

Structure-activity relationship

A slight chemical modification of a polysaccharide which is entirely devoid of antitumoral activity induced its antitumoral activity, indicating that there is a mechanism whereby the conformation of polysaccharides is recognized [31]. Although pachyman, obtained from *Poria cocos* Wolf, is a (1→3)-β-D-glucan having 9–10 branches of (1→6)-β-D-glucopyranosides and one internal (1→6)-β linkage and does not show any antitumoral activity, chemical destruction of these (1→6)-β-D-glucopyranoside linkages markedly increased its antitumoral activity. This antitumoral polysaccharide was termed pachymaran (Tab. 1). We have proposed the importance of the three-dimensional structure of polysaccharides for biological activities. Use of denaturants, such as urea, dimethylsulfoxide or sodium hydroxide, changed the specific rotation of lentinan at 589 nm (Fig. 5) and its optical rotatory dispersion in a dose-dependent manner [32]. The removal of the denaturants from the mixture of lentinan and the denaturant resulted in a return to normal values. These changes in the three-dimensional structure as a result of denaturation and renaturation were associated with reduction and recovery of the antitumoral activity and VDH, found to be T cell-mediated responses. However, induction of DT-APR, a non T cell-mediated response, was not affected by the change of the three-dimensional structure of lentinan. These results suggest that a certain three-dimensional structure is necessary for expression of T cell-mediated responses [32]. As further evidence showing the importance of the three-dimensional structure of antitumoral polysaccharides, pachyman not exhibiting an antitumoral effect can be converted to U-pachyman exhibiting a strong antitumoral activity by treatment with 8M-urea without changing its primary structure [5]. It is unclear yet whether the triple helix structure of lentinan, as deduced by X-ray analysis [33], relates to the specific three-dimensional structure necessary for its biological activities.

Genetic control of the expression of the biological activities of lentinan

According to differences in the susceptibility of mice to lentinan in the induction of DT-APR and VDH, mice used were divided into two groups, high responders and low responders, suggesting that both responses are under genetic control. However,

Table 5 - Increase of host resistance to bacteria, viruses, parasites and fungi by antitumoral polysaccharides

	Yeast glucan	**Lentinan**
Bacteria	*Pseudomonas pseudomallei* *Pseudomonas aeruginosa* *Mycobacterium leprae* *Mycobacterium tuberculosis* *Listeria monocytogenes* *Francisella tularensis* *Staphylococcus aureus*	*Mycobacterium tuberculosis* *Listeria monocytogenes*
Viruses	Hepatitis virus MHV-A 59 Herpes simplex virus I and II	*Adenovirus type 12* *Abelson virus* *VSV-encephalitis virus* Influenza A, A/PR/8/34(HINI)
Parasites	*Plasmodium berghei* *Leishmani donovani*	*Schistosoma mansoni* *Schistosoma japonicum* *Mesocestoides corti*
Fungi	*Candida albicans* *Cryptococcus neoformans*	

[28, 29, 30 and 40]

the strain distribution pattern of DT-APR was different from that of VDH induction. Analyses using F_1 combinations between a high and low responder showed that the induction of DT-APR and VDH was controlled by recessive and dominant genes, respectively. To determine the chromosomal locations of these genes, genomic DNAs of backcross mice were typed by the polymerase chain reaction-simple sequence length polymorphism (PCR-SSLP) technique using chromosome-specific microsatellite markers. Figure 6 shows the chromosomal locations of six lentinan-responsive genes. Two loci (*ltnr1* and *ltnr2*) responsible for DT-APR have been identified using 123 (SWR/J × SPR/J)F_1 × SWR/J backcross progeny derived from intercrosses between SWR/J and *Mus spretus* (SPR/J). *ltnr1* is closely linked to *D3Mit11* on chromosome 3 ($p < 0.0005$) and *ltnr2* to *D11Nds9* on chromosome 9 ($p < 0.00000$) [22]. VDH has been found to be regulated by one major gene (*Ltnr3*) and three minor genes (*Ltnr4*, *Ltnr5* and *Ltnr6*) by the same linkage analysis method using 193 segregants exhibiting the strongest VDH response of a total of 618 (MA/MyJ × AKR/J) F_1 × AKR/J backcross progeny. *Ltnr3* is closely linked to *D6Mit135* (on chromosome 6 ($p < 0.00000$) and *Ltnr4*, *Ltnr5* and *Ltnr6* to *D9Mit161* on chromosome 9 ($p < 0.00032$), *D15Mit147* on chromosome 15

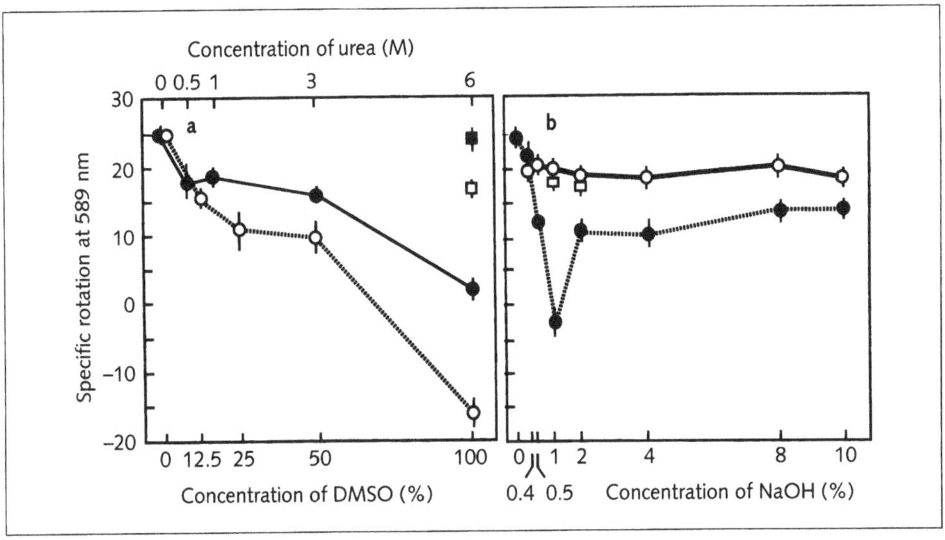

Figure 5
Denaturation and renaturation of lentinan by urea, dimethyl sulfoxide (DMSO) or sodium hydroxide (NaOH). (a) Lentinan was mixed with urea (solid circle) or DMSO (open circle) for 30 min at room temperature. Renatured lentinan was prepared by removal of urea (solid square) or DMSO (open square) through dialysis against distilled water. (b) Lentinan was denatured with NaOH by mixing at 25° C for 10 min (solid circle). Renatured lentinan was obtained by neutralization, followed by dialysis against distilled water after mixing with NaOH at 0° C for 30 min (open circle), or 25° C for 10 min (open square) [32].

($p < 0.00014$), and *D16Mit4* on chromosome 16 ($p < 0.00014$), respectively [34]. Stimulation of IL-6 production by lentinan prior to DT-APR was also suggested to be controlled by *ltnr1* and *ltnr2* [22]. Lentinan augments the skin reaction induced by bradykinin [35]. Based on a close correlation between this augmentation and VDH, the augmented skin reaction is suggested to be controlled by *Ltnr3*, *Ltnr4*, *Ltnr5* and *Ltnr6*. Further genetic analyses may provide a new tool for the elucidation of host defence mechanisms.

Clinical application of lentinan

Based on many fundamental studies, a phase III randomized control study of lentinan was carried out. Treatment with lentinan plus 5-fluoro-1-(tetrahydro-2-furyl)-uracil (tegafur) of 77 patients having advanced or recurrent gastric cancer markedly prolonged their life span, as compared with a control group treated with tegafur alone (Fig. 7) [36]. In addition to the prevention of the side effects of radiation ther-

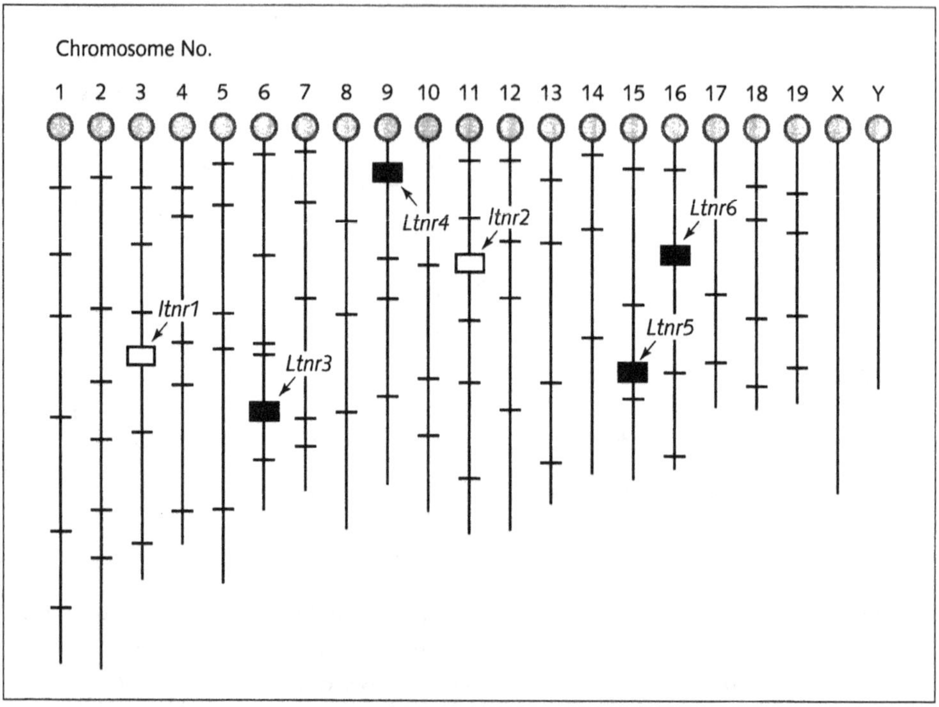

Figure 6
Chromosomal positions of 5 lentinan-responsive loci for DT-APR (open bar) and for VDH (shaded bar). Short horizontal lines show chromosome-specific microsatellite loci used for interval mapping of VDH-susceptibility loci using a PCR-SSLP technique [22, 34].

apy, combined treatment with lentinan and radiation therapy was effective against squamous cell lung cancer of hilar origin, resulting in the prolongation of their life span and the curing of ten out of 50 patients [37]. Similar results were obtained for scirrhous gastric cancer and breast, colon and esophageal cancers [38]. Considering that the cancers, as tested clinically, were either classified as advanced or recurrent, or the patients were not considered suitable candidates for surgery, these clinical results are surprising. We believe that lentinan can be used effectively in the treatment of cancer, if lentinan is used in combination with surgery and radiation at an early stage .

Conclusion

Antitumoral polysaccharides, including lentinan, are regarded as unique immunostimulants. To date, they have led to new research directions in the fields of chem-

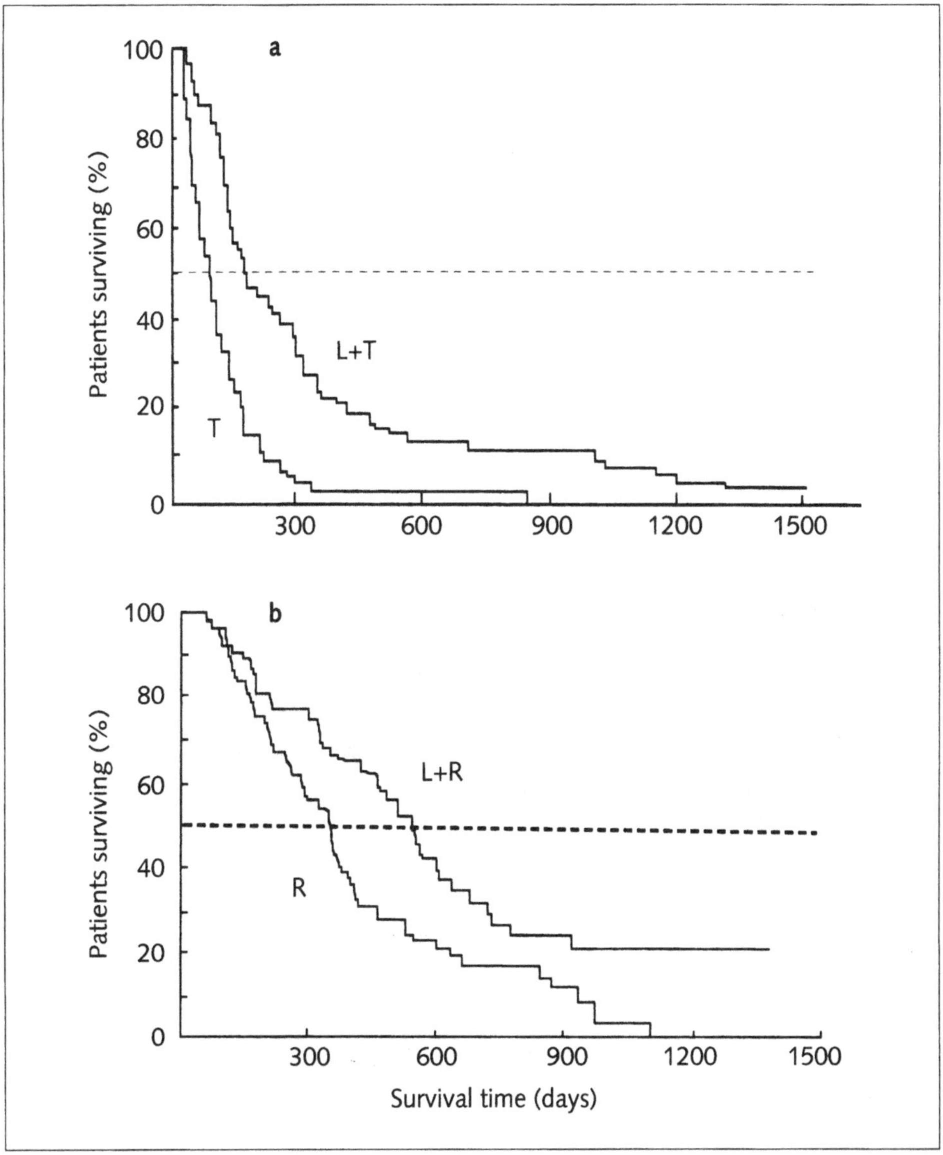

Figure 7
Clinical effect of lentinan against advanced or recurrent gastric cancer (a) and squamous cell lung cancer of hilar origin (b). Of 145 gastric cancer patients, 68 and 77 were treated with tegafur alone (T) or lentinan in combination with tegafur (L + T), respectively. Median survival periods for the two groups were 92 days (T) and 173 days (L + T) ($p < 0.01$). Fifty lung cancer patients were treated with chest irradiation (60 Gy) alone (R), and 50 with lentinan plus radiation (L + R). Median survival periods were 344 days (R) and 529 days (L + R) ($p < 0.1$) [36, 37].

istry, pharmacology, immunology and genetics. However, further studies are required for (1) the determination of the three-dimensional structure of polysaccharides necessary for their biological activities, (2) identification of lentinan-responsive genes, and (3) improvement of clinical applications, such as in the method of administration and the combination with surgery, radiation therapy and other drugs. Accumulation of such research data on antitumoral polysaccharides will result in their gaining an important position in cancer and infection chemotherapy.

Acknowledgment
We sincerely thank Dr. Yasuko Takeda for her excellent suggestions regarding the preparation of this manuscript.

References

1 Nakahara W, Tokuzen R, Fukuoka F, Whistler RL (1967) Inhibition of mouse sarcoma 180 by a wheat hemicellulose B preparation. *Nature* 216: 374–375

2 Chihara G, Maeda YY, Hamuro J, Sasaki T, Fukuoka F (1969) Inhibition of mouse sarcoma 180 by polysaccharide from *Lentinus edodes* (Berk.) Sing. *Nature* 222: 687–688

3 Chihara G, Hamuro J, Maeda YY, Arai Y, Fukuoka F (1970) Fractionation and purification of the polysaccharides with marked antitumor activity, especially lentinan, from *Lentinus edodes* (Berk.) Sing. (an edible mushroom). *Cancer Res* 30: 2776–2781

4 Sasaki T, Takasuka N (1976) Further study of the structure of lentinan, an anti-tumor polysaccharide from *Lentinus edodes*. *Carbohydr Res* 47: 99–104

5 Maeda YY, Hamuro J, Yamada YO, Ishimura K, Chihara G (1973) The nature of immunopotentiation by the anti-tumour polysaccharide lentinan and the significance of biogenic amines in its action. In: Wolstenholme GEW, Knight J (eds): *Immunopotentiation. Ciba Found. Symposium new series.* Elsevier, Amsterdam, *Excerpta Medica* 18: 259–286

6 Zákány J, Chihara G, Fachet J (1980) Effect of lentinan on tumor growth in murine allogeneic and syngeneic hosts. *Int J Cancer* 25: 371–376

7 Akiyama Y, Kashima S, Hayami T, Izawa M, Mitsugi K, Hamuro J (1981) Immunological characteristics of antitumor polysaccharides, lentinan and its analogues, as immune adjuvants. In: Aoki T, Urushizaki I, Tsubura E (eds): *Manipulation of host defence mechanisms. Excerpta Medica*, Amsterdam, 227–243

8 Shiio T, Yugari Y (1981) The anti-tumor effect of lentinan and the tumor recognition in mice. In: Aoki T, Urushizaki I, Tsubura E (eds): *Manipulation of host defence mechanisms. Excerpta Medica*, Amsterdam, 29–42

9 Suga T, Shiio T, Maeda YY, Chihara G (1984) Antitumor activity of lentinan in murine syngeneic and autochthonous hosts and its suppressive effect on 3-methylcholanthrene-induced carcinogenesis. *Cancer Res* 44: 5132–5137

10 Suga T, Yoshihama T, Tsuchiya Y, Shiio T, Maeda YY, Chihara G (1989) Prevention of tumour metastasis and recurrence of DBA/2.MC.CS-1, DBA/2.MC.CS-T fibrosarcoma, MH-134 hepatoma, and other murine tumours using lentinan. *Int J Immunotherapy* 5: 187–193

11 Maeda YY, Chihara G (1971) Lentinan, a new immuno-accelerator of cell-mediated responses. *Nature* 229: 634

12 Dresser DW, Phillips JM (1974) The orientation of the adjuvant activities of *Salmonella typhosa* lipopolysaccharide and lentinan. *Immunology* 27: 895–902

13 Dennert G, Tucker D (1973) Antitumor polysaccharide lentinan, a T cell adjuvant. *J Natl Cancer Inst* 51: 1727–1729

14 Zákány J, Chihara G, Fachet J (1980) Effect of lentinan on the production of migration inhibitory factor induced by syngeneic tumor in mice. *Int J Cancer* 26: 783–788

15 Izawa M, Ohno K, Amikura K, Hamuro J (1983) Lentinan augments the production of interleukin 3 and colony stimulating factor(s) by T cells. In: Aoki T, Tsubura E, Urushizaki I (eds): *Manipulation of host defence mechanisms. Excerpta Medica*, Amsterdam, 59–69

16 Hamuro J, Röllinghoff M, Wagner H (1978) β (1→3) glucan-mediated augmentation of alloreactive murine cytotoxic T-lymphocytes *in vivo*. *Cancer Res* 38: 3080–3085

17 Maeda YY, Chihara G, Ishimura K (1974) Unique increase of serum proteins and action of antitumor polysaccharides. *Nature* 252: 250–252

18 Maeda YY, Watanabe ST, Chihara G, Rokutanda M (1984) T-cell mediated vascular dilatation and hemorrhage induced by antitumor polysaccharides. *Int J Immunopharmac* 6: 493–501

19 Suga T, Maeda YY, Uchida H, Rokutanda M, Chihara G (1986) Macrophage-mediated acute-phase transport protein production induced by lentinan. *Int J Immunopharmac* 8: 691–699

20 Maeda YY, Chihara G (1973) Periodical consideration on the establishment of antitumor action in host and activation of peritoneal exudate cells by lentinan. *GANN* (*Jap. Cancer Res*) 64: 351–357

21 Hamuro J, Röllinghoff M, Wagner H, Seitz M, Grimm W, Gemsa D (1979) Depressed prostaglandin release from peritoneal cells induced by a T cell adjuvant, lentinan. *Z Immun-Forsch* 155: 248–254

22 Maeda YY, Takahama S, Kohara Y, Yonekawa H (1996) Two genes controlling acute phase responses by the antitumor polysaccharide, lentinan. *Immunogenetics* 43: 215–219

23 Kishida E, Sone Y, Shibata S, Misaki A (1989) Preparation and immunochemical characterization of antibody to branched β-(1→3)-D-glucan of *Volvariella volvacea*, and its use in studies of antitumor actions. *Agric Biol Chem* 53: 1849–1859

24 Oka M, Hazama S, Suzuki M, Wang F, Wadamori K, Iizuka N, Takeda S, Akitomi Y, Ohba Y, Kajiwara K, Suga T, Suzuki T (1996) *in vitro* and *in vivo* analysis of human leukocyte binding by the antitumor polysaccharide, lentinan. *Int J Immunopharmac* 18: 211–216

25 Okuda T, Yoshioka Y, Ikekawa T, Chihara G, Nishioka K (1972) Anticomplementary activity of antitumor polysaccharides. *Nature New Biol* 238: 59–60

26 Czop JK, Austen KF (1985) Generation of leukotrienes by human monocytes upon stimulation of their β-glucan receptor during phagocytosis. *Proc Natl Acad Sci USA* 82: 2751–2755

27 Hamuro J, Chihara G (1973) Effect of antitumour polysaccharides on the higher structure of serum protein. *Nature* 245: 40–41

28 White TR, Thompson RCA, Penhale WJ, Chihara G (1988) The effect of lentinan on the resistance of mice to *Mesocestoides corti. Parasitol Res* 74: 563–568

29 Irinoda K, Masihi KN, Chihara G, Kaneko Y, Katori T (1992) Stimulation of microbicidal host defence mechanisms against aerosol influenza virus infection by lentinan. *Int J Immunopharmac* 14: 971–977

30 DiLuzio NR. Chihara G (1981) Polysaccharides and related substances I. In: Hadden J, Chedid L, Mullen P, Spreafico F (eds): *Advances in Immunopharmacology.* Pergamon Press, Oxford, New York, 477–484

31 Chihara G, Hamuro J, Maeda YY, Arai Y, Fukuoka F (1970) Antitumour polysaccharide derived chemically from natural glucan (pachyman). *Nature* 225: 943–944

32 Maeda YY, Watanabe ST, Chihara C, Rokutanda M (1988) Denaturation and renaturation of a β-1,6;1,3-glucan, lentinan, associated with expression of T-cell-mediated responses. *Cancer Res* 48: 671–675

33 Bluhm TL, Sarko A (1977) The triple helical structure of lentinan, a linear β-(1→3)-D-glucan. *Can J Chem* 55: 293–299

34 Maeda YY, Takahama S, Yonekawa H (1998) Four dominant loci for the vascular responses by the antitumor polysaccharide, lentinan. *Immunogenetics* 47: 159–165

35 Takatsuki F, Namiki R, Kikuchi T, Suzuki M, Hamuro J (1995) Lentinan augments skin reaction induced by bradykinin: Its correlation with vascular dilatation and hemorrhage responses and antitumor activities. *Int J Immunopharmac* 17: 465–474

36 Taguchi T, Furue H, kimura T, Kondo T, Hattori T, Ito I, Ogawa N (1985) End-point results of a randomized controlled study on the treatment of of gastrointestinal cancer with a combination of lentinan and chemotherapeutic agents. In: Tsubura E, Urushizaki I, Aoki T (eds): *Rationale of biological response modifiers in cancer treatment. Excerpta Medica*, Amsterdam, 151–166

37 Kimura I, Ohnochi T, Konno K et al. (1993) A randomized trial of chest irradiation alone versus chest irradiation plus lentinan in squamous cell lung cancer in limited stage [in Japanese]. *Biotherapy* 7: 601–617

38 Suzuki M, Takatsuki F, Maeda YY, Hamuro J, Chihara, G (1994) Lentinan: Rationale for development and therapeutic potential. *Clin Immunother* 2: 121–133

39 Kikumoto S, Miyazima T, Kimura K, Okubo S, Komatsu N (1971) Polysaccharide produced by *Schizophyllum commune*, part II. Chemical structure of an extracellular polysaccharide. *Nippon Nogeikagaku Kaishi (Jap J Agr Chem)* 45: 162–168

40 DiLuzio NR, Williams DL, McNamee RB, Edwards BF, Kitahama A (1979) Compara-

tive tumor-inhibitory and anti-bacterial activity of soluble and particulate glucan. *Int J Cancer* 24: 773–779
41 Sasaki T, Abiko N, Sugino Y, Nitta K (1978) Dependence on chain length of antitumor activity of (1→3)-β-D-glucan from *Alcaligenes faecalis* var. *myxogenes*, IFO 13140, and its acid-degraded products. *Cancer Res* 38: 379–383
42 Whistler RL, Bushway AA, Singn PP, Nakahara W, Tokuzen R (1976) Noncytotoxic, antitumor polysaccharides. *Advan Carbohydrate Chem Biochem* 32: 235–274
43 Byram JE, Sher A, DiPietro J, von Lichtenberg F (1979) Potentiation of schistosome granuloma formation by lentinan, a T-cell adjuvant. *Am J Pathol* 94: 201–218
44 Tokuzen R (1971) Comparison of local cellular reaction to tumour grafts in mice treated with some plant polysaccharides. *Cancer Res* 31: 1590–1593

Addendum

Further polysaccharides with immunoinduced antitumoral activity have been isolated from the culture broth of *Laetisaria arvalis* [Aouadi S, Heyraud A, Seigle-Murandi F, Steimann R, Kraus J, Franz G (1991) *Carbohydrate Polymers* 16: 155–165], from the fungus *Glomerella cingulata* [Gomaa K, Kraus J, Roßkopf F, Röper A and Franz G (1992) *J Cancer Res Clin Oncol* 118: 136–140], from *Phytophthora parasitica* [Kraus J, Blaschek W, Schütz M, Franz G (1992) *Planta Medica* 58, 39-42], and *Pythium aphanidermatum* [Blaschek W, Käsbauer J, Kraus J, Franz G (1992) *Carbohydrate Res* 231: 293–307]. The polysaccharides possess a β 1→3/1→3 glucan and show antitumoral effects against allogenic, syngenic and even autologous tumors. The polysaccharides showed in the *in vivo* experiments inhibition rates of 20 to 100% at concentrations between 5 and 25 mg/kg.

Mistletoe lectins as immunostimulants (chemistry, pharmacology and clinic)

Rainer Samtleben[1], Tibor Hajto[2], Katarina Hostanska[2] and Hildebert Wagner[1]

[1]Institute of Pharmaceutical Biology, Ludwig-Maximilians-Universität Munich, Karlstr. 29, D-80333 Munich, Germany; [2]Department of Internal Medicine, University Hospital Zürich, P.O.Box 77, CH-4132 Muttenz, Switzerland

Introduction

The European mistletoe *Viscum album* L. has attracted special interest in folklore and ethnomedicine throughout the centuries. The Celtic druids used it already in their ceremonies more than 2000 years ago. Later on it was thought to be potent against epilepsy "since the mistletoe did not fall down – neither would the patient" and this belief was carried on through the middle ages. In the 16th century mistletoe was commonly used against the falling sickness as well as against illnesses of the blood circulation, heart failure, dropsy, asthma and nervous diseases [1, 2].

In 1920 Rudolf Steiner [3] deduced on an anthroposophical basis that fermented mistletoe extract had a therapeutic benefit for cancer patients. He introduced fermented mistletoe injection preparations for the treatment of some human tumors. Dissatisfaction with current cancer chemotherapy concepts led to a wide acceptance of these unconventional therapies. The popularity of the mistletoe injection preparations mainly in Central Europe strongly stimulated the investigations of their chemical constituents and possible active components. Among them the mistletoe polymers (proteins, peptides and polysaccharides) are now favourite compounds for immunostimulation. In the last 10 years it has been clearly demonstrated that the mistletoe lectins are good candidates for modulating different immunological parameters which might be beneficial for immunodeficient patients. The main active lectin (mistletoe lectin 1, *Viscum album* agglutinin 1 = VAA-1) is one of the best investigated biological response modifiers so far.

Biochemistry of the mistletoe lectins

"Lectins are sugar-binding proteins or glycoproteins of non-immune origin which are devoid of enzymatic activity towards sugars to which they bind and do not require free glycosidic hydroxyl groups of these sugars for their binding" [4]. They agglutinate cells and/or precipitate glycoconjugates [5]. Lectins are a structurally

Immunomodulatory Agents from Plants, edited by H. Wagner

diverse group of proteins capable of binding mono-, di- or oligosaccharides with considerable specificity. They are found in different organs of nearly all organisms and serve to mediate cellular regulation and biological recognition events. Recent developments support the idea that some of the plant lectins are involved in the defense mechanisms of these plants [6–8]. The first lectin described by Stillmark in 1888 was ricin [9] which is structurally closely related to the toxic lectins from the European mistletoe *Viscum album* L.

The hemagglutinating activities of mistletoe extracts were first detected by Krüpe [10], Bird [11] and Pardoe et al. [12]. Affinity chromatography was the method of choice to purify these lectins. The different matrices used were fixed erythrocytes [13], immobilized immunoglobulins [14], or agarose gels [15–17]. The European mistletoe contains different lectins which can be separated into two subgroups with different sugar specificities [17]. The mistletoe lectin 1 (VAA-1) is best inhibited by galactose and its derivatives whereas lectin 2 (VAA-2) is N-acetylgalactosamine specific in close analogy to the lectins from castor bean *Ricinus communis* L. or jequirity bean *Abrus precatorius* L. [17]. There is still some confusion on the number and nomenclature of the different mistletoe lectins. Samtleben et al. [17] separated the agglutinins into only two groups (VAA-1, VAA-2) in close analogy to the other toxic plant lectins. Franz and coworkers [18] described three different types of lectins (ML1, ML2, ML3). Structurally, and as far as the sugar binding specificity is concerned, VAA-1 corresponds to ML 1 and VAA-2 to ML 3. Whether the mistletoe lectin 2 (ML 2) according to the definition of Franz et al. with a sugar specificity for galactose and N-acetylgalactos- amine is an independent lectin or an isolectin form of VAA-1 or VAA-2 is still a matter of controversy [18]. In the following, only the generally accepted three letter code for lectins is used for the mistletoe agglutinins (VAA).

Very recently a novel, totally different lectin has been isolated from the mistletoe by Peumans et al. [19]. On the basis of its structure and specifity towards oligomers of N-acetylglucosamine it belongs to the widespread family of chitin-binding plant lectins and was preliminary named *Viscum album* chitin binding agglutinin (Visalb-CBA). At present one can only speculate about the possible involvement of Visalb-CBA in the therapeutic effects of mistletoe preparations. A similar chitin-binding lectin from the rhizomes of stinging nettle (*Urtica dioica*) is a potent superantigen in mice [20] (see Tab. 1).

The mistletoe lectins belong to the interesting family of toxic plant lectins: ricin, abrin, modeccin and volkensin. They share a similar protein structure, subunit organization and considerable sequence homology [17]. The native lectins from *Viscum album* L. are composed of two dissimilar subunits: the A-chain with ribosome-inactivating activity in a cell free extract and the slightly larger B-chain, which possess the galactose (VAA-1) or N-acetylgalactosamine (VAA-2) binding activity. Both subunits are connected by disulfide bonds to form the holotoxin. Under physiological conditions VAA-1 forms a dimer by non-covalent interactions.

Table 1 - Biochemical properties of the different mistletoe lectins

Lectin	VAA 1 (ML 1)	VAA 2 (ML 3)	VAA ? (ML 2)	VisalbCBA
Mol.mass	63 kDa	60 kDa	60 kDa	ca. 10 kDa
Subunits	2	2	2	no
A-chain	31 kDa	29 kDa	28 kDa	
B-chain	34 kDa	32 kDa	30 kDa	
Specificity	Gal>GalNAc	GalNAc>Gal	Gal=GalNAc	$(GluNAc)_n$
Glycosylation	yes	yes	yes	n.d.
Toxicity to mice, i.p.	28 µg/kg	55 µg/kg	1.5 mg/kg	n.d.

n.d., not determined

Structure of the mistletoe lectins:

VAA-1: $[A_I - S - S - B_I]_2$ VAA-2: $A_{II} - S - S - B_{II}$

These proteins are potent inhibitors of eukaryotic protein synthesis. They function as N-glycosidases to remove a specific adenine residue, A_{4324} in rat liver, from 28S rRNA [21–23] leading to an impaired ability of ribosomes to bind elongation factors. These ribosome inactivating proteins (RIPs) have been generally grouped into two types. Type 1 RIPs consist of a single peptide chain and have a molecular mass of 23–32 kDa. They exhibit a typical alkaline pI of 8.0 to 10.0. Type 2 RIPs consist of an A chain, which is essentially equivalent to a type 1 RIP, disulfide linked to a lectin like B chain that binds the RIP to cell surfaces and facilitates entry of the A chain into the cytosol. Thus, the type 2 RIPs are potent cell toxins whereas the type 1 RIPs are most active in a cell-free translation system.

The toxic plant lectins are commonly classified according to their monosaccharide specificity (Gal or GalNAc). Both α- and β-galactosyl residues are recognized equally well. From the galactosyl disaccharides tested the highest affinity to VAA-1 is found with Galβ(1–2)Gal or Galβ(1–3)Gal. Polymers having ten or more terminal galactosyl residues have a 500-fold higher affinity to VAA-1 than Gal [24].

Mistletoe lectins have been extensively analyzed for their primary structure. Only the complete amino acid sequence of the A chain of mistletoe lectin 1 (VAA-1) has been determined thus far [25] but the data show a great homology with other ribosome inactivating proteins such as abrin a or ricin D with 111 and 103 amino acid residues conserved, respectively.

The complete amino acid sequence of the VAA-1 A-chain is [25]:

Y E R L R L R V T H Q T T G E E Y F R F I T L L R D Y V S S G S F S N E I P L L R Q
25
S T I P V S D A Q R F V L V E L T N Q G Q D S V T A A I D V T N A Y V V A Y Q A G
50 75
D Q S Y F L R D A P R G A E T H L F T G T T R S S L P F N G S Y P D L E R Y A G H
100
R D Q I P L G I D Q L I Q S V T A L R F P G G S T R T Q A R S I L I L I Q M I S E A A
125 150
R F N P I L W R Y R Q Y I N S G A S F L P D V Y M L E L E T S W G Q Q S T Q V Q H
175 200
S T D G V F N N P I R L A I P P G N F V T L T N V R D V I A S L A I M L F V C G E R
225 250
P S S S.

The plant-derived ribosome inactivating proteins are widely distributed throughout the plant kingdom. They may be found in virtually all parts of a plant and may accumulate to significant amounts. RIPs exist in multigene families on plant genomes [26, 27].

In using RIPs for therapy, protein purity is an important issue that may be resolved by expression of cloned genes. Another reason for expression of cloned genes is to be able to control the type and extent of glycosylation. If used as a therapeutic agent, RIPs that are naturally glycosylated may be cleared from the circulation by binding of the sugar moiety through mannose-dependent recognition in the liver.

The initial cloning experiments for the misteletoe lectin VAA-1 were done by Zinke et al. [28]. Expression vectors containing either the A-chain coding region or the B-chain coding region were constructed. Expression studies in *E. coli* gave insoluble inclusion bodies which were subjected to purification and, after renaturation, fully functional active A- and B-chains were obtained which could be coupled *in vitro* to yield the active holotoxin. Although a more prominent GalNAc-specifity was found for the recombinant mistletoe lectin (rVAA), the biological activities (MOLT4-cytotoxicity, RIP-activity, induction of apoptosis, induction of cytokine secretion in PBMC) are not altered. The recombinant (non-glycosylated) VAA-1 A-chain was found to be about three times less active as a protein biosynthesis inhibitor in a cell-free translation system than the A-chain from plant material [29].

Immunomodulatory effects of VAA-1 *in vitro*

Cytotoxic and apoptotic effects of VAA-1

The cytotoxic and apoptotic activity of lectins may represent a conserved mechanism in elimination of altered cells. As a member of the type 2 RIPs, VAA-1 has been

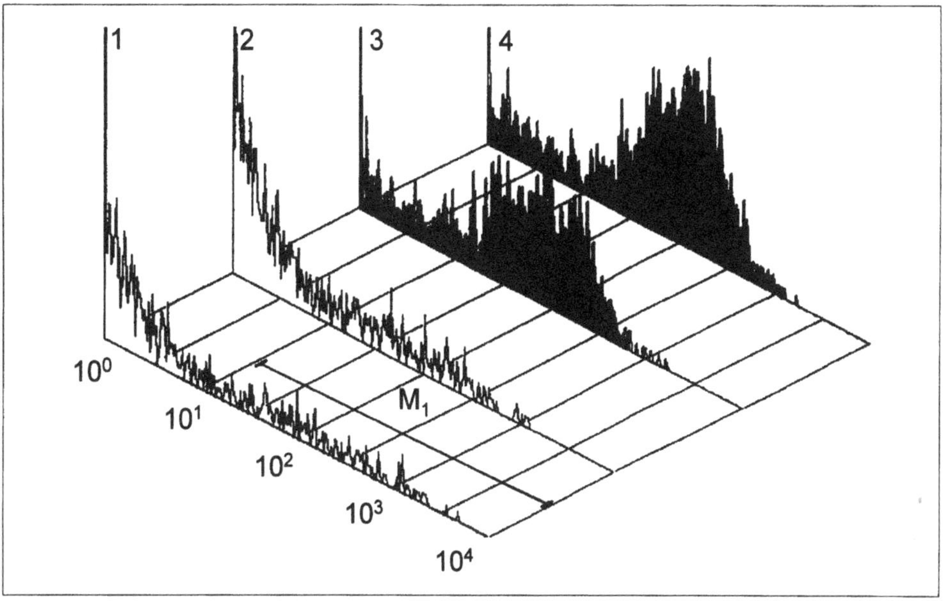

Figure 1
Representative flow-cytometric histograms of VAA-1-induced apoptotic effect by the TUNEL assay in culture of 1x10⁶/well human PBL incubated with medium (1), 0.1% sodium azide (2), 100 ng/ml VAA-1 (3) and 1 µg/ml VAA-1 (4) for 24 h. x-axis represents the logarithmic scale of green fluorescence intensity (FITC) and the y-axis the number of cells. Percentages of end-labelled apoptotic cells in the region M_1 were 8% (1), 9.3 % (2), 45.6 % (3) and 57 % (4), respectively. Region M_1 was set using sample (1) as control.

shown to induce cytotoxic effects in cultures of various eukaryotic cells *in vitro* [23, 30–34]. In cultures of human peripheral blood mononuclear cells (PBMC) incubated with VAA-1 for 24 h, the cell viability was found to be significantly affected above 10 ng/ml lectin concentration [35]. Recently, there is growing evidence that VAA-1-induced cell killing is mediated by induction of apoptosis [31, 36]. In a 24 h culture of human peripheral lymphocytes, in the presence of various concentrations of VAA-1 (between 1 µg/ml and 1 ng/ml), flow cytometric investigations with propidium iodide (PI) in hypotonic buffer and quantitative assessment of DNA breaks with terminal deoxynucleotydil transferase (TdT)-mediated dUTP-digoxigenin nick end-labeling (TUNEL) assay [37] revealed a dose-dependent VAA-1 induced apoptosis above 10 ng/ml lectin concentration (Fig. 1). Isolated A-chain showed the similar apoptotic effect as the whole lectin molecule. B-chain, however, was not effective [37].

These results suggest that inhibition of protein synthesis by the ribosome-inactivating A-chain can be responsible for the whole lectin molecule-induced apoptosis.

In a culture of U-937 promonocytes, VAA-1 (30–100 ng/ml) caused an increase in cytosolic Ca^{2+} concentration which is also a signal for apoptosis [38]. In addition, the same concentrations of VAA-1 enhanced the histamine (H1) and complement (C5a) induced raises in cytosolic Ca^{2+} concentration which play an accelerating role in the regulation of apoptosis [38]. Not only lectins with RIP activity cause apoptosis. *Griffonia simplicifolia* 1 B_4 and wheat germ agglutinin also trigger programmed cell death in cultures of various cell lines [39]. The triggering of apoptosis by lectin-sugar interactions raises the question whether this is solely an *in vitro* phenomenon or whether it has some biological significance *in vivo* and therefore it may be interesting to research its therapeutic potential.

Lectin-induced gene expression and secretion of proinflammatory cytokines

The effects of VAA-1 on the cellular mechanisms of the human immune system are not fully understood. It has been suggested that lectin-induced proinflammatory cytokines such as interleukin (IL)-1, IL-6 and tumor necrosis factor (TNF)-α are, at least in part, involved in its immunomodulatory potency [40]. After 24 h incubation of PBMC with non-cytotoxic concentrations of VAA-1 (10 ng/ml and 1 ng/ml), mRNA expression and secretion of a panel of cytokines were evaluated by reverse polymerase chain reaction (rPCR) and by ELISAs, respectively [35]. The lectin induced expression of IL-1α, IL-1β, IL-6, TNFα, interferon-(IFN)-γ, granulocyte-monocyte colony stimulating factor (GM-CSF) and IL-10 genes, but no expression of IL-2 and IL-5 genes could be detected. These results are related to an incubation of PBMC for 24 h with serum free medium and a shorter incubation of PMBC with higher concentrations of VAA-1 induced similar TNFα gene expression [41]. After 24 h incubation, IL-1β, IL-6 and TNFα production was induced by 1 and 10 ng/ml VAA-1. IL-10 secretion was only stimulated by 1 ng/ml lectin. No IL-2 or IFNγ production could be detected.These findings suggest that the cell source of lectin-induced cytokine production is likely to reside in monocytes. This hypothesis is supported by the prevailing detection of monocyte-derived cytokines such as IL-1α, IL-1β, TNFα, and IL-10. The results are also in agreement with another observation in that the amount of TNFα released from human PBMC correlates with the percentage of monocytes in cell cultures [40]. In addition, human peripheral blood monocytes isolated from healthy donors show dose-dependent enhanced secretions of proinflammatory cytokines in the presence of VAA-1 or VAA-2 [40, 42]. Under these conditions, D-galactose, a competitive inhibitor of the binding of VAA-1 to galactoside residues on the cell membrane, caused a marked inhibition [40]. The analysis of binding of FITC-conjugated VAA-1 to leukocytes [35] showed a higher affinity to monocytes than to lymphocytes (Fig. 2).

Thus, lectin-sugar interactions on the cell surface of monocytes may be primarily responsible for the cytokine secretion induced by VAA-1. In monocyte cultures THP-1

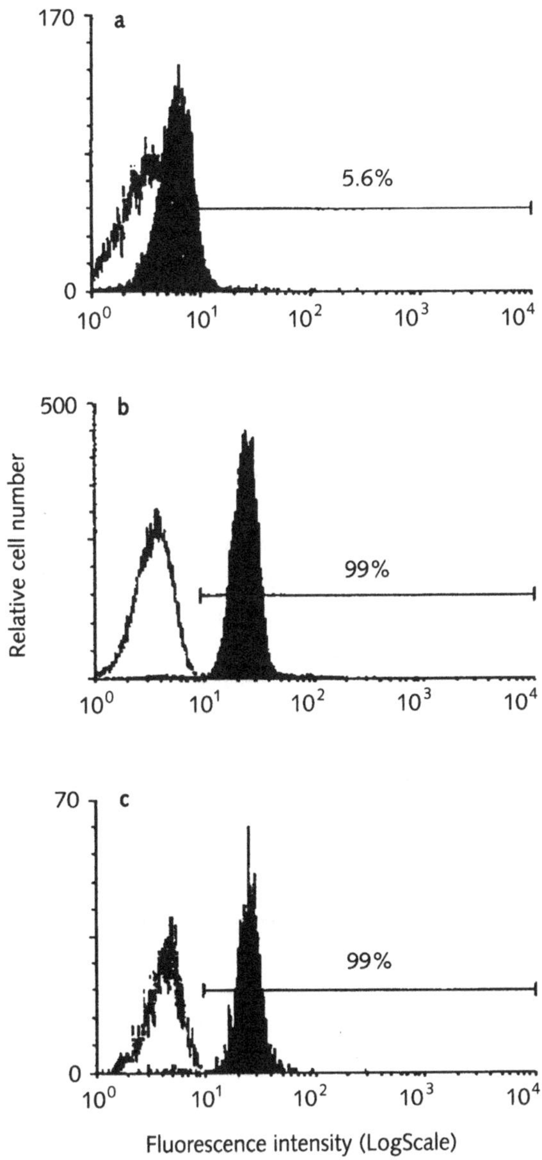

Figure 2
Binding of FITC-conjugated VAA-1 to different leukocytes in lysed whole blood of one donor as a representative example. Percentages of positively stained lymphocytes (a), granulocytes (b) and monocytes (c) are shown as a shift towards the right in comparison to fluorescence obtained with control. The percent of fluorescence-shifted cells is given in each histogram. As negative control unlabelled VAA-1 at a 100-fold concentration was used.

cells VAA-1 caused alterations in the level of the inositol phosphatases and phosphatidylinositols indicating lectin-induced signal-transducing events in monocytes [43].

In vitro effect of VAA-1 on cellular parameters of natural immunity and on hematopoietic progenitor cells

More than 12 years ago VAA-1 and its B-chain were found to stimulate the phagocytic activity of human leukocytes [44]. Similar to monocytes, granulocytes were also found to have a higher affinity to VAA-1 [35]. VAA-1 induces a stronger superoxide release from human neutrophils than other lectins [45]. Ca^{2+} entry plays a part in the activation of O_2-formation by phagocytic cells. VAA-1 has been shown to activate Ca^{2+} entry into neutrophiles indicating a galactoside-specific activation of a signal-transduction pathway [46]. Recent results indicate that an other important member of natural immunity, the NK-cells, are also stimulated by VAA-1 *in vitro*. This was in an additive manner, being enhanced by its combination with IL-2 and IL12 (*Nat Immun; in press*). Since proinflammatory events exhibit regulatory effects on bone marrow functions, the question arised as to whether VAA-1 can influence the proliferation of progenitor cells. $CD34^+$ hematopoietic progenitor cells were found to bind VAA-1 [47, 48]. $CD34^+$ cells have also been shown to bind other lectins [49, 50], but VAA-1 has a costimulatory effect on their proliferation too. In cultures of PBMC and bone marrow $CD34^+$ cells, coincubation of VAA-1 with other hematopoietic growth factors induced a dose-dependent increase in clonogenic growth. Morphological investigations of single colonies revealed that the growth of both erythroid and granulocyte/macrophage progenitor cells was stimulated [48].

***In vivo* effects of VAA-1 on cellular parameters of natural immunity in animal models and in healthy human persons**

In cancer patients the mechanisms of natural immunity, which are believed to serve as essential functions for their survival, are often significantly decreased [51, 52]. Investigations on animal models and clinical observations with extracts standardized on galactoside-binding lectin activity suggest that the immunomodulatory efficacy of VAA-1 is necessary for its beneficial effects [53–55]. Therefore, the proof of an immunomodulatory effect of VAA-1 on human subjects requires reliable and repoducible monitoring of cellular and cytokine parameters. In animal models the NK system was found a suitable tool for immunological monitoring of the effect of lectin [53, 56, 57]. NK cells are a subpopulation of lymphocytes distinct from T and B cells that have the ability to mediate cytotoxicity and cytokine production. They represent 5–15% of lymphocytes in the blood and are associated with a particular morphology, that is, the large granular lymphocyte (LGL) phenotype.

To establish the modulatory potency of VAA-1 on the natural immunity of human subjects, four randomized, double blind, crossover pilot trials were performed on healthy volunteers. In contrast to the significant lectin-induced increases in number and activity of natural killer (NK) cells observed in animal models, in the first and second trial human healthy individuals showed no significant differences between their NK responses following injection of lectin-enriched preparation or saline. However, high intrinsic fluctuations of immune parameters were observed after saline injection in the blood of healthy persons. It should not be overlooked that the biological vulnerability of NK cells has been well established in various human studies [58–60] demonstrating an association between various effects of stress and a significantly reduced NK activity. These data may help also to determine why it has often been difficult to prove the effect of a biomodulator on host defense. Due to considerable intrinsic fluctuations of these parameters, a third and a fourth double blind trial with freshly isolated VAA-1 was performed using a more rapidly detectable parameter, the priming of granulocytes, to establish the modulatory potency of VAA-1 on the natural immunity of human subjects. In addition, the frequency of LGL cells was also morphologically evaluated. Significant lectin-induced increases were found (see Tab. 2).

The results of the third and the confirmatory fourth trial suggest that priming of PMNs and LGL frequency may be suitable for immunological monitoring of VAA-1 [61]. In addition, mistletoe extracts were also able to activate the priming of granulocytes and LGL frequency [62].

Clinical trials to demonstrate immunostimulation with VAA-1 or commercially available mistletoe extracts

Change of the immune parameters in humans

In cancer patients regular subcutaneous injections (four weeks) of the optimal dose of VAA-1 (1 ng per kg body weight (bw), twice a week) yielded notable increases in the apparent numbers of certain lymphocyte subsets such as pan T cells, helper T cells and NK cells [63]. However, controlled investigations of the immunological efficacies of this plant lectin revealed several difficulties as mentioned above [61]. Still, a phase I dose-finding study in tumor patients showed significant differences between 0.2, 1 and 5 ng/kg bw doses of VAA-1 (Fig. 3). Only a 1 ng/kg dose of VAA-1 was able to increase the NK and LAK activity in peripheral blood [64].

Need for immunologically active preparations

It has been shown that the optimal dose range of VAA-1 is narrow (0.5–2 ng/kg bw) [56, 64]. Previous preclinical data demonstrate that immunologically active appli-

Table 2 - Double blind crossover trials on healthy donors

Placebo				Therapeutics			
Rel. augm. in oxidative response of PMNs		LGL/µl		Rel. augm. in oxidative response of PMNs		LGL/µl	
5 h	24 h	0 h	24 h	5 h	24 h	0 h	24 h
Third trial (n=8)							
0.92	0.85	656	472	1.94**	1.32*	540	1052*
(0.25)	(0.29)	(163)	(137)	(0.59)	(0.43)	(173)	(364)
Confirmatory trial (n=6)							
1.04	0.8	639	578	3.56**	1.84*	555	1131*
(0.31)	(0.69)	(205)	(196)	(1.33)	(0.88)	(204)	(395)

*Mean relative augmentations (95% confidence intervals) of oxidative response of circulating polymorphonuclear leukocytes (PMNs) to pretreatment values were determined 5 h and 24 h after a single subcutaneous injection of purified VAA-1 and saline. In addition, absolute numbers of LGL cells in 1 µl blood were morphologically evaluated. Statistical analysis by paired t test verified significant differences between lectin and placebo responses (*p<0.05; **p<0.01).*

cation of VAA-1 to BALB/c and nude mice can induce an antimetastatic/antitumor effect on a lymphosarcoma (RAW 117), a fibrosarcoma (L1), and a xenotransplanted leiomyosarcoma model system [53, 54]. However, small doses of VAA-1 given twice a week, which has been found immunologically active in previous studies [55, 56], failed to act on chemically-induced tumor development in the urinary bladder of rats [65]. For the interpretation of these different results a comparative immunological estimation of preparations is necessary.

The immunomodulatory effects of VAA-1 showed a bell-shaped dose-response curve in animal models [56]. Therefore, to obtain clinical benefit, it appears to be desirable to apply standardized and active preparations in an immunologically most effective application schedule. Already three of the commercially available and clinically applied mistletoe preparations have been standardized on the contents of their immunomodulatory VAA 1.

Inflammatory processes after mistletoe lectin or extract application and the cytokine release

VAA-1 has been shown to induce proinflammatory cytokines *in vitro* [35, 40]. Standardized mistletoe extracts *in vivo* induced only small and short increases in the

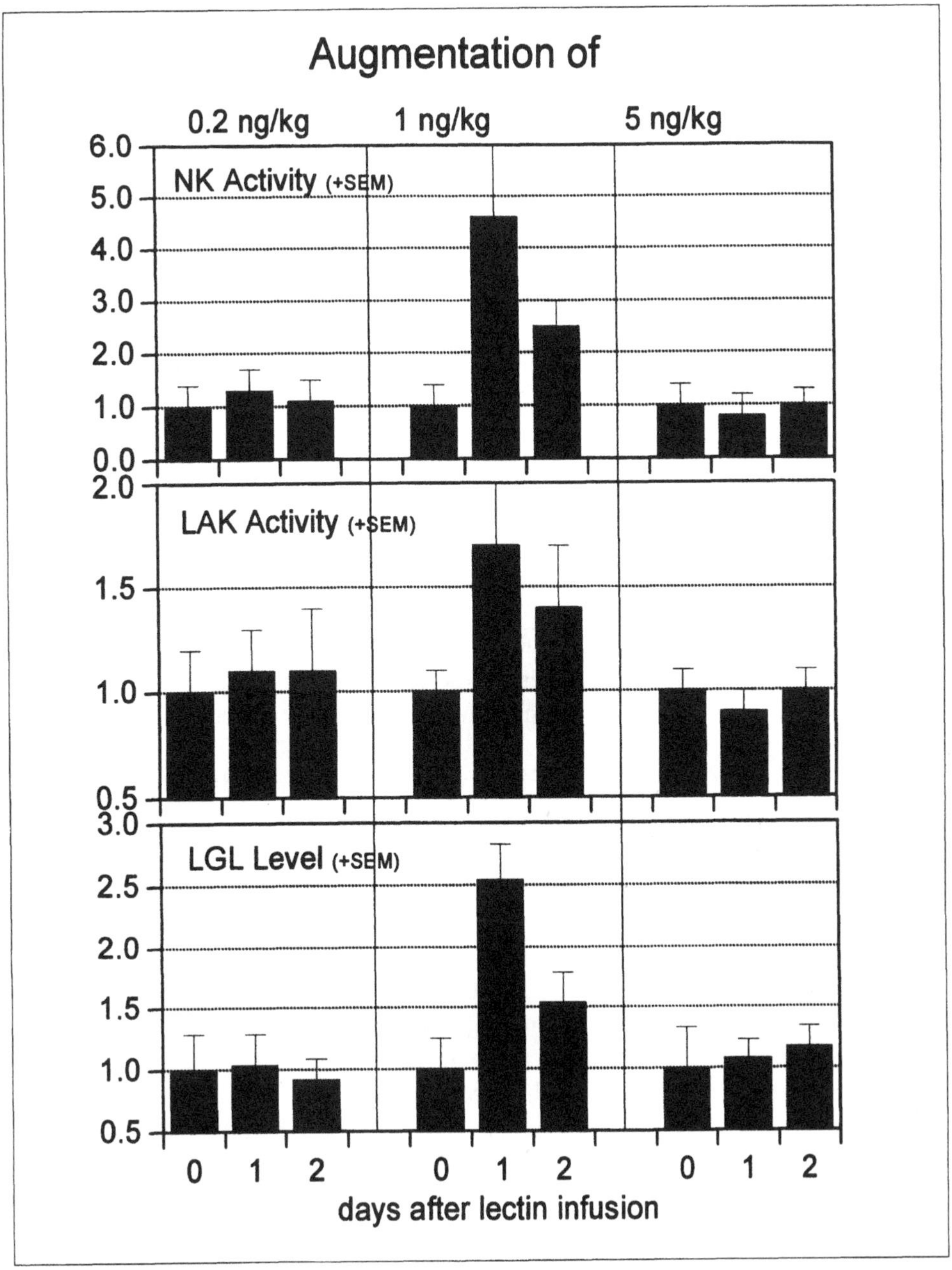

Figure 3
Relative mean augmentations (±SEM) of NK cytotoxicity, LAK activity and LGL frequency in peripheral blood of twenty cancer patients 24h and 48h after a single infusion of 0.2, 1.0 or 5.0 ng/kg bw (VAA-1). 24h after 1.0 ng/kg lectin the NK cytotoxicity, LAK activity and LGL level enhanced significantly relative to base line ($p<0.05$).

serum of tumor patients [40] indicating that these effects within physiological conditions remain without undesirable side effects (such as tumor growth stimulation etc.).

Mistletoe extracts in tumor therapy

Unvonventional therapies are very popular in the treatment of cancer, especially in Central Europe. The main motives are the "wish not to leave anything untried" and the "trust in the efficacy of the alternative treatment" [66]. In contrast to the wide application and acceptance of mistletoe extracts, controlled trials led to the conclusion that their application is not (yet) justified [67–71]. Kiene [72, 73] and Kleijnen and Knipschild [74] critically reviewed the mistletoe treatment for cancer in controlled trials in humans. As a final conclusion they recommended the use of mistletoe extracts only for cancer patients involved in these clinical trials [74].

Eleven controlled trials were analyzed (3 bronchus carcinoma, 3 mamma carcinoma, 2 colorectal carcinoma, 1 gastric cancer, 1 cervix carcinoma, 1 female genital carcinoma). Nearly all appeared to be of a very bad methodological quality. Randomization was done only in four studies. In no trial was there an attempt for double blinding. The positive results given by the corresponding authors of the trials (1 = no effect, 6 = trend for and 4 = significant positive results) were critically reevaluated and could not be confirmed.

The best trial so far was done by Dold et al. [75]. In a randomized multi-center trial they assessed the effects of Iscador® with a multivitamin preparation (as a placebo) in 408 patients with advanced non-small-cell bronchial carcinoma. The median survival time was 9.1 and 7.6 months for the Iscador® and placebo groups, respectively. The difference is not statistically significant but has a positive trend for the Iscador® group [74].

In the published trials mistletoe extracts of different origin (host tree) and mode of preparations have been used. Assuming that the lectin VAA-1 is an active component, its content in the extracts varies with the host tree, the season of mistletoe harvest, the extraction procedure, the fermentation, etc. This makes the trials no longer comparable. The demand for future clinical research and trials is the use of biologically active and reproducibly standardized preparations.

To circumvent the drawbacks of different preparations from plant material, recombinant mistletoe lectin might be the substance of choice. It can be prepared in large quantities of equal quality.The research of the recombinant form of VAA-1 may also give new clinical perspectives. Recent *in vitro* investigations with recombinant lectin revealed NK stimulatory effects in synergism with IL-2 and IL-12. Similar to plant lectin in animal models, recombinant VAA-1 was also able to stimulate the NK cell-mediated cytotoxic activity of splenocytes (*Nat Imm; in press*; Fig. 4).

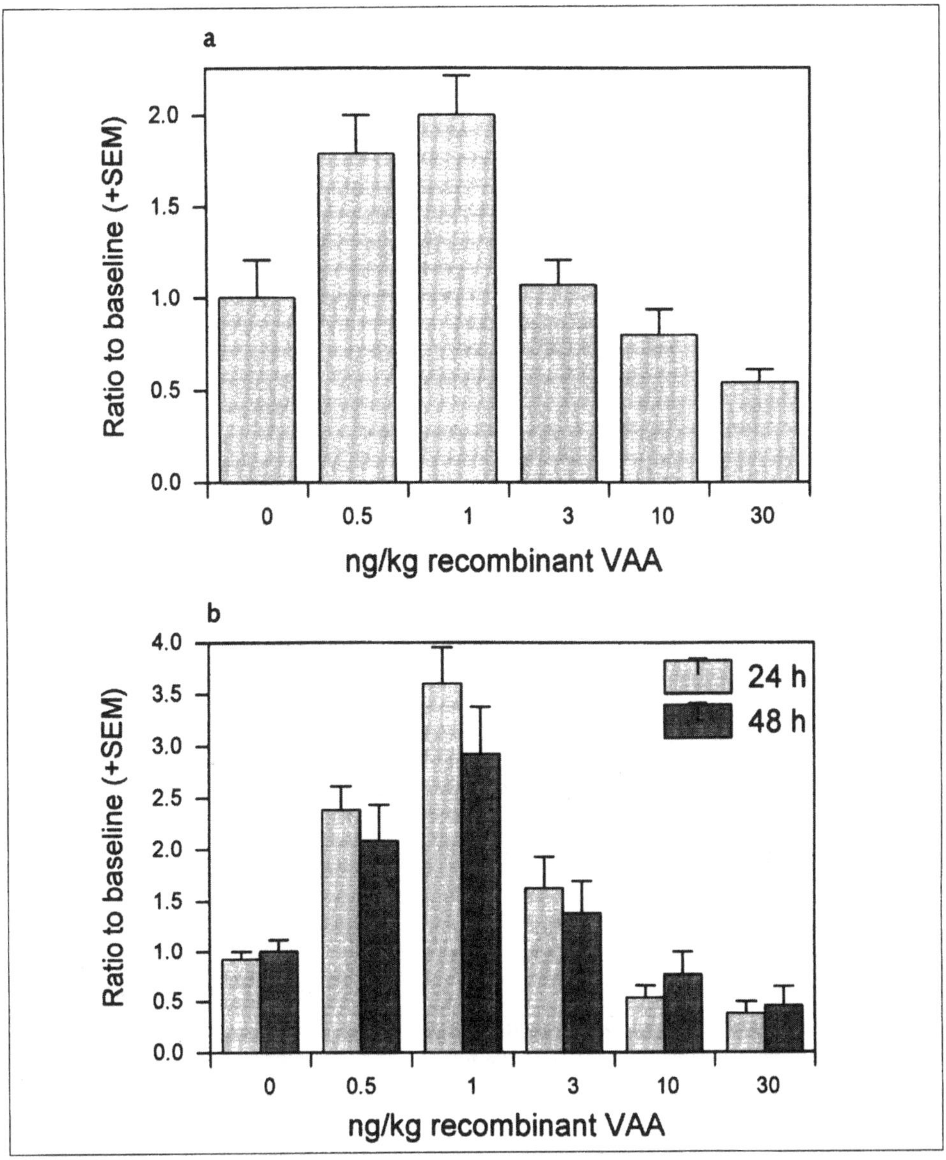

Figure 4

Immunological responses after a single intravenous injection of rVAA in rats. Six randomized groups each containing eight animals were treated once with placebo or with various doses of rVAA. Blood samples were collected before, 24 h and 48 h after a single injection. After two days all animals were sacrificed. The following parameters are shown: (a) NK-mediated cytotoxicity of splenocytes against YAC-1 cells (after 48 h) expressed in mean relative augmentations (±SEM) of lytic units ($10^7/LU_{33}$) of each group as ratios to control one; (b) mean relative enhancements (±SEM) in absolute counts of LGLs in peripheral blood.

There is still a great deal of uncertainty regarding the actual role that immunity plays in the control of human malignancy [76–79]. Until this point is settled, the role of immunostimulating mistletoe extracts will also remain open. Nevertheless, the immunosuppression that accompanies tumor development affects the patient, at least indirectly, by the predisposition to infections. It complicates the treatment and can be a major cause of mortality (e. g. in multiple myeloma patients). How to cope with opportunistic infections seems worth investigating since positive results might have therapeutic implications. Further, it has been reported that mistletoe treatment may improve the life quality of cancer patients by inducing β-endorphin release [80].

References

1 v. Tubeuf K (ed) (1923) *Monographie der Mistel.* R. Oldenbourg Verlag, München und Berlin

2 Luther P, Becker H (eds) (1987) *Die Mistel. Botanik, Lektine, medizinische Anwendung.* VEB Verlag Volk und Gesundheit, Berlin

3 Steiner R: Vortrag vom 2. April 1920, in Steiner R (ed) *Geisteswissenschaft und Medizin.* Verlag der R. Steiner Nachlassverwaltung, Dornach, 246–263

4 Goldstein IJ, Hughes RC, Monsigny M, Osawa T, Sharon N (1980) What should be called a lectin? *Nature* 285: 66

5 Kocourek J, Horejsi V (1981) Defining a lectin. *Nature* 290: 188

6 Chrispeels MJ, Raikhel NV (1991) Lectins, lectin genes, and their role in plant defense. *Plant Cell* 3: 1–9

7 Peumans WJ, Van Damme EJM (1995) Lectins as plant defense proteins. *Plant Physiol* 109: 347–352

8 Peumans WJ, Van Damme EJM (1995) The role of lectins in plant defense. *Histochem J* 27: 253–271

9 Stillmark H (1888) *Über Ricin, ein giftiges Ferment aus den Samen von Ricinus comm. L und einigen anderen Euphorbiaceen.* Thesis. Dorpat 1888

10 Krüpe M (1956) *Blutgruppenspezifische pflanzliche Eiweisskörper.* Enke, Stuttgart

11 Bird G (1958) *Erythrocyte agglutinins from plants.* PhD Thesis, London

12 Pardoe G, Bird G, Uhlenbruck G, Sprenger I, Heggen M (1970) Heterophile agglutinins with a broad spectrum specificity. 4. The nature of cell surface receptors for the agglutinins present in the seeds of *Amaranthus caudatus, Maclura aurantica, Datura stramonium, Viscum album, Phaseolus vulgaris* and *Molucella laevis. Z Immunitätsforsch* 140: 374–394

13 Luther P, Mehnert W, Graffi A, Prokop O (1973) Reaktionen einiger antikörperähnlicher Substanzen aus Insekten (Protektinen) und Pflanzen (Lektine) mit Ascites-Tumorzellen. *Acta Biol Med Germ* 31: K11–K18

14 Franz H, Haustein B, Luther P, Kuropka U, Kindt A (1977) Isolierung und Charakterisierung von Inhaltstoffen der Mistel (*Viscum album* L.). 1. Affinitätschromatographie

von Mistelrohextrakt an insolubilisierten Plasmaproteinen. *Acta Biol Med Germ* 36: 113–117

15 Lutsik M (1975) The antitumor activity of phythemagglutinin from *Viscum album* L. *Dokl Acad Sci USSR*, Ser B, No 6: 541–544

16 Ziska P, Franz H, Kindt A (1978) The lectin from *Viscum album* L. Purification by biospecific affinity chromatography. *Experentia* 34: 123–124

17 Samtleben R, Kiefer M, Luther P (1985) Characterization of the different lectins from *Viscum album* (mistletoe) and their structural relationships with the agglutinins from *Abrus precatorius* and *Ricinus communis*. In: Bog-Hansen TC, Breborowicz J (eds): *Lectins: Biology, biochemistry, clinical biochemistry*, Vol 4. DeGruyter, Berlin New York, 617–626

18 Franz H (1986) Mistletoe lectins and their A and B chains. *Oncology* 43 (Suppl 1): 23–34

19 Peumans WJ, Verhaert P, Pfüller U, Van Damme EJM (1996) Isolation and characterization of a small chitin-binding lectin from mistletoe (Viscum album). *FEBS Lett* 396: 261–265

20 Galelli A, Delcourt M, Wagner MC, Peumans W, Truffa-Bachi P (1995) Selective expansion followed by profound deletion of mature Vb8.3$^+$ T cells *in vivo* after exposure to the superantigenic lectin *Urtica dioica* agglutinin. *J Immunol* 154: 2600–2611

21 Endo Y, Mitsui K, Motizuki M, Tsurugi K (1987) The mechanism of action of ricin and toxic lectins on eukaryotic ribosomes. *J Biol Chem* 262: 5908–5912

22 Endo Y, Tsurugi K (1987) RNA-glycosidase activity of ricin A-chain. *J Biol Chem* 262: 8128–8130

23 Endo Y, Tsurugi K, Franz H (1988) The site of action of the A-chain of mistletoe lectin 1 on eukaryotic ribosomes: the RNA N-glycosidase activity of the protein. *FEBS Lett* 231: 378–380

24 Lee RT, Gabius HJ, Lee YC (1992) Ligand binding characteristics of the major mistletoe lectin. *J Biol Chem* 267: 23722–23727

25 Soler MH, Stoeva S, Schwamborn C, Wilhelm S, Stiefel T, Voelter W (1996) Complete amino acid sequence of the A chain of mistletoe lectin 1. *FEBS Lett* 399: 153–157

26 Halling KC, Halling AC, Murray EE, Ladin BF, Houston LL, Weaver RF (1985) Genomic cloning and characterization of a ricin gene from Ricinus communis. *Nucleic Acids Res* 13: 8019–8033

27 Chow TP, Feldman RA, Lovett M, Piatak M (1990) Isolation and DNA sequence of a gene encoding a-trichosanthin, a type 1 ribosome inactivating protein. *J Biol Chem* 265: 8670–8674

28 Zinke H, Eck J, Langer M, Möckel B, Baur A, Lentzen H (1996) Molecular cloning of the *Viscum album* L. (mistletoe) gene for ML-1 and characterization of the recombinant protein. *Phytomedicine* 3: Suppl 1, 25

29 Langer M, Rothe M, Eck J, Möckel B, Zinke H (1996) A nonradioactive assay for ribosome-inactivating proteins. *Anal Biochem* 243: 150–153

30 Dietrich JB, Ribereau G, Jung ML, Franz H, Beck JP, Anton R (1992) Identity of the N-

terminal sequences of the three A-chains of mistletoe (*Viscum album* L.) lectins: homology with ricin-like plant toxins and single-chain ribosome-inactivating proteins. *Anticancer Drugs* 3: 507–511
31 Janssen O, Scheffler A, Kabelitz D (1993) *In vitro* effects of mistletoe extracts and mistletoe lectins. Cytotoxicity towards tumor cells due to the induction of programmed cell death (apoptosis). *Drug Res* 43: 1221–1227
32 Stirpe F, Barbieri L, Batelli MG, Soria M, Lappi DA (1992) Ribosome-inactivating proteins from plants: present status and future prospects. *BioTechnology* 10: 405–412
33 Schumacher U, Stamouli A, Adam E, Peddie M, Pfüller U (1995) Biochemical, histochemical and cell biological investigations on the actions of mistletoe lectins I, II and III with human breast cancer cell lines. *Glycoconjugate J* 12: 250–257
34 Ribereau-Gayon G, Jung ML, Beck JP (1995) Effect of foetal calf serum on the cytotoxic activity of mistletoe (*Viscum album* L.) lectins in cell culture. *Phytother Res* 9: 336–339
35 Hostanska K, Hajto T, Spagnoli GC, Fischer J, Lentzen H, Herrmann R (1995) A plant lectin derived from *Viscum album* induces cytokine gene expression and protein production in cultures of human peripheral blood mononuclear cells. *Nat Immun* 14: 295–304
36 Büssing A, Suzart K, Bergmann J, Pfüller U, Schietzel M, Schweizer K (1996) Induction of apoptosis in human lymphocytes treated with *Viscum album* L. is mediated by mistletoe lectins. *Cancer Letters* 99: 59–72
37 Hostanska K, Hajto T, Weber K, Fischer J, Lentzen H, Sütterlin B, Saller R (1996–97) A natural immunity activating plant lectin, *Viscum album* agglutinin-I (VAA-I) induces apoptosis in human lymphocytes, monocytes, monocytic THP-1 cells and murine thymocytes. *Nat Immun* 15: 295–311
38 Wenzel-Seifert K, Lentzen H, Seifert R (1997) In U-937 promonocytes, mistletoe lectin I increases basal $[Ca^{2+}]i$, enhances histamin H1- and complement C5a-receptor-mediated rises in $[Ca^{2+}]i$, and induces cell death. *Naunyn-Schmiedeberg's Arch Pharmacol* 355: 190–197
39 Kim M, Rao MV, Tweardy DJ, Prakash M, Galili U, Gorelik E (1993) Lectin induced apoptosis of tumor cells. *Glycobiology* 3: 447–453.
40 Hajto T, Hostanska K, Frei K, Rohrdorf C, Gabius HJ (1990) Increased secretion of tumor necrosis factor α, interleukin 1, and interleukin 6 by human mononuclear cells exposed to β-galactoside-specific lectin from clinically applied mistletoe extract. *Cancer Res* 50: 3322–3326
41 Männel DN, Becker H, Gundt A, Kist A, Franz H (1991) Induction of tumor necrosis factor expression by a lectin from *Viscum album*. *Cancer Immunol Immunother* 33: 177–182
42 Ribereau-Gayon G, Dumont S, Muller C, Jung ML, Poindron P, Anton R (1996) Mistletoe lectins I, II and III induce the production of cytokines by cultured human monocytes. *Cancer Letters* 109: 33–38.
43 Walzel H, Bremer H, Gabius HJ (1993) Lectin-induced alterations in the level of phos-

pholipids, inositol phosphates, and phosphoproteins. In: Gabius HJ, Gabius S (eds): *Lectins and glycobiology*. Springer-Verlag, Berlin, 357–361

44 Metzner G, Franz H, Kindt A, Fahlbusch B, Süss J (1985) The *in vitro* activity of lectin from mistletoe (ML-I) and its isolated A and B chains on functions of macrophages and polymorphonuclear cells. *Immunobiol* 169: 461–471

45 Timoshenko AV, Gabius HJ (1993) Efficient induction of superoxide release from human neutrophils by the galactoside-specific lectin from *Viscum album*. *Biol Chem Hoppe-Seyler* 374: 237–243

46 Wenzel-Seifert K, Krautwurst D, Lentzen H, Seifert R (1996) Concanavalin A and mistletoe lectin I differentially activate cation entry and exocytosis in human neutrophils: lectins may activate multiple subtypes of cation channels. *J Leuko Biol* 60: 345–355

47 Mann KK, Andre S, Gabius HJ, Sharp G (1994) Phenotype-associated lectin-binding profils of normal and transformed blood cells: a comparative analysis of mannose- and galactose-binding lectins from plants and human serum/placenta. *Eur J Cell Biol* 65: 145–151

48 Vehmeyer K, Hajto T, Hostanska K, Könermann S, Lösert H, Saller R,Wörmann B (1998) Lectin-induced increase in clonogenic growth of hematopoietic progenitor cells. *Eur J Hematol* 60: 16–20

49 Unverzagt KL, Martinson J, Lee W, Stiff PJ, Williams S, Bender JG (1996) Identification of human erythroid progenitor cell population which express the CD34 antigen and binds the plant lectin Ulex europaeus I. *Cytometry* 23: 54–58

50 Kuemmel TA, Thiele J, Blaeser AH, Wickenhauser C, Baldus SE, Fischer R (1997) Lectin binding sites on CD34+ human hematopoietic stem cells and lymphocytes from peripheral blood: an ultrastructural post-embedding study. *Histochem J* 29: 695–705

51 Shau H, Roth MD, Golub SH (1993) Regulation of natural killer function by nonlymphoid cells. *Nat Immun* 12: 235–249

52 Karimine N, Nanbara S, Arinaga S, Asoh T, Ueo H, Akiyoshi T (1994) Lymphokine-activated killer cell activity of peripheral blood, spleen, regional lymph node, and tumor infiltrating lymphocytes in gastric cancer patients. *J Surg Oncol* 55: 179–185

53 Hajto T, Hostanska K, Steinberg F, Gabius HJ (1989) Galactoside-specific lectin from clinically applied mistletoe extract reduces tumor growth by augmentation of host defense system. *Blut* 61: 164

54 Beuth J, Ko HL, Gabius HJ, Pulverer G (1991) Influence of treatment with the immunomodulatory effective dose of the β-galactoside-specific lectin from mistletoe on tumor colonization in BALB/c-mice for two experimental model systems. *In vivo* 5: 29–32

55 Hajto T, Hostanska K, Fornalski M, Kirsch A (1991) Antitumorale Aktivität des immunmodulatorisch wirkenden Beta-galaktosidspezifischen Mistellektins bei der klinischen Anwendung von Mistelextrakten (Iscador). *Dtsch Zschr Onkol* 23: 1–6

56 Hajto T, Hostanska K, Gabius HJ (1989) Modulatory potency of the β-galactoside-spe-

cific lectin from mistletoe extract (Iscador) on the host defense system *in vivo* in rabbits and patients. *Cancer Res* 49: 4803–4808

57 Joshi SS, Komanduri KC, Gabius S, Gabius HJ (1991) Immunotherapeutic effects of purified mistletoe lectin ML-I on murine large cell lymphoma. In: Gabius S, Gabius HJ (eds): *Lectins in cancer*. Springer-Verlag, Heidelberg, 207–217

58 Levy S, Herberman R, Lippman M, d'Angelo T (1987) Correlation of stress factors with sustained depression of natural killer cell activity and predicted prognosis in patients with breast cancer. *J Clin Oncol* 5: 348–353

59 Kiecolt-Glaser JK, Glaser R, Strain E, Stout JC, Tarr KL, Holliday JE, Speicher CE (1986) Modulation of cellular immunity in medical students. *J Behav Med* 9: 5–21

60 Kiecolt-Glaser JK, Ricker D, George J, Messick G,. Speicher CE, Garner W, Glaser R (1984) Urinary cortisol levels, cellular immunocompetency, and loneliness in psychiatric inpatients. *Psychosom Med* 46: 15–23

61 Hajto T, Hostanska K, Fischer J, Lentzen H (1996) Investigations of cellular parameters to establish the response of a biomodulator: galactoside-specific lectin from *Viscum album* plant extract. *Phytomedicine* 3: 129–137

62 Hajto T, Hostanska K (1986) An investigation of the ability of *Viscum album*-activated granulocytes to regulate natural killer cells *in vivo*. *Clin Tri J* 23: 345–358

63 Beuth J, Ko HL, Gabius HJ, Burrichlet H, Oette K, Pulverer G (1992) Behaviour of lymphocyte subsets and expression of activation markers in response to immunotherapy with galactoside-specific lectin from mistletoe in breast cancer patients. *Clin Invest* 70: 658–661

64 Hajto T, Hostanska K, Herrmann R (1993) Immunomodulatory potency of mistletoe lectins in cancer patients. Results of a dose finding study. *Allergy* (Suppl) 48: 54

65 Kunze E, Schulz H, Ahrens H, Gabius HJ (1997) Lack of an antitumoral effect of immunomodulatory galactoside-specific mistletoe lectin on N-methyl-N-nitrosourea-induced urinary bladder carcinogenesis in rats. *Exp Toxic Pathol* 49: 167–180

66 Muthny FA, Bertsch C (1997) Why some cancer patients use unorthodox treatment and why others do not. *Onkologie* 20: 320–325

67 Hauser SP (1991) Unproven methods in oncology. *Eu. J Cancer* 27: 1549–1551

68 Hauser SP (1993) Klinische Anwendung von Mistelpräparaten in der Onkologie: Mistel – Wunderkraut oder Medikament? *Therapiewoche* 43: 76–81

69 Hauser SP (1997) Unproven treatments for lung cancer: a real alternative? *Atemwegs- und Lungenkrankheiten* 23: 331–335

70 Gabius HJ, Gabius S, Joshi SS, Koch B, Schroeder M, Manzke WM, Westerhausen M (1994) From ill-defined extracts to the immunomodulatory lectin: will there be a reason for oncological application of mistletoe? *Planta med* 60: 2–7

71 Gabius HJ, Gabius S (1997) Therapeutic relevance of immunomodulation by mistletoe preparations: Fact or fiction? *Int J Oncol* 11 (Suppl.): 886

72 Kiene H (1989) *Klinische Studien zur Misteltherapie der Krebserkrankung. Eine kritische Würdigung*. Dissertation. University of Witten/Herdecke

73 Kiene H (1989) Klinische Studien zur Misteltherapie Karzinomatöser Erkrankungen. Eine Übersicht. *Therapeutikon* 3: 347–353
74 Kleijnen J, Knipschild P (1994) Mistletoe treatment for cancer. Review of controlled trials in humans. *Phytomedicine* 1: 255–260
75 Dold U, Edler L, Mäurer HC, Müller-Wening D, Sakellariou B, Trendenelenburg F, Wagner G (1991) *Krebszusatztherapie beim fortgeschrittenen nicht-kleinzelligen Bronchialkarzinom.* Stuttgart, Georg Thieme Verlag
76 Sulitzeanu D (1985) Human cancer-associated antigens: present status and implications for immunodiagnosis. *Adv Cancer Res* 44: 1–42
77 Brunson KW, Goldfarb RH (1989) In: HE Kaiser (ed): *Cancer growth and progression.* Kluwer Academic Publishers, Dordrecht, 133–138
78 Sulitzeanu D (1993) Immunosuppressive factors in human cancer. *Adv Cancer Res* 60: 247–267
79 Kedar E, Klein E (1992) Cancer immunotherapy: are the results discouraging? Can they be improved? *Adv Cancer Res* 59: 245–322
80 Heiny BM, Beuth J (1994) Mistletoe extract standardized for the galactoside-specific lectin (ML-1) induces β-endorphin release and immunopotentiation in breast cancer patients. *Anticancer Res* 14: 1339–1342

Saponins as immunoadjuvants and immunostimulants

Marie-Aleth Lacaille-Dubois

Laboratoire de Pharmacognosie, Faculté de Pharmacie, Université de Bourgogne,
7, Bd Jeanne d'Arc, F-21033 Dijon Cedex, France

Introduction

Saponins are either triterpene or steroid glycosides widely distributed in the plant and animal kingdom and include a large number of biologically active compounds. Most of them have surface-active and cholesterol-binding properties.

They have been shown to exhibit a multitude of biological and pharmacological activities such as antiphlogistic, antiallergic, cytotoxic, antitumor and antitumor-promoting, antiviral, immunomodulating, antihepatotoxic, molluscicidal and antifungal activities. They are also acting on the cardiovascular, the central nervous and the endocrinal systems [1–3].

The present review focuses on the immune enhancing potential of saponins with mainly immunoadjuvant and immunostimulating properties.

Saponins as immunoadjuvants

Adjuvants (from the latin, adjuvare = to help) have been used to improve vaccine efficacy since the early 1929s. Currently many new vaccines are under development and there is a desire to find more effective adjuvants [4, 5]. Here we will give up-to-date information on specific vaccine adjuvants.

Definition of adjuvants

Traditional vaccines mainly composed of live attenuated or inactivated whole bacteria or viruses, often show unwanted side effects. New generations of vaccines will probably be composed of relevant antigen subunits derived either from the pathogen itself or prepared via molecular, biological or chemical techniques. However, formulations based on antigens or subunits bearing one or more B and T cell epitopes in a monomeric form are often weakly immunogenic when compared to traditional

Immunomodulatory Agents from Plants, edited by H. Wagner

vaccines. They need potent adjuvants or immune enhancers which increase the specific immune response to an antigen and induce immune protection [4, 6–8].

Adjuvants comprise a heterogeneous group of compounds. The only vaccine adjuvants currently licensed for human use are aluminium salts. All other adjuvants are considered experimental and must undergo special preclinical testing. Some triterpene saponins, most notably those originating from *Quillaja saponaria*, are potent immune adjuvants [9].

Saponin components for testing as adjuvants

The adjuvant activity of saponins has been known for more than 50 years [10]. Commercially available saponins frequently consist of highly heterogeneous preparations of varying composition, sometimes being little more than crude extracts of the bark of the South American soap tree, *Quillaja saponaria* (Rosaceae), which may be contamined with tannins. The major components, however, are bidesmosidic quillaic acid triterpene-saponins [10].

When used in vaccines, *Quillaja* extracts caused local reactions. This effect could be reduced by the use of purified fractions. Quil A, the pure compound QS-21 (**3**), ISCOMs and ISCOPREP 7.0.3 are the four major preparations used in experimental animal trials and in veterinary practice [11].

Quil A is a partially purified fraction, obtained through dialysis, ion exchange and gel filtration chromatography of an aqueous extract of the bark.

It is marketed as, and has been described to be, a potent adjuvant which has found widespread use in veterinary vaccines against, for example, foot and mouth disease, rabies, and in a number of experimental vaccines and in preclinical trials. Unfortunately its hemolytic activity and local counter reactions make it unsuitable for human vaccines [5]. Furthermore, Quil A is used for production of ISCOMs (immunostimulating complexes, typically composed of 0.5 % *Quillaja* saponins, 0.1% cholesterol, 0.1% phospholipid and antigen dissolved in PBS). Although side effects of Quil A were almost absent when incorporated into ISCOM, this form of vaccine is only used for veterinary vaccines and has not been approved for humans. Quil A is still a heterogeneous mixture, consisting of up to 23 different individual saponins detectable by HPLC [8]. Later, it was observed that not all saponins were active as adjuvants. A saponin termed QS III was purified from of a methanol extract of *Quillaja* bark by several chromatographic steps, it has, however, not been tested for adjuvant activity [12].

Kensil et al. (1991) have isolated four saponins from *Quillaja* bark termed QS-7, QS-17 (**1**) , QS-18 (**2**) and QS-21 (**3**) [13, 14]. They were found to be adjuvant-active, although differing in biological activities such as hemolysis and toxicity in mice. Interestingly, QS-7 and QS-21 (**3**) had lower toxicity than Quil A or QS-18 (**2**) as determinated by lethality studies in mice.

Three saponin fractions of interest (QH-A, QH-B, QH-C) have been obtained from an aqueous extract of the *Quillaja* bark by reversed HPLC according to their elution profile. The mixture of these compounds in a ratio 7:0:3 known as ISCO-PREP 7.0.3 has recently been tested as a component of a new ISCOM-adjuvanted human influenza vaccine .

Adjuvant activity has also been observed with saponins from *Gypsophila* and *Saponaria* (Caryophyllaceae) whereas it was absent with other saponin containing extracts prepared from *Soya*, *Alfalfa*, *Chenopodium quinoa* and *Glycyrrhiza* radix [15]. Since the strongest adjuvant activity was observed with saponins from *Quillaja saponaria*, we will describe the activities associated with saponins from this species.

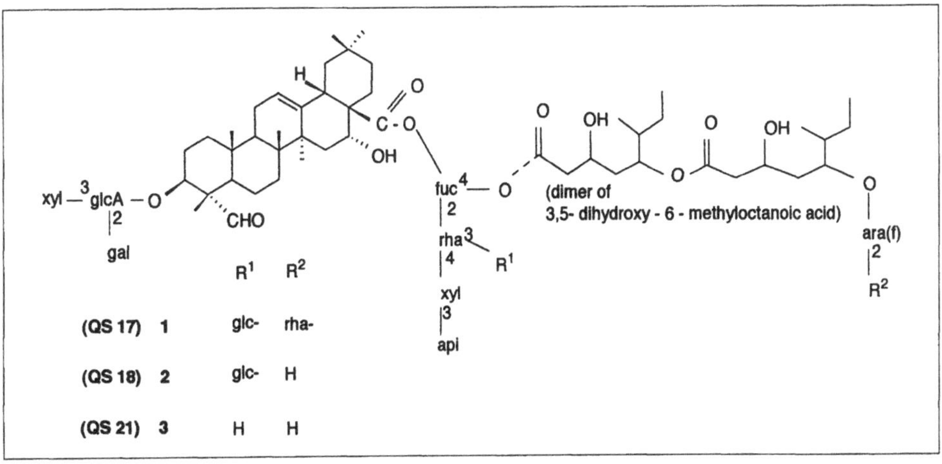

glc, β-D-glucopyranosyl; gal, β-D-galactopyranosyl; rha, α-L-rhamnopyranosyl; xyl, β-D-xylopyranosyl; ara (f), α-L-arabinofuranosyl; glcA, β-D-glucuronopyranosyl; fuc, β-D-fucopyranosyl; api, β-D-apiofuranosyl

Adjuvant properties

Much of the experimental work has been performed so far in mice models and the substances which have been tested more extensively are QuilA (as a free saponin or in ISCOM form) and QS-21 (3). Non-particulate adjuvants are compounds whose activity does not depend upon any particulate or multimeric nature (QS-21,(3)) whereas particulate adjuvants are substances that exist as microscopic particles and owe some of their adjuvant activity to this property (ISCOM) [4].

Non particulate adjuvants

Although the exact mechanism of the adjuvant effects is poorly understood it has been demonstrated that an appropriate system can direct antigens into antigen presenting cells (APCs) to generate both cellular and humoral responses [7].

Enhanced potentiation of both the humoral and cell mediated responses appears to play a major role in offering significant protection against infections in mice.

Humoral immune response

As T cells recognize antigen on APCs along with major histocompatibility complex (MHC), the form of antigen may affect its recognition by T cells and the type of T cells elicited. A MHC class II response usually leads to antibody production.

Quil A

Several studies showed the role of Quil A as an adjuvant in controlling antibody response and antibody isotypes.

For example, Quil A was shown to be superior to other adjuvants for promoting the immune response to recombinant gp120 from HIV in mice [16]. This was analyzed in terms of antibody isotypes and secretion of cytokines by lymph node cells. All the tested adjuvants induced IgG1 antibodies but Quil A induced the highest levels of IgG2a, confirming its efficacy. In mice the levels of IgG1 and IgG2a antibodies are respectively controlled by two subsets of T cells, Th2 secreting IL-4 and IL-5 cells, and Th1 secreting IFNγ and IL-2 cells. A study of the secretion of IL-5 and IFNγ by lymph node cells cultured *in vitro* together with gp120 showed that all the cultures secreted IL-5, but only those from saponin-immunized mice produced IFNγ. These results suggest that Quil A was capable of activating both Th1 and Th2 T cell subsets [16].

Non-protein antigens, such as polysaccharides and lipids, do not possess the peptide moiety necessary for binding to T cell receptor and are thus classified T independent (TI). They are unable to bind to T lymphocytes, but can bind to B cells and stimulate antibody production. Quil A was shown to markedly augment antibody responses to TI antigens, suggesting that its adjuvant effect may be, at least partly, mediated through B cells [17].

The adjuvant activity of Quil A was not only observed in mice, but also in higher species such as cats, guinea pigs, rabbits, dogs, cynomolgus macaques, sheep and cattle [9]. Effective saponin doses used for stimulation of antibody responses range from 5 μg in mice to 1 mg in cattle. A novel infected-cell vaccine administered with Quil A to cynomolgus macaques generates a strong humoral and cellular immune response to simian immunodeficiency virus (SIV) resulting in protection of animals. These results could be useful for the development of HIV vaccines [18].

Purified saponins

Saponins QS-7, QS-17 (**1**), QS-18 (**2**) and QS-21(**3**) typically induce an increase in Ag-specific IgG ELISA titers in CD-1 mice by two intradermal immunizations with bovine serum albumin (BSA) or with beef liver cytochrome b5, when used at doses ranging from 10 to 20 μg in a 0.2 ml PBS/Ag solution (see Fig. 1) [13].

Saponins also influence the Ag-specific isotype distribution. They increase titers of the three major IgG subclasses, IgG1, IgG2a and IgG2b. For some saponins, IgG2a predominated.

QS-21 (**3**) increased IgG1, IgG2a and IgG2b responses to BSA and to ovalbumin (OVA) in a dose-dependent manner. The maximum titers were observed with saponin doses > 10 μg [13, 19]. QS-21 (**3**) was shown to stimulate antigen-specific IgG2a to a number of antigens including human cytomegalovirus (HCMV) envelope glycoprotein gB [20], purified fusion protein (F) of respiratory syncytial virus (RSV) [21], feline leukemia virus (FeLV) envelope gp70 [22] and the outer surface proteins A (Osp A) and B (Osp B) of *Borrelia burgdorferi* [23].

Enhancement of immune responses to T independent antigens such as bacterial polysaccharides need the conjugation of the antigens to a carrier such as a diphteria toxin or keyhole limpet hemocyanin (KLH) in order to provide T cell help to the polysaccharide [14]. However, experiments have demonstrated that certain strains of mice had significantly enhanced serum antibody titers to an unconjugated *E. coli* polysaccharide (60 μg/dose) when QS-21 (15 μg/dose) was used. The titer increase was largely a result of increased levels of IgG2b subclass antibodies [24].

QS-21 (**3**) stimulated antibody production in several higher species including cats, guinea pigs, dogs, rhesus monkeys and baboons at doses ranging from 20 μg (cats) to 100 μg (baboons) [9].

A dose of 50μg of QS-21 (**3**) showed substantially enhancing antibody responses to recombinant HIV-1IIIB gp160 in rhesus monkeys [9, 25]. It also significantly increases serum titers of IgG1 and IgG2 to recombinant *Borrelia burgdorferi* Osp A and Osp B in dogs [26].

Cytotoxic T lymphocytes response

The induction of antigen-specific $CD8^+$ cytotoxic T lymphocytes (CTL) possessing an effector function for lysis of antigen-presenting MHC class I- expressing cells, is an important effector mechanism of cell-mediated immunity. This immune response is associated with protection against, and clearance of, infection by virus and other intracellular pathogens [9]. Wu et al. showed in 1994 the contribution of macrophages to the processing and presentation of protein antigens to $CD8^+$ T lymphocytes and the subsequent induction of CTL responses [27].

Endogenous antigens, such as viral antigens, induce antigen-specific $CD8^+$ CTL after presentation of processed antigen by the classical class I MHC pathway.

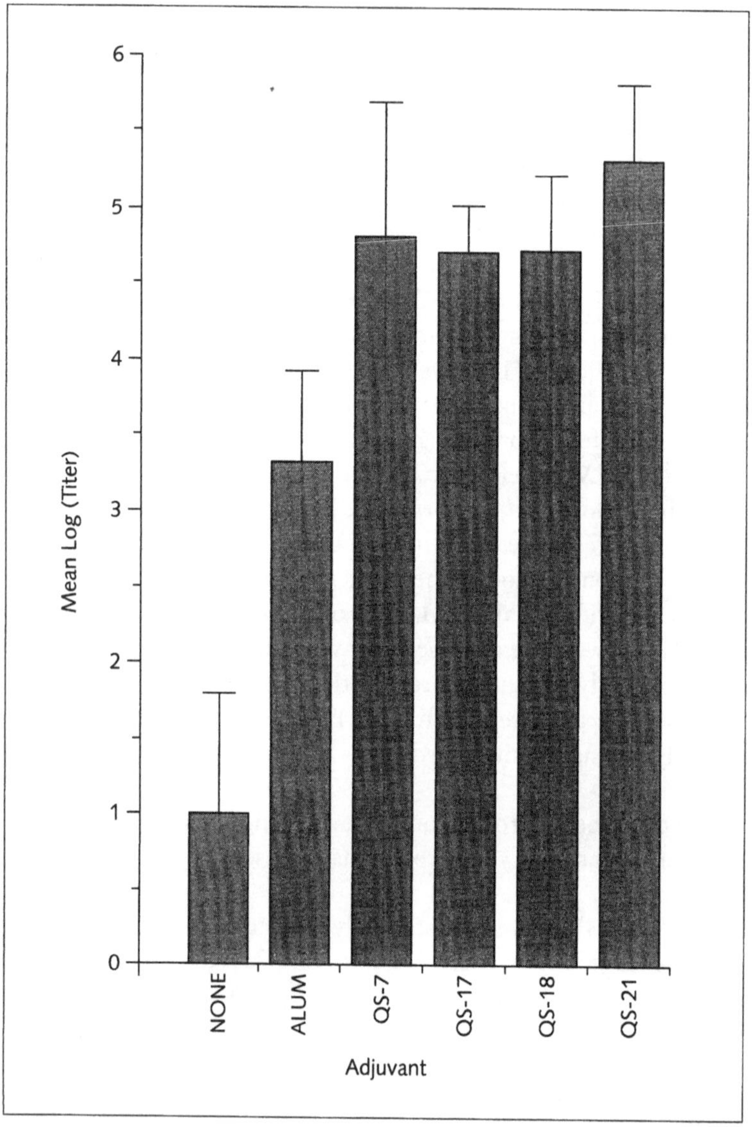

Figure 1

Adjuvant effect on stimulation of IgG: Comparison of purified Quillaja saponaria *saponins to other adjuvants. CD-1 mice (5 per group) were immunized intradermally with 10 µg cytochrome b5 and the indicated adjuvant. The alum formulation consisted of 400 µg of aluminium hydroxide per dose. All saponins (QS-7, QS-17, QS-18, and QS-21) were used at 20 µg per dose. EIA titers were determined after two immunizations. The results are expressed as the mean of log10 titers for individual mice per group. The error bar is 1 standard deviation. Reprinted from [13], with permission from The American Association of Immunologists.*

Exogenous particulate antigens are known to induce CTL after being phagocytosed by macrophages whereas exogenous soluble antigens (such as subunit vaccines) do not efficiently induce CD8$^+$ CTL and require novel strategies in order to induce a CTL response. One of these is the use of adjuvants or delivery systems that direct subunit antigens into the cytoplasm of APCs (MHC class I pathway of antigen presentation). Effective systems are saponins simply mixed with antigen or saponin-based presentation systems such as ISCOMs (immunostimulating complexes). QS-21 (3) has been shown to be a potent stimulator of CD8$^+$ CTL response to subunit antigens. HIV-1 type specific CTL responses were produced in mice after vaccination with alum-adsorbed envelope protein (HIV-1 160D) mixed with QS-21 adjuvant and were readily detected using P815 target cells infected with the vPE 8 recombinant vaccinia virus [27]. Newmann et al. (1992) [28] confirmed QS-21 mediated induction of CTLs to subunit antigen using OVA as immunogen and E.G7-OVA cells for targets (cell line that expresses OVA peptides). Doses as low as 2.5 µg of QS-21 induced a significant CTL response to native OVA after three imunizations (see Fig. 2).

QS-21 also induced CTL to HCMV gB [20] and RSV fusion protein (F) subunit antigen in mice [21].

Saponins were shown to induce antigen-specific CTL responses in non-human primates [29], such as rhesus monkeys immunized with experimental subunit vaccine formulations containing recombinant SIVmac 251 gag and env proteins combined with an aluminium hydroxide/QS-21 mixture [29].

Mode of saponin adjuvant action

The amplitude of the adjuvant effects results from a complex interplay between route of administration, time of inoculation, antigen dose, antigen constituents, adjuvant form, and host species. The *in vivo* response to an antigen has been extensively studied in order to investigate the mechanism of action and the main results are summarized below.

The adjuvant action of free saponin may not be due to a "depot" formation of the antigen at the site of injection, the major mechanism of adjuvanticity of many adjuvant formulations [9].

A formulation of *Quillaja* saponins and sheep red blood cells (SRBC) injected s.c. into the flank of mice, increased the number of cells in the draining axillary lymph nodes [9], showing that it was the immediate effect of the adjuvant action.

The role of adjuvant effects of saponins on specific T cell populations was studied by depletion of T cells experiments of QS-21 in mice [31]. In CD4$^+$ deficient mice immunized with the test antigen OVA, the antibody response to OVA was eliminated, despite the use of QS-21. Surprisingly, these mice presented a significant OVA-specific CD8$^+$ CTL response suggesting that cytokines produced by CD8$^+$ cells or macrophages were sufficient to prime the CTL response. On the contrary, immu-

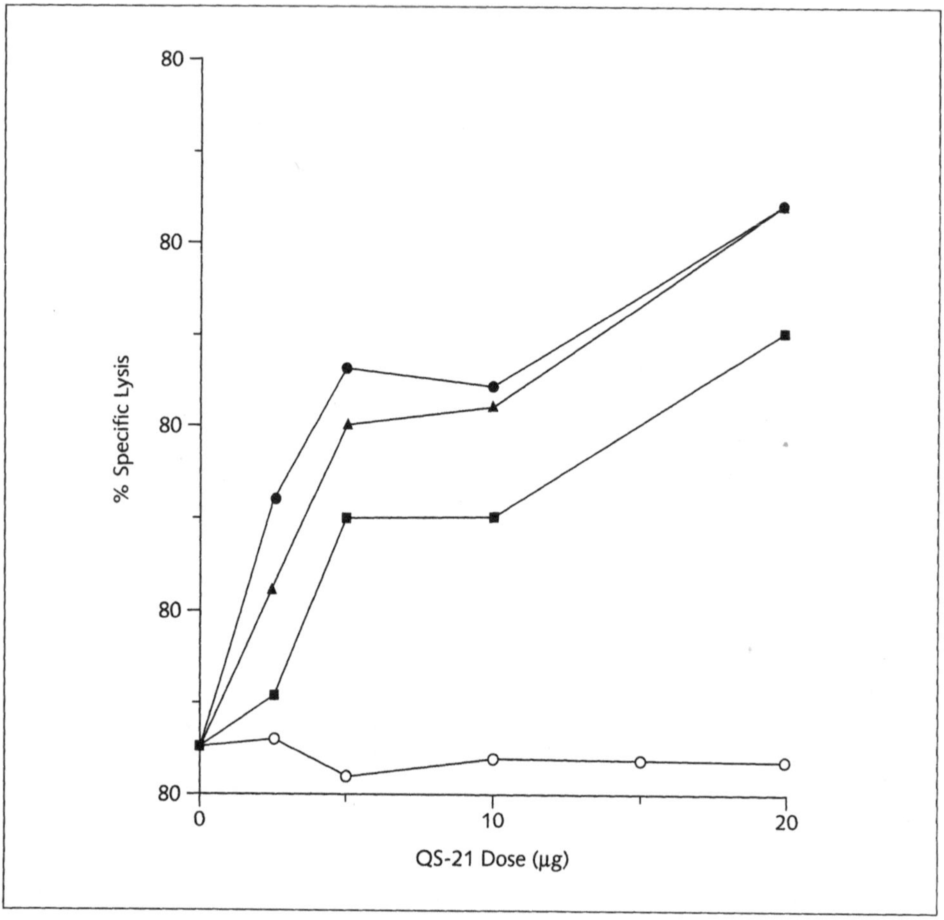

Figure 2
QS-21 dose response curve for induction of MHC Class I-restricted cytotoxic T lymphocyte response. C57BL/6 mice (10 per saponin adjuvant dose) were immunized with OVA and different doses of QS-21 by subcutaneous administration at days 0, 14, and 28. After the third immunization, splenocytes were harvested and stimulated in vitro *with OVA for use as effector cells in a CTL assay. Target cells were E.G7-OVA [Effector: Target ratio 25:1 (●), 12:1 (▲), and 6:1 (■)], and EL4 cells [Effector: Target ratio 25:1 (○)]. E.G7-OVA are EL4 cells transfected with the OVA gene. Adapted from [28], with permission from The American Association of Immunologists.*

nization of mice deficient in $CD8^+$ cells did not induce a CTL response, but elicited a significant antibody response [31].

Mice treated with silica in order to paralyse the macrophages were immunized with OVA /QS-21. The paralysis of macrophages did not allow processing and presentation of soluble exogenous antigen by the class I MHC pathway suggesting that the macrophages play a critical role as APCs in induction of QS-21-mediated $CD8^+$ CTL responses [31].

The balance between predominent antibody and cell-mediated immune responses is regulated by two subsets of $CD4^+$ cells and associated secreted cytokines. The CTL and IgG2a responses induced by *Quillaja* saponins suggest that this adjuvant induces the production of Th1 type (IL-2 and IFNγ) cytokines mediating these responses. Saponin induction of IFNγ was then demonstrated in subsequent studies. Saponin adjuvants have also been shown to influence the production of cytokines in large animals.

Toxicity in relation to the way of administration

Saponins appear to be effective adjuvants when orally administred [10]. Although intraperitoneal inocula containing 0.4 mg crude *Quillaja* saponins were often lethal, mice tolerated oral doses of 20 mg/0.4 ml without visible or histological evidence of toxicity. Mixed with saponins (10 mg), inactivated rabies vaccine stimulated serum neutralizing antibody responses significantly higher than orally-administered vaccine alone. Orally given saponins produced a marked clonal expansion of immunocompetent cells in the mesenteric lymph nodes and spleen with enhanced CTL and NK cell activities. Furthermore, T helper and B cell cooperation was increased, resulting in enhanced antibody production. Orally given saponins potentiated the protective effects of intraperitoneally administered rabies vaccine [30].

Most work on saponins as immunological adjuvants has been done following parenteral inoculation. Saponins are more toxic by parenteral (i.p. or i.v.) administration than by the oral route, presumably because of a more complete uptake by the former. Toxicity associated with Quil A has limited its development to veterinary vaccines. The maximum well tolerated i.p. dose in mice was estimated to be 25 µg. Significantly lower toxicity was observed by subcutaneous, intradermal, and intramuscular routes of administration. The toxicity of individual saponins varies considerably. For example, the major peak saponin QS-18 (**2**) was found to be toxic in mice at low doses (80% mortality within three days after i.d. injection of 125 µg) whereas QS-7 was non toxic (100% survival with 0.5 mg, the highest dose tested). A simple analogy between hemolytic activity and toxicity is not possible since QS-21 (**3**), which was shown to have a slightly higher hemolytic activity than QS-18 (**2**), was proven to be less toxic [9].

Unfractionated saponins caused moderate to severe local inflammation following s.c. injection into mouse footpad. One strategy for reducing systemic toxicity and local reactogenicity of complex mixtures, such as Quil A, is to mix the saponin with a lipid carrier such as ISCOM, or to select purified saponins with low toxicity, such as QS-21 (**3**). In general, most adjuvant formulations are combinations of immunostimulants and vehicle but QS-21 (**3**) is typically used in the absence of a carrier vehicle and it is effective in aqueous solution. It has, however, also been noted that QS-21 (**3**) is equally effective when added to aluminium hydroxide-adsorbed antigens [27].

Immunological assays

Different formulations of saponin-adjuvanted vaccines were tested for humoral and cell-mediated responses in mice. Many antigens, often including hen egg albumin (ovalbumin, OVA) as the antigen to be tested, have been used for immunizations, enzyme immunoassays, antigen-specific CTL and cellular proliferation assays [31].

Mice were immunized by s.c. injection of 0.2 ml of test formulation (25 µg of the antigen OVA and varying doses of the test adjuvants) on days 0 and 14. Mice were bled and sera collected for antibody titer determination one week after the second immunization. Several other schedules of immunization have been reported in the literature. Splenic mononuclear cells were collected two weeks after the last immunization for use as effector cells in the cytotoxic T lymphocyte assay and for the proliferation assay [32].

Measurement of antigen specific-antibodies

Antibodies produced in response to the immunizations and the relative titers of specific antibody types were measured by enzyme-linked immunosorbent assay (ELISA) [13, 16, 19, 21–25, 27, 31, 33–36, 45, 48].

Measurement of antigen-specific cellular proliferation

Proliferation assays were performed concurrently with the CTL assays to evaluate Th cell responses. Assays were run in 96-well microculture plates, using splenic mononuclear cells. In order to stimulate proliferation, Ag was added at various concentrations. After incubation at 37° C, [^{3}H]-thymidine was added to all wells 16 h prior to harvesting [25, 32]. Cellular proliferation was quantitated by standard liquid scintillation counting.

Measurement of antigen-specific CTL activity

QS-21 (**3**) was evaluated to stimulate an antigen-specific CTL response to OVA [28, 32]. After three immunizations of mice with OVA and QS-21, cytotoxic T lymphocyte responses were determined as lysis of syngeneic target lymphoma cells (EL4 and E.G7-OVA cell line), the later being EL4 cells tranfected with the complete OVA gene. The E.G7-OVA cells express an OVA peptide (amino acids 257-264) bound to MHC class I molecules on the cell surface and hence serve as target cells for specific CTL that recognize the peptide-MHC complex [31]. The lytic effector cells were immunization-primed splenocytes, stimulated from mature to functional CTL by six days culture *in vitro* together with antigen (denatured OVA) [32]. The antigen specificity of the response was shown by lack of lysis of EL4 cells. Cytotoxicity was evaluated as splenocyte lysis of ^{51}Cr-labelled target cells and the % of ^{51}Cr release due to cytotoxicity was calculated [32]. An experimental vaccine containing rHIV-1 envelope glycoprotein (HIV-1 160D) and QS-21 (**3**) has also been evaluated to stimulate an antigen-specific CTL response to HIV-1 viral proteins. Effector CTL cells were generated by culture of pooled splenic mononuclear cells from two to five immunized mice with 18 III B peptide. Murine P815 cells which only express Class I MHC Ag were used as target cells. They were infected with either recombinant vaccinia virus (vPE8) containing the HIV-1 IIIB gp120 gene or control vaccinia virus [27]. The production of serum esterase by Ag-activated splenic mononuclear cells, indicating the maturation of CTL, was used as a secondary measure of CTL activity [27].

Structure/function relationships

The structure of QS-21 (**3**) is that of a quillaic acid substituted at position three by a branched trisaccharide and at position 28 by a linear tetrasaccharide and a dimeric fatty acyl group (3,5-dihydroxy-6-methyloctanoic acid) attached to the 4-position of the first sugar of the tetrasaccharide (fucose) by an ester linkage. A further sugar (arabinofuranose) is attached to the fatty acyl group.

The saponins QS-17 (**1**), QS-18 (**2**) and QS-21 (**3**) differ predominantly in the terminal monosaccharides of the glycosidic side chains. All show similar dose-response curves for antibody production. It therefore seems that differences in terminal residues are not critical for this function. Periodate oxidation of QS-18, however, eliminated the adjuvant activity, indicating that a certain configuration of the carbohydrate chain was essential for antibody production [9]. The alkaline hydrolysis of QS-21 (**3**) yielded the deacylated saponin DS-1. This compound did not stimulate antibody production to BSA or OVA. Further, DS-1 did not induce a CTL response towards OVA, demonstrating that both of those QS-21-mediated immune responses were eliminated by deacylation of the triterpene glycoside. The fatty acid domain alone does not stimulate antibody or CTL responses. These results suggest the importance of the acyl group in QS-21 (**3**) for the immunoadjuvant activity [32]. Interestingly, it was observed that the acyl group on QS-21 (**3**) migrates between the 4-hydroxyl and the 3-hydroxyl of the fucose in aqueous solution. This migration apparently does not affect the adjuvant activity [9].

The immunostimulant activity of some adjuvants is influenced by their surface-active properties. They may influence antigen processing/presentation to antigen-presenting cells (APCs) such as macrophages [32]. It is possible that the effect of QS-21 for induction of CTL may act through interaction of this adjuvant with membranes of APCs so that the antigen is directed into the cytoplasm. The absence of induction of CTL by the deacylated QS-21 supports this hypothesis. The deacylation of QS-21 markedly influences its surface-active properties suggesting the important contribution of the fatty acid domain to these properties.

Derivatives prepared by modification at the carboxyl group of glucuronic acid were active for antibody stimulation and CTL induction. Derivatives prepared by modification of the aldehyde function were inactive for both responses suggesting that this group may be involved in the adjuvant mechanism. The loss of adjuvant activity was not necessarily due to the loss of surface activity (CMC and hemolytic titers were high) but to a cellular interaction via Schiff base formation [33].

In order to determine whether there exists a correlation between surface activity and adjuvant activity, several studies on *Quillaja* saponins are in progress [32].

Clinical studies

Until now only the saponin adjuvant QS-21 (**3**) has entered vaccine clinical trials. Saponin mixtures causing local toxicity and hemolytic activity such as Quil A, have not yet been tested in clinical trials of human vaccines. After preclinical trials of QS-21 in rabbits, dogs, rhesus monkeys and baboons, this molecule was evaluated in phase 1 clinical trials of experimental melanoma immunotherapeutic vaccines, of HIV-1 subunit vaccines and more recently of a promising malaria vaccine [34–36].

Malignant melanoma

One area of vaccination that has received much attention lately is cancer vaccination. The use of vaccines in cancer patients differs from the traditional use of vaccines since the goal is to induce immune responses against existing tumors rather than to protect the healthy individual. As such, they are typically referred to as immunotherapeutic vaccines. In a series of studies in patients with malignant melanoma, one objective has been to construct vaccines that are effective in the production of antibodies against gangliosides often overexpressed in melanoma such as G_{M2}, G_{D2} and G_{D3}. Vaccine-induced production of G_{M2} antibodies by patients with stage III melanoma after surgery was associated with increased survival [34]. The aim of this clinical study was to determine the maximal tolerated dose of QS-21 (**3**) consistent with repeated outpatient administration and the optimal dose for induction of the antiboby response to G_{M2} [34]. The vaccine G_{M2+}KLH (G_{M2} conjugated with the carrier keyhole limpet haemocyanin) adjuvanted with various doses of QS-21 (**3**) (10, 50, 100 and 200 µg/ml) was shown to be very effective in patients with AJCC stage III or IV melanoma after surgery. It induced a much higher titer, a longer-lasting IgM antibody response against G_{M2} and a consistent IgG response. It also induced the highest titer anti-KLH response. The results suggested that the conjugate G_{M2}-KLH + QS-21 vaccine elicited significant T cell help. QS-21, at any of the doses used, resulted in a qualitatively different immune response to G_{M2} ganglioside. The results of this phase 1 trial showed that the 100 µg and 200 µg doses of QS-21 (3) induce the optimal antibody response against G_{M2} (see Tab. 1) and that the 100 µg dose is better tolerated. Namely, there was a clear increase in local and systemic toxicity with progression from 100 to 200 µg.

Table 1 - Serological response of patients after vaccination with G_{M2}-KLH plus various doses of QS-21

		Peak ELISA titre against G_{M2}			
Vaccine		Pretreatment		After treatment	
G_{M2}-KLH+ QS-21 (μg)	No. of patients	IgM	IgG	IgM	IgG
0	6	20, 0 (5)[a]	0 (6)	160 (2), 80 (2), 40, 0	40, 0 (5)
10	4	0 (4)	0 (4)	1280, 640, 320, 80	80, 20 0 (2)
50	6	20, 0 (5)	0 (6)	640, 320 (2), 160, 80	80 (3), 40 (2), 20
100	6	40, 0 (5)	0 (6)	5120, 1280 (3), 160, 80	2560, 640, 320, 80, 40 (2)
200	6	320, 20, 0 (04)	0 (6)	5120, 1280 (3), 320 (2)	1280 (2), 640 (2), 320, 80

[a] *One patient had a pretreatment peak titre ELISA response of 1/20. The number in parentheses indicates the number of patients with a given response. In this case, five patients had no detectable G_{M2} antibodies. Adapted from [34], with permission from Elsevier Science.*

Since no serious toxicity was observed at doses < 100 μg of QS-21, this vaccine approach is attractive for augmenting the immunogenicity of other gangliosides, such as G_{D2} and G_{D3} and to determine the effects of ganglioside antibodies on the course of melanoma [35].

Malaria

A recent clinical study has been carried out in order to develop a vaccine effective in preventing infection with malaria [36].

So far, the candidate vaccines are poorly immunogenic and have been ineffective in preventing infection. A vaccine containing the circumsporozoite protein of *Plasmodium falciparum* together with adjuvants has been developed in order to enhance the immune response.

In this trial the antigen tested is a hybrid in which the circumsporozoite protein is fused to hepatitis B surface antigen, HBsAg. Three formulations of this antigen have been tested in human volunteers who have never been exposed to malaria-causing pathogens. One of these formulations consisted of the antigen in an oil-in-water emulsion plus the immune stimulants monophosphoryl lipid A and QS-21. Twenty two vaccinated subjects and six unimmunized controls underwent a challenge consisting of bites from mosquitoes infected with *P. falciparum*. Six out of seven individuals receiving the QS-21-containing formulation were protected against malaria infection when challenged with the parasite, whereas only one out of seven or two out of seven individuals receiving the other formulations were protected. Malaria developed in all six control subjects. The cellular mechanisms explaining the protection obtained with the QS-21 formulation have so far not been identified. It might be due to an optimal stimulus of T cells recruited after challenge to eliminate liver-stage parasites by an enhanced local release of IFNγ.

AIDS

A phase I clinical study is in progress with healthy subjects receiving an AIDS vaccine in order to compare the adjuvants QS-21 and aluminium hydroxide. No significant side effects were observed in 100 healthy volunteers who received the QS-21 vaccine formulation. However no immunogenicity data are yet available for these formulations [14].

Particulate adjuvants (ISCOMs)

Definition and history

The acronym ISCOMs was derived from the ability of these submicron particles to act as immunostimulating complexes in animals when used in vaccines initially prepared from membrane proteins of parainfluenza-3, measles and rabies viruses [37]. The ISCOMs were shown to induce a wide range of protective immune mechanisms. They were described as highly effective forms for viral antigen presentation, as potent enhancers of both B and T (Th and CTL) cell mediated immune responses having less side effects, and as inducers of secretion of various cytokines [38]. Morein et al. in 1984 were the first to describe ISCOMs [37]. The basic requirements for the production of these complexes were established in 1988, while the first ISCOM-based vaccine (equine influenza vaccine for horses) was sold. The demonstration of ISCOMs inducing a CTL response (against HIV-1) appeared in 1990. Whereas preclinical toxicology studies on ISCOMs started in 1994, the first human phase 1 clinical trials were performed in 1995 with an influenza ISCOM-based vaccine.

ISCOMs structure and composition

The ISCOM is a cage-like 30–40 nm particle formed through hydrophobic interactions between amphipathic molecules and the complexes formed by *Quillaja* saponin, cholesterol and phospholipids such as phosphatidylcholine or ethanolamine [8]. The amphipathic molecules are derived from cell walls and membranes from a variety of viruses, bacteria and parasites. The basic ISCOM which is formed in the absence of envelope protein is termed ISCOM matrix or empty ISCOM. The addition of phospholipids is necessary in order to provide a certain flexibility of the

ISCOM matrix, making the incorporation of the protein antigen into the structure possible. This stable construction offers the advantage of reduction of the required antigen and adjuvant doses and resulted in enhanced immune responses.

Quil A has been the major saponin mixture used for ISCOM work to date. The major modification to ISCOM technology has been the use of three HPLC-fractions of *Quillaja saponaria* bark aqueous extract named QH-A, QH-B and QH-C [47]. The ratio 7:0:3 for these fractions known as ISCOPREP 7.0.3. has been recently tested as a component of a new ISCOM-adjuvanted human influenza vaccine.

Preparation of the ISCOMs

For the incorporation of viral membrane proteins into the ISCOM matrix, virus particles are usually solubilized with detergent, in order to obtain them in non-complexed monomeric forms.

In the presence of phospholipids, cholesterol and Quil A, ISCOMs spontaneously form when the detergent is removed [39, 40]. Generally good results are obtained when cholesterol, aqueous protein solution and Quil A are mixed together in a ratio of 1:1:5 (w/w/w), respectively [41].

Immunogenicity of ISCOMs

ISCOM technology has been used to enhance the immunogenicity of the surface proteins of several types of viruses. Immunization with viral antigen incorporated into the ISCOM matrix results in the induction of high-titer virus-specific antibodies that persist for long periods of time [41]. Such B cell responses have been observed with many viruses, including feline leukemia virus (FeLV), human immunodeficiency (HIV), hepatitis-B virus (HBV), measles virus and influenza virus. Several possible mechanisms may contribute to the efficient B cell responses after immunization with ISCOMs. One of them could be related to a strong Th-cell response, resulting in the release of soluble factors that activate B cells. In addition to the induction of Th-cells, the induction of CTLs has been shown to contribute to protection against disease in many virus systems [42, 43].

Mode of action of ISCOMs

It seems that antigen targeting and presentation functions, as well as immunomodulation, may explain the adjuvant activity of ISCOMs but current studies on cytokines will complete this explanation.

Antigen targeting

In vitro studies indicate that ISCOMs containing antigen adhere to and are taken up rapidly by peritoneal macrophages and other APCs leading to more effective presentation of the antigen to T cells. *In vivo* studies with an intraperitoneal injection of mice with labelled influenza antigen in ISCOMs resulted in relatively high levels of retained antigen in draining lymph nodes and in the spleen. Some local inflammatory responses were observed such as short-lived neutrophil accumulation in the peritoneal cavity. ISCOM do not appear to function through a depot effect. Release of "inflammatory" cytokines such as IL-1, IL-6, TNFα, and GM-CSF from mouse peritoneal cells pulsed with ISCOMs *in vitro* has been reported [38].

Antigen presentation

The stimulation of antigen-specific CTLs with several viral proteins including influenza A, RSV and HIV-1 incorporated into ISCOMs have been shown *in vivo* [43]. It has been suggested that ISCOMs can deliver antigens after passing them through either the plasma or endosomal membranes of APCs, directly into the cytosol for proteolytic degradation and loading of MHC class I in the endoplasmic reticulum for CTL induction [38]. The hydrophobic nature of the ISCOM structure and the inclusion of saponins that can penetrate into cholesterol membranes may explain its apparent capacity to pass antigen through membranes.

In addition, degradation of antigen must occur within endosomes for MHC class II loading due to the known potency of ISCOM in the induction of DHT, Th1 and Th2 (indicated respectively by IgG2a and IgG1) responses in mice [45].

Immune modulation

The capacity of adjuvants to stimulate cytokine production by APCs is important for the initiation of the immune response. As indicated above, ISCOMs induce "inflammatory cytokines" such as IL-1 and IL-6 from macrophages or monocytes. Compared with adjuvants known as IL-1 inducers, the formulation denominated QH-7.0.3 flu-ISCOMs was as efficient as the most potent IL-1 inducer, i.e. lipopolysaccharide (LPS) and superior to cholera toxin and muramyldipeptide [46]. Furthermore, flu-Ag in ISCOMs-primed T cells had the capacity to secrete high concentrations of IL-2 and IFNγ after antigen stimulation *in vitro*.

ISCOM vaccine assays

Quality control

To allow the use of ISCOMs in human vaccines, it is necessary to determine the immunological properties and toxicity of chemically defined components and to characterize and validate the production process [38, 47].

In the ISCOMs containing Quil A, the determination of the level of Quil A in the final vaccine is of great importance due to the potential toxic effects of excessive doses as seen in mice or rats. When i.m. administered to mice, ISCOMs containing 90 µg of Quil A were well tolerated with less reactogenicity than a 15 µg dose of free Quil A. However, doses of 50 and 100 µg of Quil A incorporated into ISCOM were lethal when i.p. injected into mice. Despite the toxicity of HIV-1 ISCOMs observed in mice, this vaccine was used safely in rhesus monkeys.

Lethality studies of three *Quillaja* HPLC-fractions, QH-A, QH-B, QH-C in ICR mice showed higher toxicity associated with QH-B (7/10 deaths at 400 μg) than with QH-A or QH-C (0/10 deaths at 400 μg for both) or when QH-C was incorporated into ISCOM matrix (0/10 deaths at 800 μg) [38]. These results explained that these fractions were added in a ratio of 7:0:3 in the new ISCOM-adjuvanted influenza vaccine.

Evaluation of the immunogenicity

A broad range of assays including specific antibody level determinations (using ELISA, immoprecipitation, virus neutralization), lymphocyte proliferation, DHT, CTL and cytokine assays (e.g. IFNγ) have been used to assess the in vivo effect of ISCOMs vaccines [38].

A number of studies have also assessed the capacity of the ISCOM vaccines to induce protection from challenge (assessed by survival, weight loss, virus isolation and clearance kinetics) [38]. Protection studies with experimental ISCOMs vaccine have been performed in various animal species[39, 40]. The most relevant results were obtained with ISCOMs containing viral antigens such as herpes (HSV-1), pseudorabies (PrV), bovine herpes virus type I (BHV-1), cytomegalovirus (CMV), Epstein Barr Virus (EBV) and rubella. Since 1992 the major areas of interest have been Retroviridae (HIV-1, -2, SIV, FIV and FeLV) and Orthomyxoviridae (various strains of influenza) [44]. For ISCOM vaccination, i.m. and s.c. routes of administration have mainly been used.

Preclinical trial

Neither ISCOMs nor ISCOM matrix were included in a HIV clinical trial but they were included in a recent European SIV trial in macaque monkeys [38]. This trial showed that SIV ISCOM vaccine were capable of fully protecting monkeys (3/3) against challenge with homologous SIV grown in a human cell line.

Another study showed that 3/4 macaque monkeys were protected from an i.v. challenge with ten monkey infectious doses of a simian cell grown, cell-free HIV-2 for up to 18 months post-vaccination with an HIV-2 ISCOM vaccine.

Since 1988, a licensed veterinary ISCOM-based influenza vaccine (containing Quil A < 300 μg/dose) for protecting horses from equine influenza has been produced and shown safe during tests [38].

The first data available on the potential use of influenza virus ISCOMs in a non-human primate model showed that this form of antigen presentation not only induced more antibody and T cell responses than classical subunit vaccines, but also provided absolute protection against a homologous challenge infection [48].

Many animal toxicological and pharmacological testings have been carried out on influenza-ISCOM vaccine made with ISCOPREP 7.0.3. Based on these studies it has been concluded that it will be safe to administer this vaccine i.m. to healthy adult volunteers. Prior to this clinical trial a phase I safety evaluation with ISCO-MATRIX will be undertaken by an Australian research group [38].

Saponins as immunostimulants

Immunostimulants are compounds which are administered in order to increase the resistance of an organism against pathogens or tumors. They generally stimulate, in a non-antigen dependent manner, the function and efficiency of the non-specific immune system to counteract microbial infections or immunosuppressive states [49]. Furthermore, they are effective prophylactically as well as therapeutically. A panel of standardized *in vitro* assays used to evaluate this activity was described by Wagner and Jurcic in 1991 [50].

Many saponins have been proven to be able to modify non-specific (both humoral and cellular) immune functions *in vitro* in a non-antigen-dependent manner. Here we will present a brief review on their influence on lymphocytes, macrophages, and granulocytes together with their influence on the liberation of cytokines and the activation of NK cells. Few *in vivo* studies have been performed in order to prove the significance of saponins as immunostimulants.

In vitro activities

Mitogenic effect on lymphocytes

Mitogenic effects of endotoxin free substances were screened with the lymphocyte transformation test. In this test the rate of lymphocyte proliferation was quantified by determination of the incorporation of [^{3}H]-thymidine into the DNA of human lymphocytes. Stimulation of lymphocytes was measured with or without coincubation of lectins as mitogens such as concanavalin A (ConA) and phytohemagglutinin (PHA). Saponins such as crude *Quillaja* saponins, quillayanin, Quil A and glycyrrhizic acid (4) have the capacity to induce cell proliferation in lymphocyte cultures at very low concentrations [51]. Induction of B cell proliferation was obtained with crude saponin, T cell proliferation with Quil A, and quillayanin and glycyrrhizic acid equally stimulated both T and B lymphocytes. The selective proliferation of subtypes of lymphocytes correlated with restimulation responses by polyclonal mitogens (ConA, PHA), and lipopolysaccharide (LPS).

The oleanolic acid triterpene-saponins of *Randia dumetorum* [52] have been shown to significantly enhance the proliferation of T lymphocytes in a concentration range of 1 µg to 100 ng/ml (saponin mixture), 100 ng to 10 pg/ml (5, 6), 100 ng to 1 ng/ml (7), and 10 ng to 10 pg/ml (8) respectively.

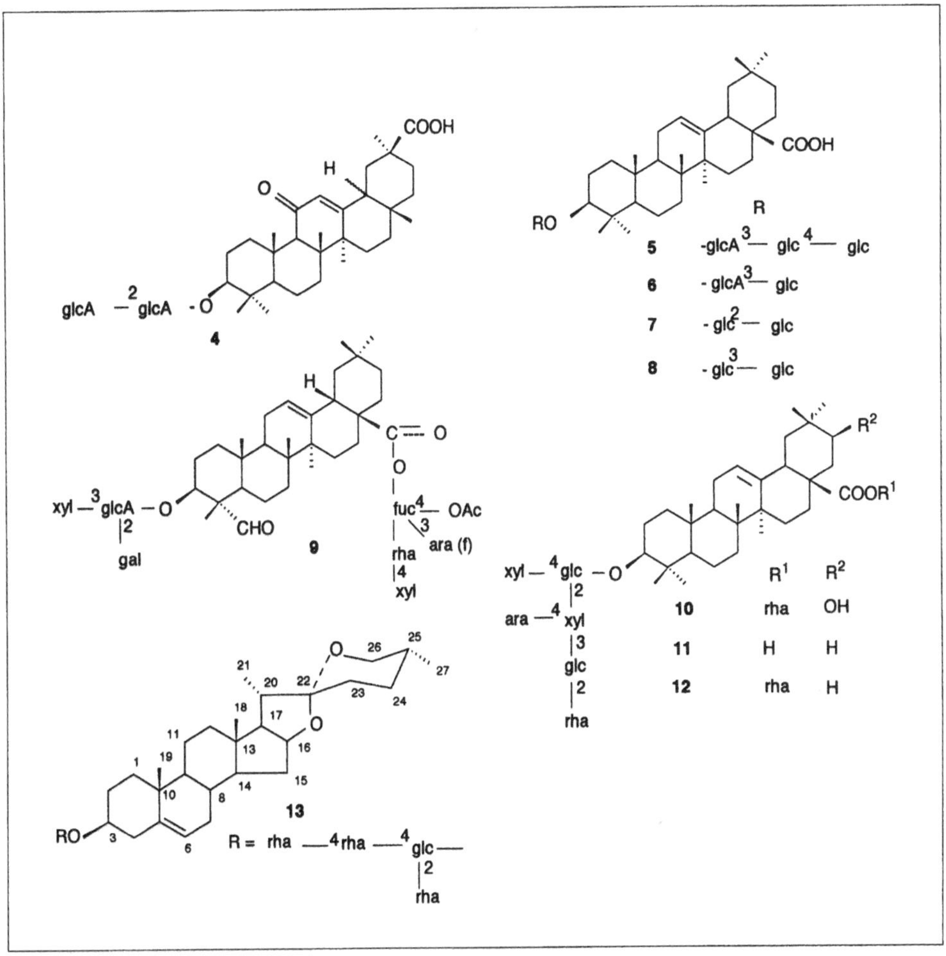

glc, β-D-glucopyranosyl; gal, β-D-galactopyranosyl; rha, α-L-rhamnopyranosyl; xyl, β-D-xylopyranosyl; ara, α-L-ararbinopyranosyl; ara (f), α-L-arabinofuranosyl; hba, β-hydroxy-butyric acid; glcA, β-D-glucuronopyranosyl; fuc, β-D-fucopyranosyl; api, β-D-apiofuranosyl

A new acylated gypsogenin heptaglycoside (**9**) from *Acanthophyllum squarrosum* showed a concentration-dependent immunomodulatory effect in the *in vitro* lymphocyte transformation test [54]. At high concentrations (10 µg/ml), the saponin showed an immunosuppressive effect (60%) whereas the same compound displayed immunostimulating activity at very low concentrations (10 pg/ml). In the concentration range of 100 pg/ml–1 pg/ml, compound **9** exerted a synergic effect on ConA.

New glycosides of oleanolic acid and machaerinic acid (**10–12**) isolated from *Mimosa tenuiflora* showed a significant mitogenic effect on murine normal lymphocytes (thymocytes and splenocytes) cultured *in vitro*. In this study, the saponins at low concentration (10 µM) were more active on T lymphocytes than on B lymphocytes. Furthermore, they exhibited a synergistic effect with ConA on activation of thymocytes and with LPS on the activation of splenocytes [55].

At the concentrations of 0.03 and 0.16 µM, formosanin-C, a diosgenin tetraglycoside (**13**) from *Paris formosana*, dose-dependently enhanced the proliferative response of human peripheral whole blood to PHA, as shown by evaluated ^{3}H-thymidine incorporation. Formosanin-C also significantly increased the proliferation of Con-A-stimulated lymphocytes at concentrations of 0.1 and 0.01 µM and inhibited this response at concentrations of 1 and 10 µM [56].

Recently, cycloartane triterpene glycosides (**14–21**) from the roots of *Astragalus melanophrurius* [57] were shown to stimulate human lymphocyte proliferation in the concentration range of 0.01–10 µg/ml. At higher concentrations (100–200 µg/ml) inhibition of thymidine incorporation was observed.

Saikosaponin d (**22**) from *Bupleurum* radix, which itself has no mitogenic activity, decreased the spleen cell proliferative response to T cell mitogen (ConA) at a concentration of 0.1 µM, while increasing the response to B cell mitogen (LPS) at the same concentration [58].

Ginsenoside Rg1 (**27**) from *Panax ginseng* also exerted a direct mitogenic effect when applied *in vitro* to microcultures of thymus cells. Again, this effect was greater with a lower dose (25 µg/ml) while a higher dose of Rg1 (50 µg/ml) had no significant effect on thymocytes [59].

The proliferation of murine spleen cells was increased by virgaureasaponin E (**34**) isolated from *Solidago virgaurea* in a dose-dependent manner at very low concentrations (0.01 µg/ml–0.1 ng/ml) [69]. Furthermore, virgaureasaponin E (**34**) showed by flow cytometric investigations, T cell and B cell selective mitogen effects at 0.001 µg/ml and 0.01 µg/ml, respectively [69]. These effects were only known in the case of glycyrrhizin (**4**) [51].

Activation of macrophages

The influence of saponins on immunological functions of macrophages was investigated in a chemiluminescence assay and an assay for induction of cytotoxic macrophages. Addition of saikosaponin d (**22**) (0.5 µM) to mouse peritoneal macrophages remarkably induced the chemiluminescence in response to PHA, in contrast to the lack of effect at 0.1 µM [58]. An increase in phagocytosis was detected after treatment with saikosaponin b2 (**24**) (0.1 µM) for 24 h *in vitro*, while a suppression of phagocytosis was observed following treatment with other saikosaponins (0.5 µM) [58]. Ginsenoside Re (**28**) and glycyrrhetic acid significantly stimulated phagocytosis of murine bone marrow macrophages, but not that of human monocytes and granulocytes [69].

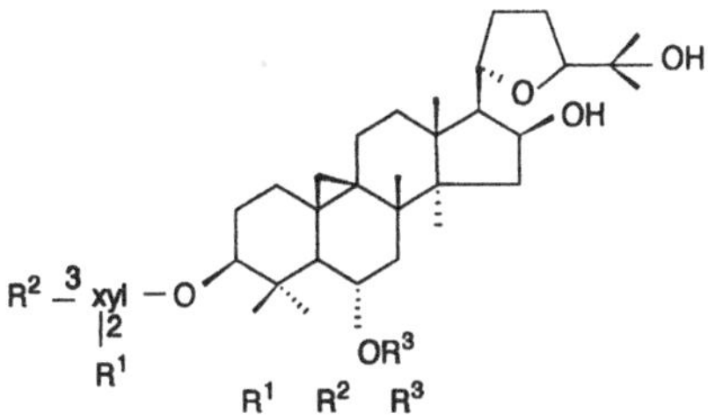

	R^1	R^2	R^3
14	Ac	Ac	xyl
15	Ac	Ac	glc
16	Ac	H	glc
17	H	H	xyl
18	H	H	glc
19	glc	H	glc

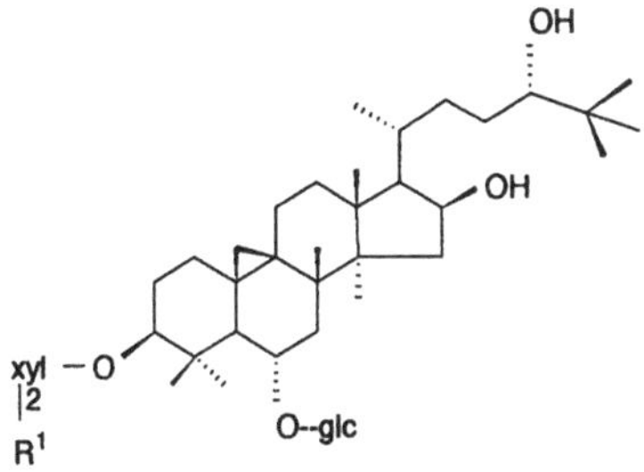

20 $R^1 = H$

21 $R^1 = glc$

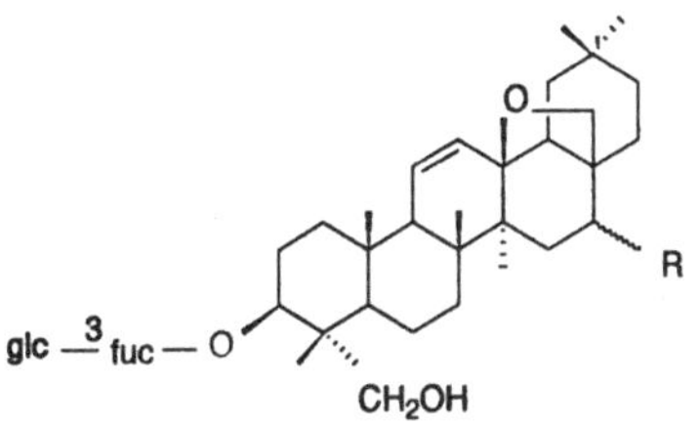

22 R = α - OH

23 R = β - OH

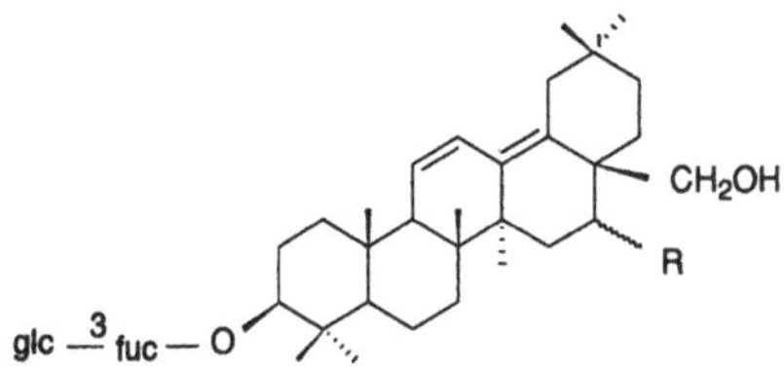

24 R = α - OH

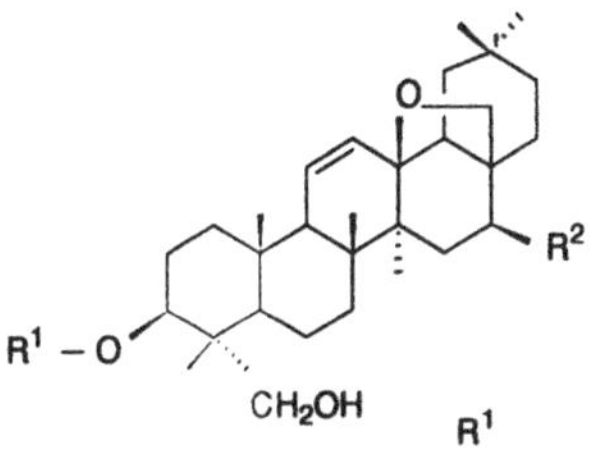

	R^1	R^2
25	glc —3 fuc (2 — glc)	OH

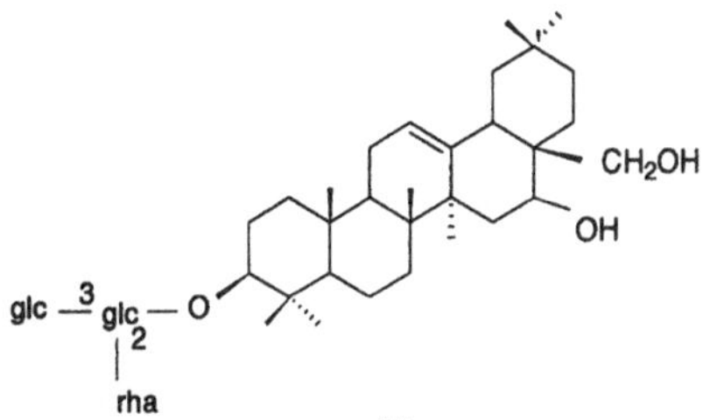

26

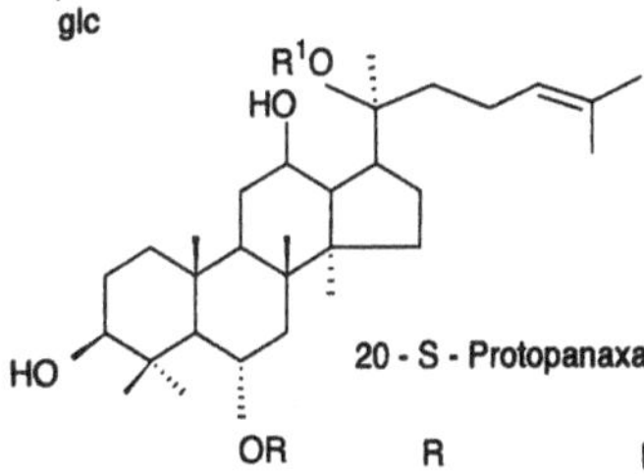

20 - S - Protopanaxatriol

	R	R^1
27	glc-	glc-
28	rha 2 - glc-	glc-

Ginsenoside Re (**28**) and glycyrrhizin (**4**) were able to induce significantly cytotoxic macrophages. After priming with IFNγ and incubating with the saponins the induced cytototoxic macrophages directly killed P 815 tumor cells. Macrophages incubated with glycyrrhizin (0.01 μg/ml) removed 80 ± 30% of the tumor cells and when they were incubated with ginsenoside Re (1 μg/ml), they killed 80 ± 10% of the tumor cells [69].

Activation of granulocytes

In an *in vitro* granulocyte test system according to Brandt, the *Dodonea* saponins (**29–30**) showed a dose-dependent enhancement of phagocytosis up to 25%, while a phagocytosis-independent increase of luminescence of 65% was seen in the chemiluminescence test [53].

In the granulocyte phagocytosis test, a saponin fraction from *Bupleurum fruticosum* showed a 57% stimulation of phagocytosis at a concentration of 1 μg/ml, whereas the main saponin saikogenin F 3-O-triglycoside (**25**) was inactive [60]. The ineffectiveness of this compound could be explained by the fact that the aglycone saikogenin F possesses the same 16β-OH configuration as saikosaponin-a (**23**), which was found to be less effective than saikosaponin-d (16α-OH) (**22**) in the macrophage activation assay [61]. In a concentration range of 10–100 μg/ml, the acylated tetraglycosides of quillaic acid from *Silene jenisseensis* (**31**, **32**) showed a significant enhancement of granulocyte phagocytosis (70%–37%) [62]. Similar results were obtained with a new acylated saponin from *Silene fortunei* [63].

Effect on the production of cytokines

Some triterpene-saponins described in the literature showed the ability to activate cytotoxic macrophages, cytotoxic T cells and NK cells and further to release cytokines like IFNγ, IL-2 and TNFα. Among them, virgaureasaponin E (**34**) was able to release TNFα from murine bone marrow macrophages. The growth inhibition of TNFα-sensitive L 929 fibroblasts was 70 ± 20% [69]. The *in vitro* effect of ginsenoside Rg1 (**27**) on IL-1 production by peritoneal macrophages has been investigated. The results showed that the lower dose of ginsenoside Rg1 (**27**) (25 μg/ml) induced a higher production of IL-1 than the higher dose (50 μg/ml) [59].

An *in vitro* study involving stimulation of IL-1 production by test drugs demonstrated that saikosaponin-d (**22**) had the strongest activity, while saikosaponin-a (**23**), its 23-O-acetyl derivative, and the crude saponin mixture only showed moderate activity. In these oleanene-type triterpenoids, evidence suggested that the C-16 OH is important for biological activity while saikosaponin-d (**22**) (having an ether linkage between C13 and C28, 16α-OH) demonstrated a much stronger effect than the others [61]. Among the saponins tested by Plohmann et al. (1997), no substance induced the release of IL-2 from murine spleen lymphocytes [69].

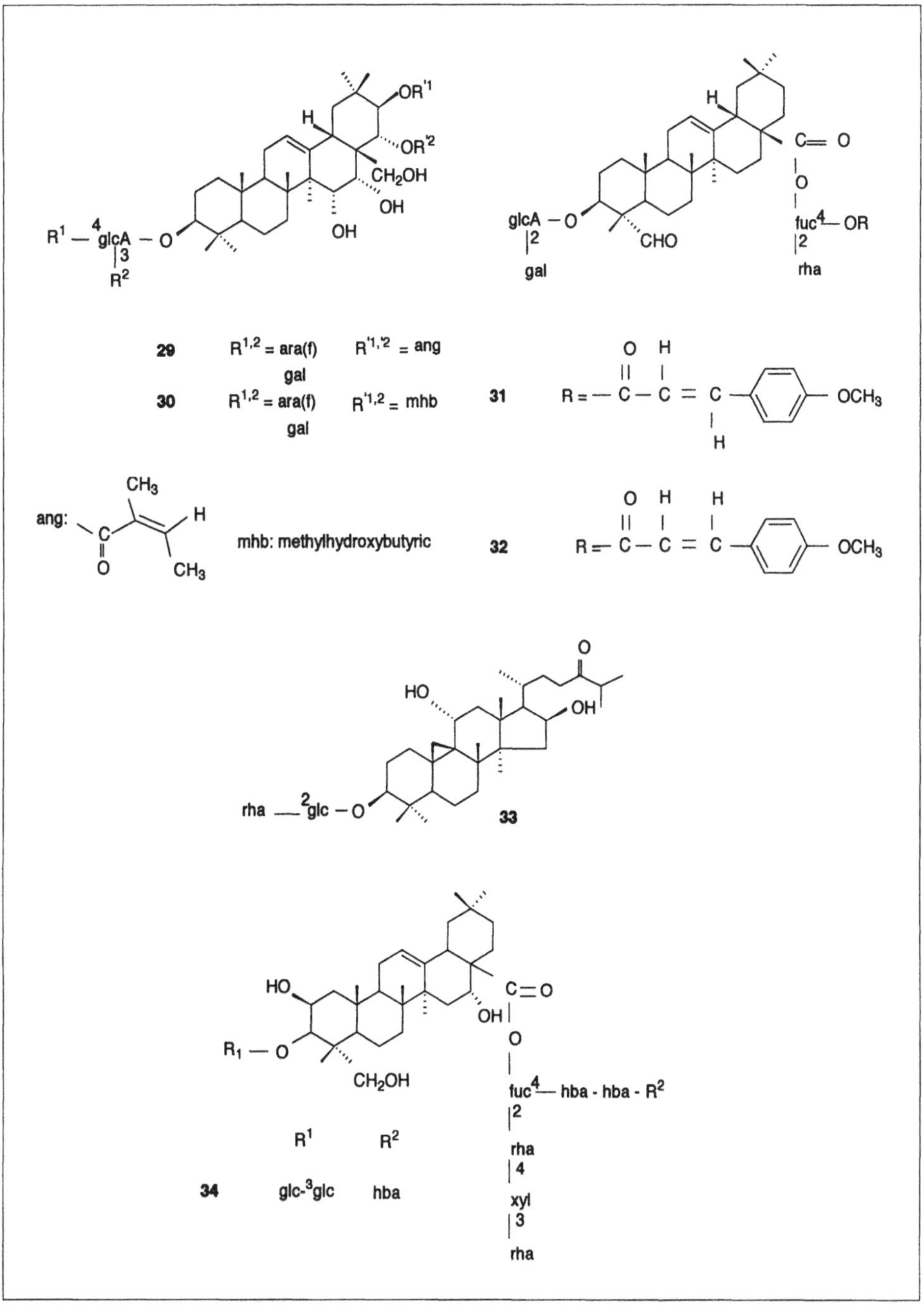

glc, β-D-glucopyranosyl; gal, β-D-galactopyranosyl; rha, α-L-rhamnopyranosyl; xyl, β-D-xylopyranosyl; ara (f), α-L-arabinofuranosyl; fuc, β-D-fucopyranosyl; glcA, β-D-glucuronopyranosyl; hba, β-hydroxy-butyric acid; api, β-D-apiofuranosyl

Formosanin-C (**13**) enhanced the responsiveness of granulocyte-macrophage colony-forming cells (GM-CFC) to mouse fibroblast cell (L929) conditioned medium at a very low concentration of 0.01 μM. This effect may be mediated by directly stimulating GM-CFC proliferation and/or stimulating production of granulocyte-macrophage colony stimulated factor (GM/CSF) [56].

In vivo activities

Curculigosaponin G (**33**), a new cycloartane type triterpene saponin from the rhizomes of *Curculigo orchioides* was shown to significantly promote proliferation of spleen lymphocytes in mice ($p < 0.01$) but no marked influence on antibody formation was seen ($p > 0.05$) [65].

Saikosaponin-d (**22**) injected i.m. in mice increases the phagocytic activities of peritoneal macrophages such as spreading activity, phagocytosis, lysosomal enzyme activity (acid phosphatase) and intracellular killing activity against living yeast [61, 66]. Chemiluminescence of macrophages isolated from mice treated with saikosaponin-d (**22**), stimulated by opsonized zymosan and PMA, was also enhanced [67]. IL-1 production by the cells was increased in a dose-dependent manner [67]. This work also shows an augmentation of lymphoproliferative responses to stimulation with T or B cell mitogens after *in vivo* treatment with saikosaponin-d [67].

The saikosaponins-a (**23**), -d (**22**), -f (**26**) and the crude saponin mixture from the roots of *Bupleurum kaio* demonstrated an immunomodulatory activity in mice [68]. Mice were injected i.p. with drugs to assess immune responses weekly over a four week period. According to the levels of IgA, IgM and IgG in serum, the activity of B cell stimulation in mice treated with saikosaponins-a and -d was promoted week by week. This was correlated with an enlargement of the spleen, the functional organ for maturation of immature B cells. Furthermore, the saikosaponins and the crude mixture enhanced thymus function at an early phase and gradually decreased at a late phase whereas the Th/Ts (T helper/T suppressor) ratio rose to a maximum at an early phase and then decreased. It was also shown that the IL-2 level of mice in each drug-treated group was significantly higher than that of the control group throughout the test period [68].

The literature described the *in vivo* activity of saponins on the liberation of cytokines. For example, interferon was detected in blood of mice after i.v. administration of glycyrrhizin (**4**) [64].

Formosanin C (**13**), given i.p. to mice at doses of 1–2.5 mg/kg induced NK cell activation and interferon production, retarded the growth of transplanted MH 134-mouse hepatoma and potentiated the activity of 5-fluorouracil against this mouse tumor. These results suggest that formosanin C might display an immune-induced antitumor activity [56].

The *in vivo* antitumoral effect of Virgaureasaponin E (**34**) in the mouse tumor models (sarcoma 180 and DBA2/MC.SC-1 fibrosarcoma models) could be due, at least in part, to an immunostimulant activity [69]. The ability of virgaureasaponin E (**34**) to reduce the tumor size by stimulating the immune system could be a consequence of stimulated immune parameters detected in *ex vivo* assays (proliferation and phagocytosis of bone marrow macrophage cells, release of TNFα in the blood of mice treated with the saponin after LPS induction) [69].

Summary

This review provides a summary of recent data concerning immunostimulating properties of saponins. In the first part the saponins of *Quillaja saponaria* bark are described as possessing a potential usefulness as immunoadjuvants, increasing the immunogenicity of many vaccines. From this crude extract of triterpene glycosides, a partially purified fraction (Quil A), a pure isolated saponin (QS-21) and a mixture of defined entities (ISCOPREP 7.0.3) have been obtained. Saponins induced strong Th1 and Th2 responses as well as moderate CTL responses to some non-replicative protein antigens. Quil A is extensively used as an adjuvant in veterinary vaccines but so far not in human trials due to overt toxicity. Quil A and ISCOPREP 7.0.3 are used for the production of immune stimulating complexes (ISCOMs). These submicroscopic particles composed of saponin, cholesterol, phospholipid and antigen are powerful adjuvants inducing strong Th1 and Th2 responses, good targeting and presentation as well as excellent CTL responses. ISCOMs have not shown hemolytic activity at normally administred doses. The side-effects of Quil A were almost absent when Quil A was incorporated into ISCOMs. The basis of the adjuvant activity of these agents has so far not been completely clarified, but they could influence the manner in which the carrier particles interact with the cell membrane, or with membranes of cytoplasmic vesicles of antigen presenting cells. Studies in human Phase I clinical trials of a therapeutic melanoma vaccine, a prophyllactic HIV-1 subunit vaccine, and a malaria vaccine containing QS-21 provided encouraging results, but more extensive proof of inocuity and demonstration of protective efficacy will be required before any new adjuvant reaches the market in the form of a licensed vaccine.

The second part of this review summarizes the immunostimulating effects of saponins, which stimulate, in a non-antigen dependent manner, the function and efficiency of the non-specific immune system. The mitogenic effect of saponins on lymphocytes, the activation of macrophages, the activation of granulocytes and the effect of saponins on the production of cytokines have been shown in several *in vitro* assays. *In vivo* activities have been confirmed with *Curculigo* saponins, saikosaponins, glycyrrhizin, and formosanin C, showing the potential of saponins as immunostimulant compounds. Furthermore, studies showed that formosanin C and virgaureasaponin E might display antitumor activity in association with modulation of the immune system.

This review showed that many recent studies have evaluated the influence of saponins on immune responses proving their importance as immunostimulants. Based on preclinical and clinical observations, it appears that the *Quillaja* saponins, especially QS-21 may have great benefits as adjuvants in commercial vaccines.

References

1 Lacaille-Dubois MA, Wagner H (1996) Biological and pharmacological activities of saponins. *Phytomedicine* 4: 363–383

2 Waller GR, Yamazaki K (eds) (1996) *Saponins used in traditional and modern medicine ACS symposium on saponins: chemistry and biological activity* (Chicago, 1995). Plenum Press, New York

3 Hostettmann K, Marston A (1995) *Saponins.* Cambridge University Press, Cambridge,

4 Cox JC, Coulter AR (1997) Adjuvants – a classification and review of their mode of action. *Vaccine* 15: 248–256

5 Gupta RK, Siber GR (1995) Adjuvants for human vaccines – current status, problems and future prospects. *Vacc*ine 13: 1263–1276

6 Bomford R (1992) Adjuvants for viral vaccines. *Reviews in Medical Virology* 2: 169–174

7 Zhao Z, Leong KW (1996) Controlled delivery of antigens and adjuvants in vaccine development. *J Pharm Sci* 85:1261–1270

8 Kersten GFA (1990) Aspects of ISCOMs: Analytical, pharmaceutical and adjuvant properties. Thesis, National Institute for public health and environmental protection, Biltoven, The Netherlands and the department of Pharmaceutics, University of Utrecht, The Netherlands

9 Kensil CR (1996) Saponins as vaccine adjuvants. *Critical Reviews in Therapeutic Drug Carrier-Systems* 13: 1–55

10 Campbell JB, Peerbaye YA (1992) Saponin. *Res Immunol* 143: 526–530

11 Vogel FR, Powell MF (1995) Compendium of vaccine adjuvants and excipients. In: MF Powell, MJ Newmann (eds): *Vaccine design: The subunit and adjuvant approach.* Plenum Press, New York, 141–228

12 Higuchi R, Tokimitsu Y, Komori T (1988) An acylated triterpenoid saponin from *Quillaja saponaria. Phytochemistry* 27: 1165–1168

13 Kensil CR, Patel U, Lennick CK, Marciani D (1991) Separation and characterization of saponins with adjuvant activity from *Quillaja saponaria* Molina Cortex. *J Immunol* 146: 431–437

14 Kensil CR, Wu JY, Soltysik S (1995) Structural and immunological characterization of

the vaccine adjuvant QS 21. In: MF Powell, MJ Newmann (eds): *Vaccine design: The subunit and adjuvant approach*. Plenum Press, New York, 525–541

15 Bomford R, Stapleton M, Winsor S, Beesley JE, Jessup EA, Price KR, Fenwick GR (1992) Adjuvanticity and ISCOM formation by structurally diverse saponins. *Vaccine* 10: 572–578

16 Bomford R, Stapleton M, Winsor S, Mcknight A, Andronova T (1992) The control of antibody isotype response to recombinant human immunodeficiency virus gp 120 antigen by adjuvants. *AIDS Res Human Retroviruses* 8: 1765–1771

17 Flebbe LM, Braley-Mullen H (1986) Immunopotentiation by SGP and Quil A. II. Identification of responding cell populations. *Cell Immunol* 99: 128–139

18 Stott EJ, Chan WL, Mills KHG, Page M, Taffs F, Cranage M, Greenaway P, Kitchin P (1990) Preliminary report: protection of cynomolgus macaques against simian immunodeficiency virus by fixed-infected cell vaccine. *Lancet* Dec 22/29: 1538–1541

19 Kensil CR, Newman MJ, Coughlin RT, Soltysik S, Bedore D, Recchia J, Wu JY, Marciani DJ (1993) The use of stimulon adjuvant to boost vaccine response. *Vaccine Res* 2: 273–281

20 Britt W, Fay J, Seals J, Kensil, C (1995) Formulation of an immunogenic human cytomegalovirus vaccine: responses in mice. *J Infect Dis* 171: 18–25

21 Hancock GE, Speelman DJ, Frenchick PJ, Mineo-Kuhn MM, Baggs RB, Hahn DJ (1995) Formulation of the purified fusion protein of respiratory syncytial virus with the saponin QS-21 induces protective immune responses in Balb/c mice that are similar to those generated by experimental infection. *Vaccine* 13: 391–400

22 Clark N, Kushner NN, Barrett CB, Kensil CR, Salsbury D, Cotter S (1991) Efficacy and safety field trials of a recombinant DNA vaccine against feline leukemia virus infection. *J Amer Veterin Med Assoc* 199: 1433–1443

23 Ma J, Bulger PA, vR Davis D , Perilli-Palmer B, Bedore DA, Kensil CR, Young EM, Hung CH, Seals JR, Pavia CS et al (1994) Impact of the saponin adjuvant QS-21 and aluminium hydroxide on the immunogenicity of recombinant OspA and Osp B of Borrelia burgdorferi. *Vaccine* 12: 925–932

24 White AC, Cloutier P, Coughlin RT (1991) A purified saponin acts as an adjuvant for a T-independent antigen. *Immunobiol of Proteins and Peptides* VI, 207–210

25 Newmann MJ, Wu JY, Coughlin RT, Murphy CL, Seals JR, Wyand, MS, Kensil CR (1992) Immunogenicity and toxicity testing of an experimental HIV-1 vaccine in non human primates. *AIDS Res Human Retroviruses* 8: 1413–1418

26 Coughlin RT, Fish D, Mather TN, Ma J, Pavia C, Bulger P (1995) Protection of dogs from lyme disease with a vaccine containing outer surface protein (Osp)A, Osp B, and the saponin adjuvant QS-21. *J Infect Dis* 171: 1049–1052

27 Wu JY, Gardner, BH, Murphy CI, Seals JR, Kensil CR, Recchia J, Beltz GA, Newman GW, Newman MJ (1992) Saponin adjuvant enhancement of antigen-specific immune responses to an experimental HIV-1 vaccine. *Vaccine* 148: 1519–1525

28 Newman MJ, Wu JY, Gardner BH, Munroe KJ, Leombruno D, Recchia J, Kensil CR,

Coughlin RT (1992) Saponin adjuvant induction of ovalbumin-specific CD8+ cytotoxic T lymphocyte responses. *J Immunol* 148: 2357–2362
29 Newman MJ, Munroe KJ, Anderson CA, Murphy CI, Panicali DL, Seals JR, Wu JY, Wiand MS, Kensil CR (1994) Induction of antigen-specific killer T lymphocyte responses using subunit SIV mac251 gag and env vaccines containing QS-21 saponin adjuvant. *AIDS Res Human Retroviruses* 10: 853–861
30 Chavali SR, Barton LD, Campbell JB (1988) Immunopotentiation by orally-administered *Quillaja* saponins: effects in mice vaccinated intraperitoneally against rabies. *Clin Exp Immunol* 74: 339–343
31 Wu JY, Gardner BH, Kushner NN, Pozzi LAM, Kensil CR, Cloutier PA, Coughlin RT, Newman MJ (1994) Accessory cell requirements for saponin adjuvant-induced class I MHC antigen restricted cytotoxic T-lymphocytes. *Cell Immunol* 154: 393–406
32 Kensil CR, Soltysik S, Wheeler DA, Wu JY (1996) Structure/function studies on QS-21, a unique immunological adjuvant from *Quillaja saponaria* in: GR Waller , K Yamasaki (eds): Saponins used in traditional and medicinal medicine. Plenum Press, New York, 165–172
33 Soltysik S, Wu JY, Recchia J, Wheeler DA, Newman MJ, Coughlin RT, Kensil CR (1995) Structure/function studies of QS-21 adjuvant: assessment of triterpene aldehyde and glucuronic acid roles in adjuvant function. *Vaccine* 13: 1403–1410
34 Livingston PO, Adluri S, Helling F, Yao TJ, Kensil CR, Newman MJ, Marciani D (1994) Phase 1 trial of immunological adjuvant with a GM2 ganglioside-keyhole limpet haemocyanin conjugate vaccine in patients with malignant melanoma. *Vaccine* 12: 1275–1280
35 Helling F, Zhang S, Shang A, Adluri S, Calves M, Koganty R, Longenecker BM, Yao TJ, Oettgen HF, Livingston PO (1995) GM2-KLH conjugate vaccine: increased immunogenicity in melanoma patients after administration with immunological adjuvant QS-21. *Cancer Res* 55: 2783–2788
36 Stoute JA, Slaoui M, Heppner DG, Momin P, Kester KE, Desmons P, Wellde BT, Garçon N, Kazych U, Marchand M et al (1997) A preliminary evaluation of a recombinant circumsporozoite protein vaccine against *Plasmodium falciparum* malaria. *N Engl J Med* 336: 86–91
37 Morein B, Sundquist B, Höglund S, Dalsgaard K, Osterhaus A (1984) Iscom, a novel structure for antigenic presentation of membrane proteins from enveloped viruses. *Nature* 308: 457–462
38 Barr IG, Mitchell GF (1996) ISCOMs (immunostimulating complexes): The first decade. *Immunol Cell Biol* 74: 8–25
39 Morein B, Lövgren K, Höglund S, Sundquist B (1987) The ISCOM: an immunostimulating complex. *Immmunol Today* 8: 333–338,
40 Claassen I, Osterhaus A (1992) The iscom structure as an immune-enhancing moiety: experience with viral systems. *Res Immunol* 143: 531–541
41 Rimmelzwaan GF, Osterhaus AD (1995) A novel generation of viral vaccines based on the ISCOM matrix. In: MF Powell, MJ Newmann (eds): *Vaccine design: The subunit and adjuvant approach*. Plenum Press, New York, 543–558

42 Villacres-Eriksson M (1993) *Induction of immune response by ISCOMs*. Doctor Thesis, University of Uppsala

43 Takahashi H, Takeshita T, Morein B, Putney S, Germain RN, Berzofsky JA (1990) Induction of $CD8^+$ cytotoxic T cells by immunization with purified HIV-1 envelope protein in ISCOMs. *Nature* 344: 873–875

44 Höglund S, Dalsgaard K, Lövgren K, Sundquist B, Osterhaus A, Morein B (1989) Iscoms and imunostimulation with viral antigens. In: JR Harris (ed): *Subcellular biochemistry*, Vol 15. Plenum Publishing Corporation, New York, 39–68

45 Lövgren Bengtsson K, Sjölander A (1996) Adjuvant activity of iscoms; effect of ratio and co-incorporation of antigen and adjuvant. *Vaccine* 14: 753–760

46 Behboudi S, Morein B, Villacres-Eriksson M (1996) In vitro activation of antigen-presenting cells (APC) by defined composition of *Quillaja saponaria* Molina triterpenoids. *Clin Exp Immunol* 105: 26–30

47 Rönnberg B, Fedaku M, Morein B (1995) Adjuvant activity of non toxic *Quillaja saponaria* Molina components for use in ISCOM matrix. *Vaccine* 13: 1375–1382

48 Rimmelzwaan GF, Baars M, van Beek R, van Amerongen G, Lövgren-Bengtsson, K, Claas EC, Osterhaus AD (1997) Induction of protective immunity against influenza virus in a macaque model: comparison of conventional and iscom vaccines. *J Gen Virol* 78: 757–765

49 Wagner H, Proksch A (1985) Immunostimulatory drugs of fungi and higher plants. In: H Wagner, H Hikino, NR Farnsworth (eds): *Economic and medicinal plant research*. Academic Press, London, 1: 113–151

50 Wagner H, Jurcic K (1991) in: Hostettmann K (eds): *Methods in plant biochemistry*. Academic Press, London, 195–217

51 Chavali SR, Francis T, Campbell BJ (1987) An *in vitro* study of immunomodulatory effects of some saponins. *Int J Immunopharmacol* 9: 675–683

52 Dubois MA, Benze S, Wagner H (1990) New biologically active triterpene-saponins from *Randia dumetorum*. *Planta Med* 56: 451–455

53 Wagner H, Ludwig C, Grotjahn L, Khan MSY (1987) Biologically active saponins from *Dodonea viscosa*. *Phytochemistry* 26: 697–701

54 Lacaille-Dubois MA, Hanquet B, Rustaiyan A, Wagner H (1993) Squarroside A, a biologically active triterpene saponin from *Acanthophyllum squarrosum*. *Phytochemistry* 34: 489–495

55 Jiang Y, Weniger B, Haag-Berrurier M, Anton R, Beck JP, Italiano L (1992) Effects of saponins from *Mimosa tenuiflora* on lymphoma cells and lymphocytes. *Phytotherapy* Res. 6: 310–313

56 Wu RT, Chiang HC, Fu WC, Chien KY, Chung YM, Horng LY (1990) Formosanin-C an immunomodulator with antitumor activity. *Int Immunopharmacol* 12, 777–786

57 Calis I, Yürüker A, Tasdemir D, Wright AD, Sticher O, De Luo Y, Pezzuto JM (1997) Cycloartane triterpene glycosides from the roots of *Astragalus melanophrurius*. *Planta Med* 63: 183–186

58 Ushio Y, Abe H (1991) The effects of saikosaponin on macrophage functions and lymphocyte proliferation. *Planta Med* 57: 511–514
59 Keranova B, Neychev H, Hadjivanova C, Petkov VD (1990) Immunomodulating activity of ginsenoside Rg1 from *Panax ginseng*. *Japan J Pharmacol* 54: 447–454
60 Guinea MC, Parellada J, Lacaille-Dubois MA, Wagner H (1994) Biologically active triterpene saponins from *Bupleurum fruticosum*. *Planta Med* 60: 163–167
61 Kumazawa Y, Takimoto H, Nishimura C, Kawakita T, Nomoto K (1989) Activation of murine peritoneal macrophages by saikosaponin A, saikosaponin D and saikogenin D. *Int J Pharmacol* 11: 21–28
62 Lacaille-Dubois MA, Hanquet B, Cui ZH, Lou ZC, Wagner H (1997) Jenisseensosides C and D, biologically active acylated triterpene saponins from *Silene jenisseensis*. *Phytochemistry* 45: 985–990
63 Lacaille-Dubois MA, Hanquet B, Cui ZH, Wagner H (1997) Structure and bioactivity of a new saponin from *Silene fortunei*. *Annual meeting of the Society for Medicinal Plant Research*, Regensburg, Germany, September, 7–11, 1997, Abstract book G 18
64 Abe N, Ebina T, Ishida N (1982) Interferon induction by glycyrrhizin and glycyrrhetinic acid in mice. *Microbiol Immunol* 26: 535–539
65 Xu JP, Xu RS, Li XY (1992) Four new cycloartane saponins from *Curculigo orchioides*. *Planta Med* 58: 208–210
66 Ushio Y, Abe H (1991) Effects of saikosaponin-D on the functions and morphology of macrophages. *Int J Immunopharmac* 13: 493–499
67 Ushio Y, Oda Y, Abe H (1991) Effect of saikosaponin on the immune responses in mice. *Int Immunopharmac* 13: 501–508
68 Yen MH, Lin CC, Yen CM (1995) The immunomodulatory effect of saikosaponin derivatives and the root extract of *Bupleurum kaio* in mice. *Phytotherapy Res* 9: 351–358
69 Plohmann B, Bader G, Hiller K, Franz G (1997) Immunomodulatory and antitumoral effects of triterpenoid saponins. *Pharmazie* 52: 1–10

Garlic as an immunostimulant

Eikai Kyo[1], Naoto Uda[1], Shigeo Kasuga[1], Yoichi Itakura[1] and Hiromichi Sumiyoshi[2]

[1]Pharmacology and Safety Assessment Laboratory of Institute for OTC Research;
[2]OTC Development Department, Wakunaga Pharmaceutical Co., Ltd., 1624 Shimokotachi, Koda-cho, Takata-gun, Hiroshima 739-11, Japan

Introduction

For over 5000 years, garlic has acquired a worldwide reputation in folklore as a formidable prophylactic and therapeutic medicinal agent [1–3]. More than three thousand publications in this century have confirmed the efficacy of this herb in the prevention and treatment of a variety of diseases, acknowledging and validating the traditional uses.

Many favorable biological and pharmacological effects associated with the consumption of garlic preparations have been reported experimentally and clinically. Garlic has been shown to reduce risk factors of cardiovascular diseases, i.e. lowering serum cholesterol and triglycerides, inhibiting blood coagulation, improving blood circulation and lowering blood pressure [1, 4–11]. Many *in vitro* and *in vivo* studies have suggested possible cancer-preventive effects of garlic preparations and their respective constituents [12–16]. In 1990, the US National Cancer Institute initiated the Designer Food Program in order to determine which foods played an important role in cancer prevention, and they concluded that garlic may be the most potent food having cancer preventive properties [17].

In addition to the above pharmacological activities, garlic has been shown to be a possible biological response modifier. Weisberger and Pensky first reported the augmentation of tumor immunity by garlic [18], and subsequently a variety of immuno-stimulatory effects of garlic have been reported. Since certain diseases can be caused by immune dysfunction, modification of immune functions by garlic may contribute to the treatment and prevention of diseases. Thus, some pharmacological effects of garlic might be mediated through immune modifications. In this chapter, immunostimulatory effects of garlic including our findings using "aged garlic extract" (AGE) are described.

AGE was manufactured by Wakunaga Pharmaceutical Co., Ltd. by the following steps: Briefly, garlic cloves (*Allium sativum*) were sliced and soaked in a water-ethanol mixture and naturally extracted/aged for more than 10 months at room temperature. AGE used for the studies contained approximately 15% of solid mate-

Immunomodulatory Agents from Plants, edited by H. Wagner

rials and 0.1% (calculated on the dried basis) of S-allylcysteine, a marker compound for standardization.

In vitro and *in vivo* studies

Stimulatory effects on immuno-responding cells

A series of *in vitro* and animal studies have revealed that garlic significantly stimulates a variety of immuno-responder cells including T and B lymphocytes, macrophages and natural killer (NK) cells, i.e. enhancement of antibody production, lymphokine release, lymphocyte proliferation, phagocytosis, and NK and lymphokine activated killer (LAK) activities [19–28]. Our recent findings on the immuno-stimulatory activities of AGE are summarized in Table 1.

Phagocytosis

The enhancement of phagocytosis by garlic has been studied extensively. Hirao et al. first reported that AGE at doses of 10 to 1000 μg/ml stimulated, dose-dependently, glucose utilization by the isolated macrophages of mice and that administration of an AGE fraction (5 to 50 mg/kg) significantly increased the carbon clearance in the blood of mice [20]. Lau's group reported a series of studies using the chemiluminescence assay. Phagocytic activity of the peritoneal, spleen and lymph node cells in mice were stimulated by AGE administration [21]. Interestingly, among the four commercial garlic preparations, AGE showed the strongest stimulation of phagocytic activity in the cultured macrophage cell line, whereas two garlic preparations did not show any effect at all [22]. This observation suggests that the manufacturing process could affect the activities of garlic preparations.

Proliferation of spleen cells

AGE and its fractions have been shown to enhance the proliferation of spleen cells [20, 23, 24]. AGE showed a dose-dependent enhancement and the maximum, approximately two-fold, enhancement was observed at a concentration of 1.25 (v/v)%. In combination with other mitogens, AGE augmented ConA and phytohemagglutinin (PHA)-induced lymphocyte proliferation, but not pokeweed mitogen (PWM) and lipopolysaccharide (LPS). Furthermore, IL-2-induced proliferation was significantly augmented by addition of AGE and its fractions.

Cytokine production

AGE significantly increased IL-2, tumor necrosis factor α (TNFα) and interferon γ

Table 1 - Effects of AGE on immune functions in vitro

Immune functions		Effect of AGE	Methods
Proliferation	–	++	MTT assay
	+ ConA	+	MTT assay
	+ PWM	–	MTT assay
	+ LPS	–	MTT assay
	+ IL-2	++	MTT assay
Cytokines release	IL-2	++	ELISA
	TNFα	++	ELISA
	IFNγ	++	ELISA
NK Activity		++	^{51}Cr release
Phagocytosis		++	Latex beads

++, strong up-regulation; +, weak up-regulation; –, ineffectiveness
AGE was added to the culture medium at the final concentration of 10 μl/ml.

MTT assay [49]: C57BL/6 spleen cells (2 ×10^6 cells/well) were cultured in the presence or absence of AGE in a 96-well microtiter plate (NUNC) under 5% CO_2/95% air at 37°C. In the combination assay with mitogens, ConA (2 μg/ml, Honen Corporation, Japan), PWM (1 μg/ml, Honen Corporation, Japan), LPS (1 μg/ml, Sigma) or recombinant IL-2 (10 ng/ml, Biosource International, USA) was added before starting cultivation. Following 3 days incubation, WST-1 reagent (Dojin Corporation, Japan) was added to each well and incubated for a further 3 h [50]. The A_{450} of the incubated mixture was determined using a microplate reader (Bio-Rad).
Cytokines release: C57BL/6 spleen cells (1 ×10^7 cells/ml) were cultured in the presence or absence of AGE in a 24-well plate (NUNC) under 5% CO_2/95% air at 37°C. After 3 days incubation, released cytokines (IL-2, TNFα and INFγ) in the medium were measured using ELISA (Genzyme Duo-set™ ELISA bulk kit, USA).
NK activity: 1.5 ×10^6/100 μl of spleen T cells and 1.5 ×10^4/50 μl of ^{51}Cr-labeled YAC-1 cells were cultured in the presence or absence of AGE in a NUNC round-bottom micro-plate. After 4 and 24 h incubation, the mixture was centrifuged and the released ^{51}Cr in the supernatant was counted in a gamma-counter and the cytotoxicity was determined.
Phagocytosis: The peritoneal cells (10^6 cells/200 μl) were preincubated in the presence or absence of AGE for 3 h under 5% CO_2 at 37°C, and then the fluorescent-labeled latex beads solution (1:100 dilution, 0.75 μYG, Polyscience, USA) was added [51]. After one hour incubation, the cells were centrifuged, washed with PBS, and fixed in 2.5% buffered formalin solution. Macrophages that phagocytoised more than 10 latex beads were counted using Improved Neubauer (Erma, Japan), and the phogocytic activity was determined as the number of activated macrophages per 100 cells [52].

(INFγ) release from mouse spleen cells, and the maximum increase was approximately three-fold for IL-2, 9.5-fold for TNFα and 1.8-fold for INFγ, respectively [24]. Furthermore, a protein fraction of AGE has been shown to significantly augment Con A-induced IL-2, TNFα and INFγ release, and IL-2-induced TNFα and INFγ release from human peripheral lymphocytes [23]. Aqueous garlic extract was also reported to increase *in vitro* IL-1 and 2 production in human peripheral blood mononuclear cells [25].

NK cell and LAK activities

AGE (0.25–1.0 v/v %) treatment enhanced approximately two-fold the NK cell activity of the T cell fraction of mouse spleen cells against mouse lymphoma (YAC-1) [24]. A protein fraction of AGE (2.5–10 μg/ml) also enhanced approximately two-fold the NK cell activity against YAC-1 (unpublished data). Morioka et al. reported that a protein fraction of AGE enhanced the cytotoxicity of human peripheral blood lymphocytes against both NK-sensitive K562 and NK-resistant M14 cell lines [23]. A more remarkable enhancement was observed when a protein fraction was administered together with a suboptimal dose of IL-2 (10 U/ml); combination treatment of a protein fraction (5 μg/ml) plus IL-2 for 72 h generated lymphokine-activated killer activity equivalent to that produced by 100 U/ml IL-2 alone against M14.

Antibody production

Garlic has been shown to increase antibody production [26]. The administration of garlic powder increased the number of red blood cell hemolytic plaque-forming cells in normal mice [27] and AGE prevented the decrease of hemolytic plaque-forming cells in thymectomized mice [28].

These data indicate that garlic and AGE can modulate not only the cell-mediated immune response but also the humoral immune response through the stimulation of a variety of immuno-responder cells.

Anti-tumor activities through immuno-modulation

Garlic has been shown to be an effective biological response modifier in the control of bladder transitional cell carcinoma. Lau et al. reported that both intralesional and intravesical administration of garlic extract on Day 1 and/or 6 after the transplantation of MBT2 murine bladder carcinoma into the mouse bladder significantly reduced the incidence and size of tumors, showing that garlic was more effective than Bacillus Calmette-Guerin (BCG), the common treatment for this carcinoma [29, 30]. Histologically, infiltration of macrophages, neutrophils and lymphocytes into the tumors was observed in the mice treated with garlic extract, whereas only a few lymphocytes and neutrophils were found in the control group. An increase in spleen weight was also noted in the garlic administered group. Riggs et al. also reported that the growth of subcutaneously transplanted MBT2 carcinoma was significantly inhibited by garlic extract injection into the transplantation site [31]. Furthermore, they demonstrated the effectiveness of systemic administration of garlic. Garlic extract was administered orally by adding it to drinking water at concentrations of 5, 50 and 500 mg/100 ml. The tumor volume was significantly reduced in 50 mg/100 ml garlic administered groups. In addition to the reduction of tumor volume, mice receiving 500 mg/ml of garlic extract had a significant decrease in motility. Currently, immunotherapy with BCG is the most effective treatment for superficial bladder carcinoma, but treatment-related toxicity may limit its use in some patients. An alternative treatment using garlic may be effective for patients who fail to respond to BCG immunotherapy.

Using transplantable tumor models as shown in Figure 1a, we determined the effect of AGE on tumor growth. AGE showed growth inhibitory effects on both Sarcoma-180 and Lewis lung carcinoma LL/2 inoculated mice. As shown in Figure 1b, at week three, the tumor size of Sarcoma-180 and LL/2 was 393 ± 48 mm^3 and 1685 ± 161 mm^3 in the control group, respectively, indicating that LL/2 is fast growing, about three times as fast as Sarcoma-180. Growth inhibition by AGE was approximately 50% in Sarcoma-180 and 20% in LL/2, and a significant difference from the control was detected at week three for both of these. Moreover, we measured NK cells and killer cell activities against YAC-1 and Sarcoma-180, respectively, using spleen cells prepared from Sarcoma-180-bearing mice at week three. Significant increases in NK cell and killer cell activities were observed in spleen cells prepared from AGE administered mice (Fig. 1c).

Current cancer therapies, such as surgical excision, radiotherapy and anti-cancer agent administration, are limited, and alternative treatments are needed for patients who fail to respond to these therapies. The modification of immune function may be the most promising alternative for controlling cancer, in particular the stimulation of non-specific immune response and cell-mediated immunity because cancer cells are hardly recognized as alien substances by the immune system. Although further investigations are necessary, presently available data suggest that garlic may provide a new and effective form of cancer therapy through immune stimulation.

Restoration of stress-induced immune suppression

Psychological and physical stresses have been shown to suppress immune functions. Yokoyama et al. reported that the AGE preparation containing vitamin B_1 and B_{12} restored physical stress-induced immune suppression in mice [32]. Restraint stress

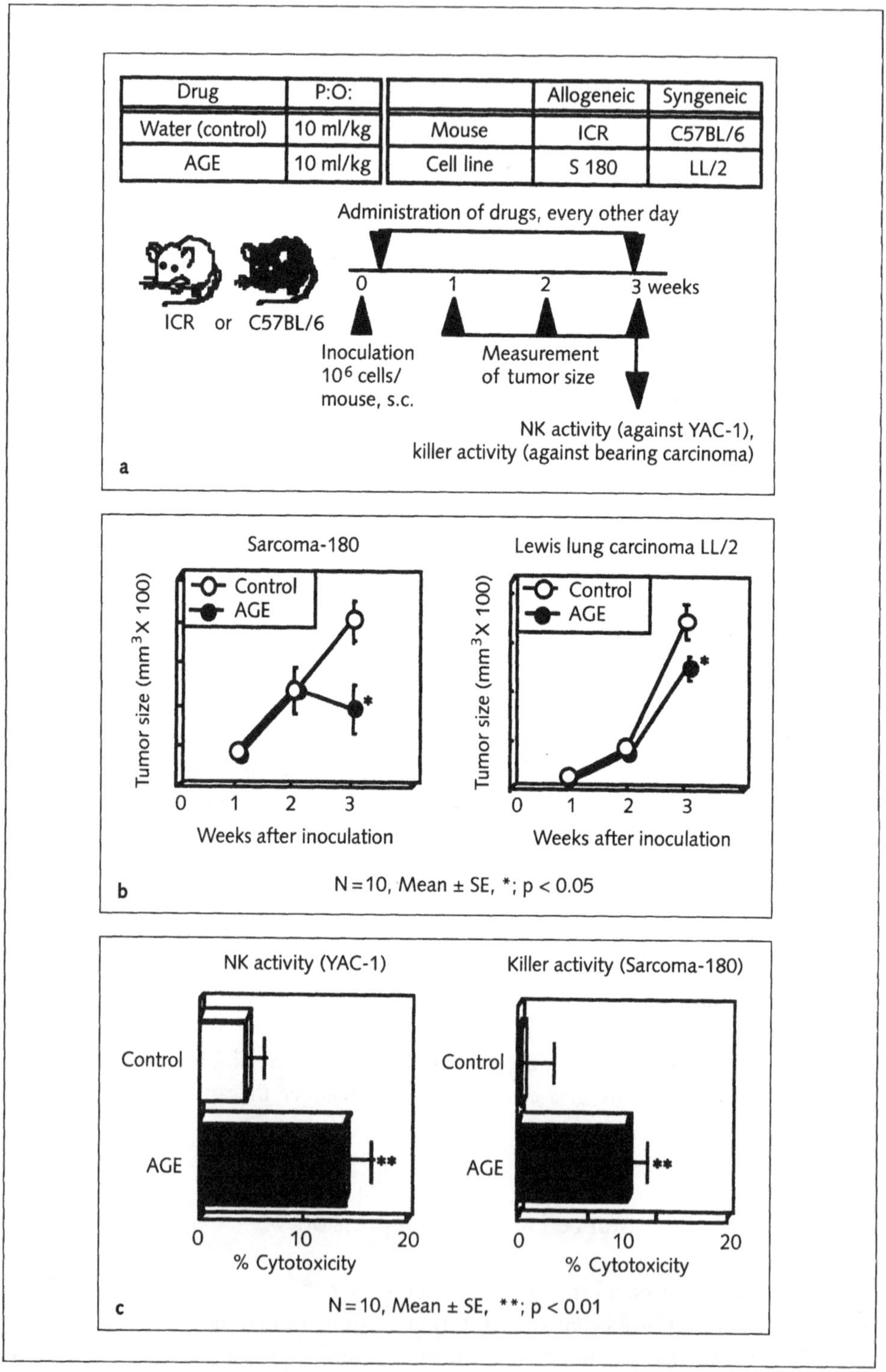
Drug
P:O:
Water (control)
10 ml/kg
AGE
10 ml/kg
Allogeneic
Syngeneic
Mouse
ICR
C57BL/6
Cell line
S 180
LL/2
Administration of drugs, every other day
0
1
2
3 weeks
ICR or C57BL/6
Inoculation
10⁶ cells/
mouse, s.c.
Measurement
of tumor size
NK activity (against YAC-1),
killer activity (against bearing carcinoma)
a
Sarcoma-180
Lewis lung carcinoma LL/2
Control
AGE
Tumor size (mm³X 100)
0
1
2
3
Weeks after inoculation
N=10, Mean ± SE, *; p < 0.05
b
NK activity (YAC-1)
Killer activity (Sarcoma-180)
Control
AGE
0
10
20
% Cytotoxicity
N=10, Mean ± SE, **; p < 0.01
c

(12 h/day) for four consecutive days markedly reduced the numbers of red blood cell hemolytic plaque-forming cells and antibody titer. Oral administration of the AGE preparation at doses of 20, 200 and 2000 mg/ml dose-dependently restored stress-induced decreases in hemolytic plaque-forming cells and antibody titer.

Recently, we determined the effect of AGE on immune suppression caused by psychological stress using a communication box. After four days of psychological stress, a decrease in spleen weight, spleen cells and hemolytic plaque-forming cells was observed in the control mice. As shown in Table 2, AGE significantly prevented the decreases in spleen weight and cells, and restored the reduction of hemolytic plaque-forming cells caused by the stress.

Anti-allergic effect

A number of reports have revealed the relationship between foods and allergic responses. Raw garlic has also been shown to cause contact dermatitis and occupational asthma [33–35]. However, Tanaka et al. reported that *Allium* vegetables, including garlic, inhibit the release of β-hexosaminidase, which is correlated with histamine release, in rat basophilic leukemia cells (RBL-2H3), suggesting an anti-allergic effect [36]. We have also found that AGE has an anti-allergic property [37]. The histamine release in rat basophil cell line RBL-2H3 was induced by mouse anti-TNP monoclonal antibody and TNP-BSA hapten carrier complex. AGE added to the culture medium at doses of 1.25, 2.5 and 5.0 v/v% significantly inhibited the

Figure 1
Anti-tumor effects of AGE
(a) Experimental procedure for anti-tumor assay. In the allogenic system, 10^6 cells of Sarcoma-180 in 100 μl of PBS were subcutaneously inoculated into the backs of ICR male mice. In the syngenic system, 10^6 cells of Lewis lung carcinoma cell line LL/2 in 100 μl of PBS were subcutaneously inoculated into the backs of C57BL/6 male mice. After 24 h carcinoma cell inoculation, water (control, 10 ml/kg) and AGE (10 ml/kg) were orally administered every other day (total 11 administrations). The tumor size was measured once a week using a micrometer, and the volume was calculated. Three weeks after the inoculation, NK and killer activities of spleen cells in Sarcoma-180-bearing mice were determined against YAC-1 cells and Sarcoma-180 cells, respectively.
*(b) Anti-tumor activities of AGE. Values are given as percent of control (mean ± SE (n = 10)). Asterisks denote significant difference from the control: *, p < 0.05.*
*(c) Enhancement of NK and killer cells activities in Sarcoma-180-bearing mice by AGE. Values are given as (mean ± SE (n = 10)). Asterisks denote significant difference from the control: **, p < 0.01.*

Table 2 - Anti-psychological stress of AGE

Group	Spleen weight (mg)	Number of spleen cells ($\times 10^6$)	Number of PFC ($/10^7$)
Normal	87.0 ± 2.9	69.1 ± 2.8	112.9 ± 8.1
Stress control	70.1 ± 2.3^{**a}	46.6 ± 2.7^{**a}	56.6 ± 7.8^{**a}
AGE	82.9 ± 3.8^{**b}	58.6 ± 4.5^{*b}	98.2 ± 14.6^{*b}

Values are mean ± SE (n = 10); $^{**a}p < 0.01$ versus normal; $^{*b}p < 0.05$, $^{**b}p < 0.01$ versus stress control

The communication box was used to provide psychological stress. The box consisted of small compartments (10 × 10 cm) equipped with either an electric foot-shock floor or a non-shock floor, and the electric shock and the non-shock floor were placed reciprocally. A mouse (sender) placed on an electric shock floor made emotional responses when charged with electricity to the floor for 10 sec at intervals of 50 sec and a mouse (responder) placed in a non-shock floor were exposed only to psychological stress. The electric current for the shock was increased stepwise from 1.6 mA to 2.0 mA at the rate of 0.2 mA per 1 h over 3 h. Sender mice were changed daily to naive mice in order to avoid reduced emotional responses to the electric shock due to adaptation to repeated exposures. Responder mice were daily administered with either AGE (10 ml/kg) or water (control) one hr prior to the 3 h emotional stress for 4 days. On day 1, responder mice were immunized with sheep red blood cells (SRBC, 1 × 10^8) after the 3 h stress. After the last day of stress exposure, the spleen weight and number of spleen cells were measured and the number of anti-SRBC plaque-forming-cells (PFC) were assayed.

antigen specific histamine release by 50, 80 and 90 %, respectively (Fig. 2). Oral administration of AGE (10 ml/kg) also decreased 25–45% of the ear swelling used as an index of IgE-mediated skin reaction, that was caused by intravenous administration of anti-TNP IgE antibody and subsequent picryl chloride painting on the ear, in mice (Fig. 3). The late phase reaction was induced first by the picryl chloride challenge to the abdominal skin and then secondly by a challenge to the ear seven days later. Repeated oral administration of AGE at 0, 4 and 16 h after the second picryl chloride challenge inhibited the antigen specific ear swelling by 55% (Fig. 4). Interestingly, among the single AGE administrations, only four h after the second picryl chloride challenge was a decrease in ear swelling noted.

These data suggest that garlic, particularly AGE, may directly and/or indirectly modify the functions of mast cells, basophils and activated T lymphocytes which play a leading role in allergic cascade reactions including inflammation.

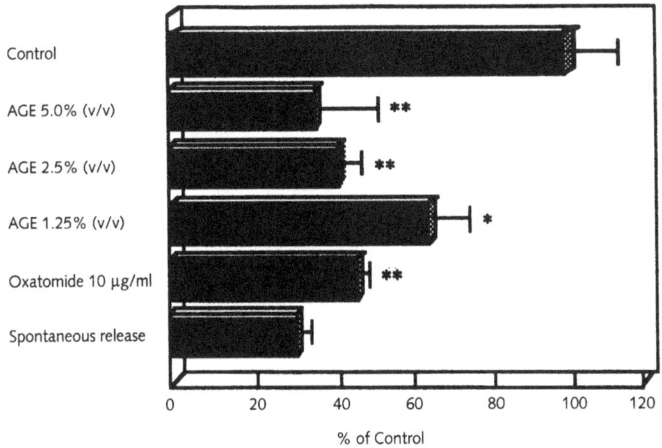

Figure 2
Inhibition of histamine release in basophil cells by AGE
*Rat basophil cell line RBL-2H3 (2×10^5 cells/ml) was inoculated in 24 well plates (Falcon). After 24 h incubation, the basophil cells were washed twice with PBS(–), and 0.3 ml of the culture supernatant containing anti-TNP mouse monoclonal IgE antibody produced by IGEL-2a mouse hybridoma was added. Since the mouse and rat IgE protein have more than 95% homology, anti-TNP mouse monoclonal IgE antibody can occupy the IgE receptors of RBL-2H3 cells. After 3 h incubation, cells were again washed twice with PBS(-). AGE or Oxatomide (positive control) and 0.3 ml of TNP-BSA (10 mg/ml tyrode solution) as the hapten-carrier antigen to induce the histamine release were added and incubated for a further one hour. Released histamine in the supernatant from RBL-2H3 cells was measured by the o-phtalaldehyde method. In this system, the histamine release in the culture medium induced by the antigen-antibody specific interaction was 116 ± 7 ng/ml, which corresponded to 25% of total histamine in RBL-2H3 cells, and the spontaneously released histamine was 36 ± 4 ng/ml. Values are given as percent of control (mean ± SE ($n = 6$)). Asterisks denote significant difference from the control: *, $p < 0.05$, **, $p < 0.01$.*

Anti-arthritic effect

Shah and Vohora reported that steam-distilled garlic oil administered orally at a dose of 2.5 mg/kg body weight inhibited formaldehyde-induced arthritis in rats by 26% [38]. Moreover, the anti-arthritic effect of garlic was enhanced when combined with boron, suggesting a synergistic action.

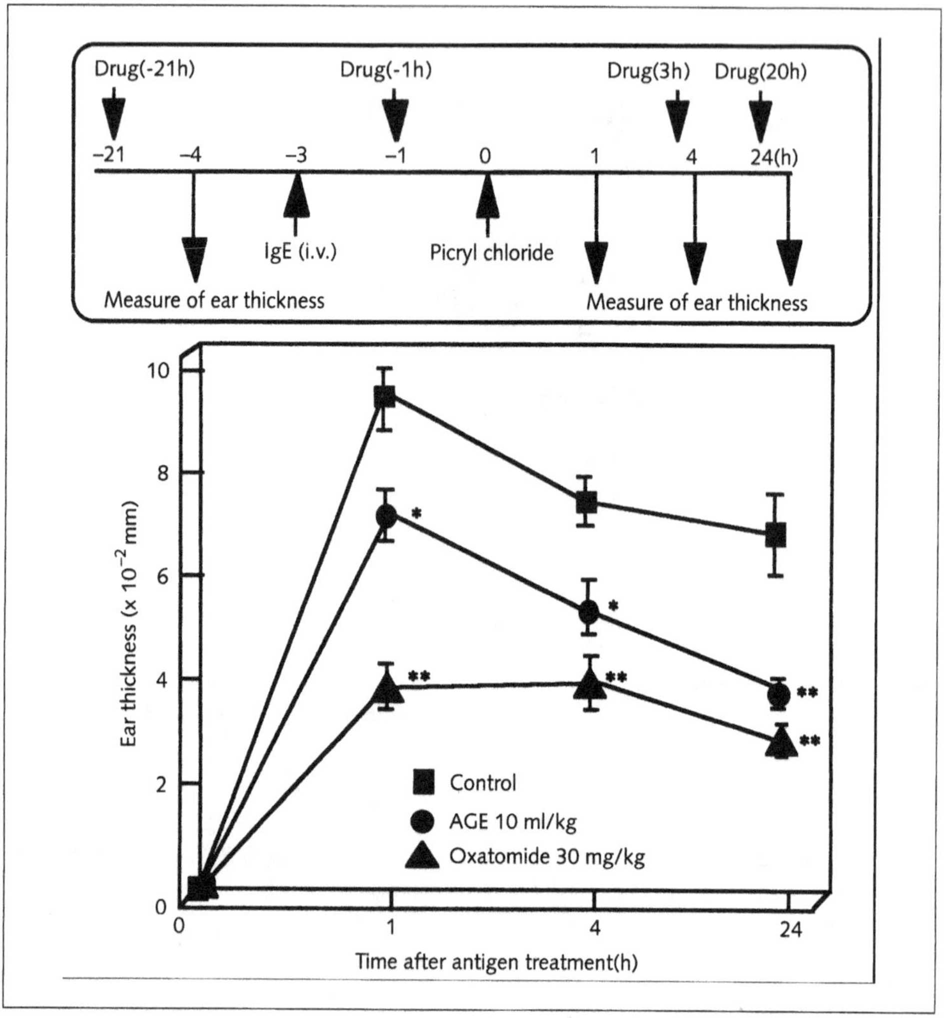

Figure 3

Suppression of IgE mediated antigen specific skin reaction by AGE

*BALB/c male mice were intravenously administered with anti-TNP IgE antibody ascites (PCA titer was 1:4800, 0.5 ml/mouse). After three hours, 0.3% picryl chloride (15 µl/ear) in the acetone and olive oil mixture (4:1) was painted on both sides of the right pinna. Since picryl chloride binds to the amino groups of protein, the conjugates work as a hapten-carrier antigen which react with anti-TNP IgE antibodies which bind to the mast cell IgE receptors and subsequently induce spongiotic changes in the ear skin. AGE and oxatomide as a positive control were orally administered at 21 and 1 h prior and 3 and 20 h after the picryl chloride treatment. Thickness of the ear was at 4 h prior and 1, 4 and 24 h after the picryl chloride treatment. Each point represents the mean ± SE (n = 10). Asterisks denote significant difference from the control: *, $p < 0.05$, **, $p < 0.01$.*

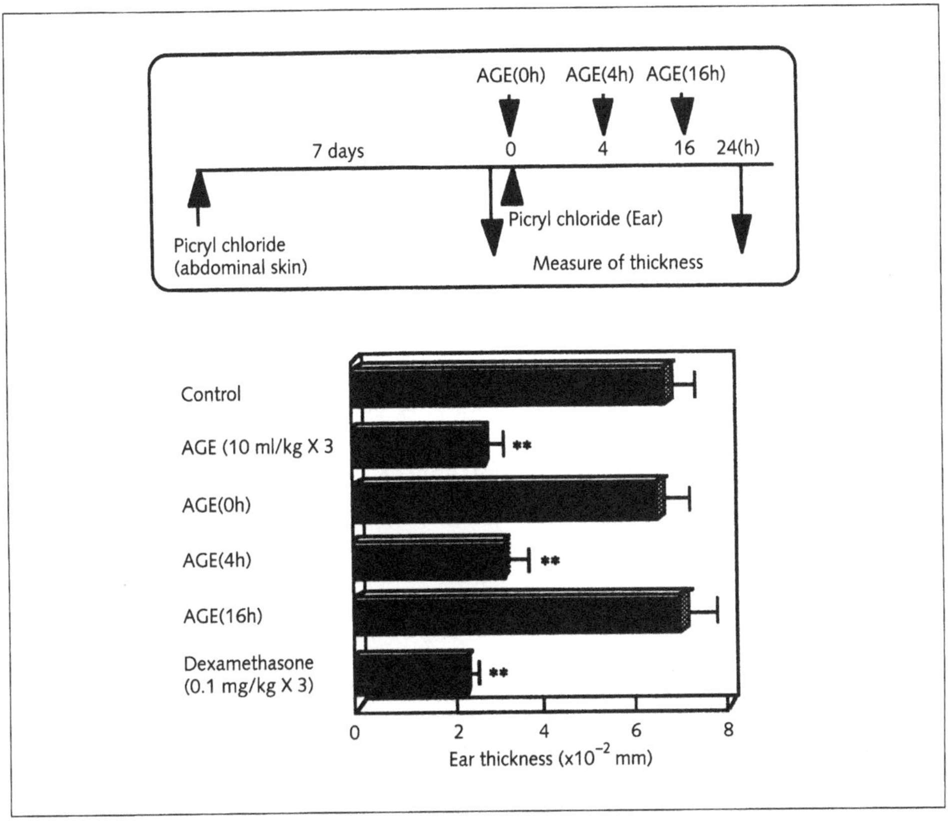

Figure 4
Suppression of antigen specific late phase reaction by AGE
*7% picryl chloride (100 µl/mouse) in ethanol was rubbed onto the abdominal skin of BALB/c male mice. Seven days later, 1% picryl chloride (10 µl/ear) in the acetone and olive oil mixture (4:1) was painted on both sides of the right ear pinna. AGE and dexamethasone as a positive control were orally administered three times at 0, 4 and 16 h after the second picryl chloride treatment. AGE was also administered once at 0, 4 or 16 h. Thickness of the ear was at 1 h prior and 24 h after the second picryl chloride treatment. Each point represents the mean ± SE (n = 10). Asterisks denote significant difference from the control: **,*

Anti-infectious and other effects

Traditional use of garlic for prevention of the common cold could be associated with the stimulation of immune functions. Nagai reported a preventive effect of the AGE preparation against influenza virus (AO/PR 8 strain) infection [39]. Oral administration of the AGE preparation for ten days prior to pernasal virus inoculation exhibited preventive activity as effective as vaccine treatment. A non-specific factor, which had a broad preventive activity against influenza viruses, was detected in the mouse serum after AGE administration.

Tadi et al. reported an effect of AGE on *Candida albicans* clearance from the blood [40]. 24 h after a *Candida albicans* injection (1×10^6), mice treated with saline yielded a colony count of 3,500/0.5 ml blood, whereas mice treated with AGE at a dose of 0.1 ml/mouse yielded only 400 colonies. At 48 h, the saline-treated group had 1400 colonies, but no colony was found in the AGE-treated mice, indicating stimulation of phagocytic activity.

The suppression of T cell-mediated immunity by UV radiation appears to be a prerequisite for the outgrowth of UV-induced tumors in mice and is also manifested by an impaired ability to respond to contact sensitizing agents. Feeding AGE improved the impairment of contact hypersensitivity in hairless mice exposed to UVB (280–320 nm) radiation [41]. The modulation of UV-induced immunosuppression by AGE has been suggested to involve antagonism of the role of cis-urocanic acid, a natural photoproduct believed to participate as an immunogenic mediator.

Human studies

Preliminary studies in humans using a powdered preparation have demonstrated positive effects on immunoreactions and phagocytosis [42]. In geriatric subjects, the garlic administration (600 mg/day) for three months induced significant increases in the percentage of phagocytosing peripheral granulocytes and monocytes when tested ex vivo for their ability to engulf *Escherichia coli* bacteria. The cell counts of lymphocyte cell subpopulations were also increased.

The stimulation of NK cell activity by garlic has been demonstrated in healthy subjects and AIDS patients. After three weeks administration of raw garlic (0.5 g/kg/day) and the AGE preparation (1800 mg/day), NK cell activity against the K562 tumor cell line was significantly enhanced in healthy volunteers, suggesting the superiority of AGE over raw garlic [43, 44]. In the AIDS patient study, AGE was administered at doses of 5 g/day for the first six weeks and 10 g/day for the next six weeks. After six weeks, six out of seven patients had a normal range of NK cell activity, and all had normal activity after 12 weeks [45]. An improvement in helper/suppresser ratio was also observed. Furthermore, during the administration period, improvement of diarrhoea, genital herpes, candidiasis and pansinusitis was also noted.

Active constituents

The efficacy of aqueous garlic extract and its thiosulfinate and polar fractions on immune functions has been evaluated using human peripheral blood cells *in vitro*

[25]. The thiosulfinate fraction increased NK cell activity, whereas the aqueous extract had no effect and the polar fraction decreased NK cell activity slightly. IL-1 production was stimulated by aqueous extract and the polar fraction, but not the thiosulfinate fraction. IL-2 production was stimulated by the aqueous extract and both fractions at a dose of 0.4 mg/ml, however, the thiosulfinate fraction at doses of 0.8 and 1.6 mg/ml and the polar fraction at a dose of 1.6 mg/ml significantly decreased the production. Furthermore, blasogenesis was inhibited by the aqueous extract and both fractions.

Feng et al. reported an immune stimulatory effect of diallyl trisulfide (DATS) [46]. DATS at concentrations of 3.125–12.5 μg/ml augmented the activation of T lymphocytes by Con A, whereas it showed an inhibitory effect at a high concentration (50 μg/ml). Although DATS inhibited nitric oxide production in macrophages, it also enhanced hydrogen peroxide production and cytotoxicity against tumor cell lines.

The immuno-stimulation of the AGE fractions has been evaluated. Glucose utilization in macrophages was stimulated by a protein fraction, but not the low molecular weight and sugar fractions [20]. Furthermore, as already mentioned, a protein fraction of AGE has been shown to have a variety of immune stimulatory effects, such as enhancement of phagocytosis, NK activity, proliferation and lymphokine release.

At present, a limited number of studies on immune stimulatory constituents in garlic were reported and the active principle(s) is far from conclusive. A variety of constituents in garlic may contribute to its effects, i.e. since the immune system involves several types of immuno-responder cells, different constituents may affect different responders. For example, our recent results suggest that AGE contains two types of SH-compounds; one stimulates interleukin-2 release from mouse spleen cells and the other suppresses the release (unpublished data).

Recently, a mannose-specific lectin was isolated from garlic cloves [47, 48]. Since some lectin has been shown to have an immune stimulatory property, it could be interesting to study the activity of garlicís lectin on immune functions.

Conclusion

Recent advanced technologies are clarifying the important roles of immune functions in disease progression. Immune dysfunction may result in infectious diseases and cancer, and hyper immune reactions may cause auto-immune diseases including allergy and rheumatoid arthritis. Thus, the development of an immune modifier, which stimulates necessary functions and suppress unnecessary functions, is truly desired.

A variety of herbs have been traditionally used to prevent and treat diseases. Presently, their pharmacological activities, particularly stimulation of immune functions, has been the focus of alternative medicine. Currently available data strongly suggest that garlic may be a promising candidate as an immune modifier, which maintains the homeostasis of immune function, and warrants further studies to elucidate its application.

References

1 Lau BHS, Adetumbi MA, Sanchez A (1983) *Allium sativum* (garlic) and atherosclerosis. *Nutr Res* 3: 119–128
2 Adetumbi MA, Lau BHS (1983) *Allium sativum* (garlic) – a natural antibiotic. *Med Hypotheses* 12(3): 227–237
3 Essman EJ (1984) The medicinal uses of herbs. *Fitoterapia* 55: 279–289
4 Fenwick GR, Hanley AB (1985) The genus Allium-Par 2. *Crit Rec Food Sci* 22: 273–377
5 Ernst E (1987) Cardiovascular effects of garlic (*Allium sativum*): a review. *Pharmatherapeutica* 5: 83–89
6 Klendler BS (1987) Garlic (*Allium sativum*) and onion (*Allium cepa*): a review of their relationship to cardiovascular disease. *Prevent Med* 16: 670–685
7 Kleijnen J, Knipschild P, ter Riet G (1989) Garlic, onion and cardiovascular risk factors. A review of the evidence from human experiments with emphasis on commercially available preparations. *British J Clin Pharmacol* 28: 535–544
8 Warshafsky S, Kamer RS, Sivak SL (1993) Effect of garlic on total cholesterol, a meta-analysis. *Ann Int Med* 119: 599–605
9 Silagy CA, Neil HA (1994) A meta-analysis of the effect of garlic on blood pressure. *J Hypertensions* 12: 463–468
10 Sendl A (1995) *Allium sativum* and *Allium ursinum*: Part 1: Chemistry, analysis, history, botany. *Phytomedicine* 4: 323–339
11 Reuter HD (1995) *Allium sativum* and *allium ursinum*: Part 2: Pharmacology and medicinal application. *Phytomedicine* 2: 73–91
12 Sumiyoshi H, Wargovich MJ (1989) Garlic (*Allium sativum*): a review of its relationship to cancer. *Asia Pacific J Pharmacol* 4: 133–140
13 Dausch JG, Nixon DW (1990) Garlic: a review of its relationship to malignant disease. *Preventive Medicine* 19: 346–361
14 Dorant E, van den Brandt PA, Goldbohm RA, Hermus RJ, Sturmans F (1993) Garlic and its significance for the prevention of cancer in human: a critical review. *British J Cancer* 67: 424–429
15 Yang CS, Wang ZY, Hong JY (1994) Inhibition of tumorigenesis by chemicals from garlic and teas. In: Jacobs MM (ed): *Diet and cancer: Markers, prevention, and treatment.* Plenum Press, New York, 113–122
16 Ip C, Lisk DJ, Scimeca JA (1994) Potential of food modification in cancer prevention. *Cancer Res* 54: 1957s–1959s
17 Caragay AB (1992) Cancer-preventive foods and ingredients. *Food Technol* 4: 65–68

18 Weisberger AS, Pensky J (1957) Tumor-inhibiting effects derived from an active principle of garlic (*Allium sativum*). *Science* 126: 1112–1114
19 Brosche T, Platt D (1993) Zur immunomodulatorische Wirkung von Knoblauch (*Allium sativum* L.). *Med Welt* 44: 309–313
20 Hirao Y, Sumioka I, Nakagami S, Yamamoto M, Hatono S, Fuwa T, Nakagawa S (1987) Activation of immunoresponder cells by the protein fraction from aged garlic extract. *Phytother Res* 1: 161–164
21 Lau BHS (1989) Detoxifying, radio-protective and phagocyte-enhancing effects of garlic. *Int Clin Nutr Rev* 9: 27–31
22 Lau BHS, Lau MD, Yamasaki T, Gridley DS (1991) Garlic compounds modulate macrophage and T-lymphocyte functions. *Mol Biother* 3: 103–7
23 Morioka N, Sze LL, Morton DL, Irie RF (1993) A protein fraction from aged garlic extract enhances cytotoxicity and proliferation of human lymphocytes mediated by interleukin-2 and concanavalin A. *Cancer Immunol Immunother* 37: 316–322
24 Kyo E, Uda N, Suzuki A, Kakimoto M, Ushijima M, Kasuga S, Itakura Y (1997) Immuno-modulation and anti-tumor activities of Aged Garlic Extract. *Phytomedicine* 5 (4): 259–267
25 Burger RA, Warren RP, Lawson LD, Hughes BG (1993) Enhancement of *in vitro* human immune function by *Allium sativum* L. (garlic) fraction. *Int J Pharmacogn* 31: 169–174
26 Gupta JB, Godhwani JL (1984) Modification of immunological response by garlic, guggal, and tumeric in albino rats. *Indian J Pharmacol* 16: 62–63
27 Arzamastsev EV (1993) Immunomodulating properties of garlic powder. Unpublished data presented at the International Conference “New Mechanism for Preventive and Therapeutic Actions of Garlic”, Nuremberg, 11–22 January
28 Zhang YX, Saito H, Nishiyama N (1994) Ameliorating effect of aged garlic extract (AGE) on learning behaviours in thymectomixed senescence accelerated mouse (SAM). In: Takeda T (ed): *The SAM model of senescence*. Excerpta Medica, Amsterdam 451–454
29 Lau BHS, Woolley JL, Marsh CL, Barker GR, Koobs DH, Torrey RR (1986) Superiority of intralesional immunotherapy with corynebacterium parvum and allium sativum in control of murine transitional cell carcinoma. *J Urol* 136: 701–705
30 Marsh CL, Torrey RR, Woolley JL, Barker GR, Lau BHS (1987) Superiority of intralesional immumotherapy with corynebacterium parvum and allium sativum in control of murine bladder cancer. *J Urol* 137: 359–362
31 Riggs DR, DeHaven JI, Lamm DL (1997) Allium sativum (garlic) treatment for murine transitional cell carcinoma. *Cancer* 79: 1987–94
32 Yokoyama K, Uda N, Takasugi N, Fuwa T (1986) Anti-stress effects of garlic extract preparation containing vitamins (Kyoleopin) and ginseng-garlic preparation containing vitamin b1 (Leopin-five) in mice. *Oyo Yakuri* (*Appl Pharma*) 31: 977–984
33 Lembo G, Balato N, Patruno C et al (1991) Allergic contact dermatitis due to garlic (*Allium sativum*). *Contact Dermatitis* 25: 330–331
34 McFadden JP, White IR, Rycroft RJG (1992) Allergic contact dermatitis from garlic. *Contact Dermatitis* 27: 333–334

35 Lybarger JA, Gallagher JS, Pulver DW et al (1982) Occupational asthma induced by inhalation and ingestion of garlic. *J Allergy Clin Immunol* 69: 448–454

36 Tanaka Y, Kataoka M, Konishi Y, Nishimune T, Takagaki, Y (1992) Effects of vegetable foods on b-hexosaminidase release from rat basophilic leukemia cells (RBL-2H3). *Jpn J Toxicol Environ Health* 38: 418–24

37 Kyo E, Uda N, Kakimoto M, Yokoyama K, Ushijima M, Sumioka I, Kasuga S, Itakura Y (1997) Anti-allergic effects of Aged Garlic Extract. *Phytomedicine* 4 (4): 335–340

38 Shah SA, Vohora SB (1990) Boron enhances antiarthritic effects of garlic oil. *Fitoterapia* 61: 121–126

39 Nagai K (1973) Experimental studies on the preventative effect of garlic extract against infection with influenza virus. *Kansenshogaku-zassi* (*Jpn J Infect Disease*) 47(9): 321– 325

40 Tadi PP, Teel RW, Lau BHS (1990) Anticandidal and anticarcinogenic potentials of garlic. *Int Clin Nutr Rev* 10: 423–429

41 Reeve VE, Bosnic M, Rozinova E, Boehm-Wilcox C (1983) A garlic extract protects from ultraviolet B (280–320 nm) radiation-induced suppression of contact hypersensitivity. *Photochem Photobiol* 58(6): 813–817

42 Brosche T, Platt D (1994) Knoblauchtherapie und zelluläre Immunabwehr im Alter. *Z Phytother* 15: 23–24

43 Kandil O, Abdullah TH, Elkadi A (1987) Garlic and the immune system in humans: its effect on natural killer cells. *Fed Proc* 46: 441

44 Kandil O, Abdullah TH, Tabuni AM, Elkadi A (1988) Potential role of *Allium sativum* in natural cytotoxicity. *Arch AIDS Res* 1: 230–231

45 Abdullah TH, Kirkpatrick DV, Carter J (1989) Enhancement of natural killer cell activity in AIDS with garlic. *J Oncol* 21: 52–53

46 Feng ZH, Zhang GM, Hao TL, Zhou B, Zhang H, Jiang ZY (1994) Effect of diallyl trisulfide on the activation of T-cell and macrophage-mediated cytotoxicity. *J Tongji Med Univ* 14: 142–147

47 Smeets K, Van Damme EJ, Verhaert P, Barre A, Rouge P, Van Leuven F, Peumans WJ (1997) Isolation, characterization and molecular cloning of the mannose-binding lectins from leaves and roots of garlic (*Allium sativum* L.). *Plant Mol Biol* 33(2): 223–234

48 Gupta A, Sandhu RS (1997) A new high molecular weight agglutinin from garlic (*Allium sativum*). *Mol and Cell Biochem* 166(1–2): 1–9

49 Mosmonn T (1983) Rapid colorimetric assay for cellular growth and survival: Application to proliferation and cytotoxicity assays. *J Immunol Methods* 65: 55–63

50 Ishiyama M, Shiga M, Sasamoto K, Mizoguchi M, He PG (1993) A new sulfonated tetrazolium salt that produces a highly water-soluble formazan dye. *Chem Pharm Bull* 41: 1118–1122

51 Stewart CC, Lehnert BE, Steinkamp JA (1986) *in vitro* and *in vivo* measurement of phagocytosis by flow cytometry. *Methods in Enzym* 132: 183–192

52 Rosenstreich DL, Blake JT, Rosenthal AS (1971) The peritoneal exudate lymphocytes. I. Differences in antigen responsiveness between peritoneal exudate and lymph node lymphocytes from immunized guinea pigs. *J Exp Med* 134: 1170–1186

Immunostimulants in Ayurveda medicine

Sharadini A. Dahanukar, Urmila M. Thatte and Nirmala N. Rege

Ayurveda Research Centre, Dept. of Pharmacology and Therapeutics, Seth GS Medical College, Parel, Mumbai 400 012, India

Introduction

Ayurveda is the traditional medicinal system of India and is believed to have originated over six thousand years ago. It is a science that describes ways to remain healthy as well as methods to treat disease. The name itself means "Knowledge (Veda) of Life (Ayu)". Although Ayurveda gives equal emphasis to diet and life-style, drugs (and among these, plants) form an important mainstay in the therapy [1].

The beginnings of immunology can be traced back to the ancient folk observation that a person who recovers once from a disease does not get it again. However, the formal use of the word 'immunity' (from the Latin word *immunitas* meaning being exempt from service of the state!), in the context in which we use it today, dates back to AD 39–65 when Roman Marcus Annaeus Lucanus described it in one of his poems [2]. The concept of modulating this immunity with chemicals is however very recent – having gained importance in the late 20th century.

Ayurveda was described centuries before this. Hence, it is only natural that Ayurveda does not mention the terms "immunostimulants" or "immunomodulators". The original Ayurvedic texts, like Charaka and Sushruta Samhita [3, 4], are written in Sanskrit, the classical language of ancient India. Thus, translation and interpretation of terms which may mean "immunostimulant" or "immunomodulator" have been the major source of research material for many scientists.

It is interesting to briefly examine some concepts of health described in Ayurveda before discussing the scientific data available on the relevant plants. This will make it simpler to appreciate why these plants have been selected for further study as potential immunomodulators by modern researchers.

Ayurvedic concept of health

Human physiology is described in Ayurveda [5] in terms of the five basic elements (*panchamahabhuta*) which form all matter on earth. These are *akash* (space), *vayu*

Immunomodulatory Agents from Plants, edited by H. Wagner

(wind), *jal* (water), *prithvi* (earth) and *agni* (fire). Health revolves around the tripod of *dosha* (humours), *dhatu* (tissues) and *mala* (metabolic end products). Each of these are made up of specific basic elements which confer on them their unique properties characteristic of those elements. There are three *doshas*. The first is *vata* which is the lightest, being formed of space (*akash*) and wind (*vayu*). This is the controlling force and mainly influences movement. The second, named *pitta* and consisting of fire (*agni*) and water (*jal*), is fiery and is responsible for enzymatic and metabolic activity. The last is *kapha*, which is made of earth (*prithvi*) and water (*jal*) and is consequently heavy and sedating. It controls secretions and anabolic activities. These three *doshas* have to be in harmony for a person to be in a state of positive health. The tissues (*dhatus*) are broadly described to be of seven types. These are arranged in a hierarchial fashion beginning with *rasa* (plasma) followed by (in their hierarchial order) *rakta* (blood), *mamsa* (muscle), *medya* (fat), *asthi* (bone), *majja* (marrow) and *shukra* (germinal tissues). These tissues derive their health from properly digested food which is assimilated into the *rasadhatu*. The qualities of *rasadhatu* influence the health of subsequent *dhatus*. This explains the preoccupation of Ayurvedic physicians with diet and the importance of drugs that act on the rasadhatu (*rasayanas*) which would in turn influence the actions of all tissues.

Ayurvedic descriptions of "immunostimulant" plants

Ayurveda does describe medicines that will "stave off diseases". In fact, the science of "prevention" is described in great detail and does not restrict itself to plants as therapeutic measures. Ayurveda also gives a lot of emphasis on the use of therapies that produce a "pro-host" effect, thus keeping a person in a state of "positive health".

The properties of plants described as "*jeevaniya*", "*balya*", "*vayasthapaniya*" or "*rasayana*" in Charaka or Sushruta Samhita suggest that they may have immunological effects. This is because, when literally translated, *jeevaniya* means "life-promoters", *balya* means "strengtheners", while *vayasthapaniya* means "agents that increase the life-span". The term *rasayana* includes all these activities. *Rasayana* plants are particularly recommended for the treatment of epidemic diseases [3] conveying that they probably promote host defences. All these plants are expected to strengthen the host so that health is promoted and diseases prevented.

Table 1 lists some of the plants described in Charaka Samhita and Sushruta Samhita having these properties.

Rasayana concept [7, 8]

The word *rasayana* literally means the path that *rasa* takes (*rasa*: the primordial *rasa-dhatu* or plasma; *ayana*: path).

Table 1 - Plants described as rasayana, jeevaniya, balya *and* vayasthapaniya *in Charaka and Sushrut Samhitas.*

Sushrut Samhita	Charaka Samhita
Rasayana	
Callicarpa macrophylla	*Acorus calamus*
Centella asiatica	*Asparagus racemosus*
Chonus calamos	*Bacopa monnieri*
Glycerrhiza glabra	*Boerhavia diffusa*
Herpestis monniera	*Centella asiatica*
Putranjiva roxburghii	*Convolvulus pluricaulis*
	Embelia ribes
	Emblica officinalis
	Ephedra gerardiana
	Glycerrhiza glabra
	Grewia hirsuta
	Leptadenia reticulata
	Piper longum
	Polygonatum verticillatum
	Polygonatum circucifollium
	Prunus cirasoldus
	Pueraria tuberosa
	Semecarpus anacardium
	Terminalia belerica
	Terminalia chebula
	Tinospora cordifolia
	Withania somnifera
Jeevaniya	
Fritillaria oxypetala	*Fritillaria oxypetala*
Glycerrhiza glabra	*Glycerrhiza glabra*
Habenaria intermedia	*Lepdtadenia reticulata*
Leptadenia reticulata	*Lilium polyphyllum*
Lilium polyphyllum	*Microstylis wallichii*
Microstylis muscitera lindi	*Microstylis muscifera*
Microstylis wallichii lindi	*Phaseolus trilobus*
Phaseoldus tribolus	*Polygonatum verticillatum*
Polygonatum verticillatum	*Polygonatum circuicifolium*
Polygonatum circucifolium	*Teraminus labialis*
Prunus cirasoidus	
Rhus succedania	

Table 1 (continued)

Sushrut Samhita	Charaka Samhita
Jeevaniya	
Teramnus labialis	
Tinospora cordifolia	
Vitis vinifera	
Balya	
Abutilon indicum	*Abutilon indicum*
Acorus calamus	*Asparagus racemosus*
Asparagus racemosus	*Bacopa monnieri*
Commiphora mukul	*Desmodium gangeticum*
Convolvulus pluricaulis	*Mucuna pruriens*
Cynodon dactilon	*Sida cordifolia*
Embelia ribes	*Teramnus labialis*
Emblica officinalis	*Terminalia chebula*
Grewia hirsuta	*Withania somnifera*
Herpestis moniera	
Premna mucronata	
Pueraria tuberosa	
Saussurea luppa	
Sida cordifolia	
Terminalia chebula	
Tinospora cordifolia	
Vayasthapaniya	
Sushrut has not classified any plants under the category of *Vayasthapaniya*.	*Asparagus racemosus*
	Boerhevia diffusa
	Centella asiatica
	Clitoria terneata
	Desmodium gangeticum
	Emblica officinalis
	Leptadenia reticulata
	Pluchea lanceolata
	Terminalia chebula
	Tinospora cordifolia

In the words of Charaka [3] with a *rasayana*, "one obtains longevity, regains youth, gets a sharp memory and intellect and freedom from diseases, gets a lustrous complexion and the strength of a horse". Sushruta [4] is more specific, describing a *rasayana* as one which "is anti-ageing, increases the life-span, promotes intelligence and memory and increases resistance to disease" (presumably infections, and therefore indicating potential immunostimulant effects).

Apart from immunostimulant activities, *rasayana* plants have also been evaluated for their anabolic, anti-stress, adaptogenic, nootropic, anti-oxidant and anti-ageing effects [8].

Jeevaniya, Balya and *Vayasthapaniya*

The *jeevaniya, balya* and *vayasthapaniya* plants also appear to have promise as immunomodulators. *Jeevaniya* drugs are those which promote life. Ayurveda says that there is a daily wear and tear in the bodily functions. This wear and tear is prevented or reversed by the *jeevaniya* group of drugs. Another definition given to the *jeevaniya* drugs by Ayurveda is "drugs necessary for life". Agents which increase the vitality of the physical body are called *balya* drugs. This vitality is believed to be the basis of life itself. *Balya* drugs could be general (e.g. *Asparagus racemosus*) or specific (e.g. *Terminalia arjuna* for the heart or iron for the blood). The *vayasthapaniya* drugs on the other hand, although mentioned as a separate class by Charaka, have not been well defined (apart from being called agents which establish or maintain youthfulness).

Today, the immune system is called the "pace-maker" of life. This is because it is hypothesised that it has a bidirectional link to several organ systems in the body and may be an important regulator, along with the nervous (somatic and autonomic) and endocrine systems, in the homeostatic mechanisms of the body, particularly during stressful situations and ageing. Hence, drugs acting on the immune system, i.e. immunomodulators, are likely to influence many systems in the body, with far-ranging effects including "strengthening" (*jeevaniya*), "vitalising" (*balya*) and "life-maintaining" (*vayasthapaniya*).

There is an overlap between these groups of the list, which is easily understood considering the central role of the immune system in the pathophysiology of many diseases. This overlap also suggests the immune system as a common target for therapeutic action.

Immunostimulant plants from Ayurveda: scientific validation

Using these leads, scientists have identified several plants which have been proved to have immunomodulating effects in experimental (*in vitro* systems and *in vivo* models) as well as clinical situations. The following paragraphs describe some of this work. It is of interest to note that all the plants described under the *rasayana* group that have been studied in some detail, reveal classical immunomodulatory effects. They produce stimulation as well as suppression of the immune system depending on the extract tested. This appears to be in accordance with the principles of Ayurveda, which advocate that *rasayanas* are essentially "normalising" agents.

Tinospora cordifolia miers (*Gulwel*)

Tinospora cordifolia is called '*amrita*' in Sanskrit, which means ambrosia. This word indicates the range of properties ascribed to *Tinospora cordifolia* by Ayurveda. The aqueous extract of this plant is widely used as a household medicine to fend off infections and the drug has acquired (in folk and traditional scientific medicines all over India) legendary fame as a medicine that has 'divine' properties.

Botany

Tinospora cordifolia Miers is a creeper which belongs to the family Menispermaceae. It is found throughout India commonly in deciduous and dry forests. It flowers in summer and Ayurveda suggests that *Tinospora cordifolia* should be harvested in the month of May which is high summer in India.

It is a glabrous, climbing shrub often growing very tall. The bark of the plant is creamy white to grey in colour, succulent, deeply cleft spirally with the space in between being spotted by large rosette-like lenticles. It sends down long, slender aerial roots with nodal swellings. The plant has sub-deltoid cordate, heart-shaped leaves. The creeper usually grows on mango or neem trees. When the stem is cut transversely, it shows a horizontal wheel-like appearance [9].

Chemistry

The chemical constituents identified in this plant include alkaloids, glycosides, sterols, lactones and fatty acids. Tinosporin, tinosporic acid and tinosporol are the alkaloids identified in the leaves of this plant. The leaves are also rich in proteins, calcium and phosphorus.

The stem is the most commonly used part of *Tinospora cordifolia* and chemicals isolated from the stem include berberine, palmitine, tembetarine, magnoflorine, choline and tinosporin. Other chemicals isolated from the stem include glycosides (like an 18-norclerodane glucoside, giloin and a furanoid diterpene glucoside) and glucosides like giloinin and gilosterol. The butanol extract of the stem has yielded the glycosides cordifoliside A, B and C [10].

Sterols such as β-sitosterol, octacosanol, heptacosanol, nonacosan-15-one and a new phenolic lignin 3-(alpha-4-dihydroxy-3-methoxy-benzyl)-4-(4-hydroxy-3-methoxy-benzyl) tetrahydrofuran have been isolated from the petroleum ether extract of the plant. The alcoholic extract has yielded δ-sitosterol as well as tinosporidine, cordifol and cordifelone. Lactones like the diterpenoid furanolactone, a clerodane derivative (5R,10R)-4R-8R dihydroxy-2S-3R:15,16-diepoxy cleroda-13 (16),14-dieno-17,12S:18,1S-dilactone, tinosporol, tinosporide and columbin have also been identified. The structures of columbin [11] and tinosporide [12] have been elucidated. A polysaccharide which is a 1-4 linked glucan with occasional branch points has been isolated from the stem [13, 14].

Ayurvedic uses

Tinospora cordifolia belongs to the *rasayana* group of drugs and regulates all three *doshas*. It is prescribed for dyspepsia, anorexia, liver disorders, dysentery and worms. It has been recommended for use in anaemia, diabetes mellitus, gout and rheumatoid arthritis. Most importantly, *Tinospora cordifolia* is described as being useful for the treatment of infections like leprosy. It has antipyretic, analgesic and anti-inflammatory properties. It is recommended as a general tonic in the convalescent period after infectious diseases [3, 4].

Pharmacological actions

The pharmacology (with respect to its immunostimulant activity in particular) of *Tinospora cordifolia* has been extensively explored by several researchers. Our group has concentrated on the immunological effects of *Tinospora cordifolia* because initial studies indicated that there may be some scientific basis for the claims in Ayurveda regarding the benefits of *Tinospora cordifolia.*

In vitro *studies*

The filtered, standardized, whole aqueous extract of the stem of *Tinospora cordifolia* was found to stimulate polymorphonuclear (PMN) cell function when incubated *in vitro*. PMN leucocytes were harvested from the peripheral venous blood of healthy volunteers, patients with obstructive jaundice and patients with tuberculosis. 1×10^6 PMN cells were incubated at 37° C for 1 h with 0.2, 0.4 and 0.8 mg/ml of *Tinospora cordifolia* (along with the same number of *Staphylococcus aureus* (in the case of healthy volunteers and patients with obstructive jaundice), or *Candida albicans* (in the case of patients with tuberculosis)) and the % phagocytosis and phagocytic index were measured by observing under a microscope a fixed and stained slide. We found that *Tinospora cordifolia* significantly stimulated the PMN cell function in normal volunteers as well as in patients with obstructive jaundice and tuberculosis. These results are summarised in Table 2.

The effects of dry stem crude extracts (DSCE) of *Tinospora cordifolia* and a related plant *Tinospora malabarica* have been shown to contain polyclonal B cell activators which are assumed to be polysaccharides. The DSCE were prepared by boiling the powdered stems in water followed by treatment with 10% trichloroacetic acid and filtration. The supernatant was further precipitated with acetone, and then fractionated on Sephadex G-200 and Sephacryl S-400 columns. The effects of these fractions were evaluated by culturing lymphocytes *in vitro* for 48 h in a 5% CO_2 environment. Proliferation was estimated by pulsing 2×10^5 cells with 1 μCi ^{3}H-thymidine for 16 h and its incorporation measured by liquid scintillation counting. It was found that DSCE was mitogenic for lymphocytes from lymph node and spleen, while thymocytes, bone marrow cells and peripheral blood cells responded poorly [15].

Mathew and Kuttan [16] have found that the methanolic extract of *Tinospora cordifolia* inhibited lipid peroxide formation and scavenged hydroxyl and superoxide radicals *in vitro*. For 100% inhibition 50 mg/ml were required. This was associated with increased bone marrow cellularity as well as an ablation of neutropenia.

Experimental in vivo *studies*

Infections

A plant with immunostimulatory potential is expected to be efficacious for the treatment of infections. The aqueous extract of *Tinospora cordifolia* has been found effective in several models of infection including normal as well as immunosuppressed animals. This work has been extensively reviewed elsewhere [17, 18].

Briefly, *Tinospora cordifolia* reduced mortality associated with intra-abdominal sepsis following caecal ligation. Thus, as compared to a mortality of 66–100% on the fifth day after surgery in untreated rats, 15 days of pretreatment with *Tinospora cordifolia* alone reduced mortality to 33% and further to 16.6% when combined with metronidazole and gentamicin [19]. This effect was reported to be associated with improved macrophage function. Furthermore, the aqueous extract of *Tinospora cordifolia* was found to be devoid of *in vitro* antimicrobial activity against *Bacillus subtilis*, *Bacillus cereus*, *Staphylococcus aureus*, *Pseudomonas aeruginosa* and *Escherichia coli*. Sera obtained from rats (n = 10 each) orally treated with the aqueous extract of *Tinospora cordifolia* in doses of 100 and 200 mg/kg were also found to have no antibacterial activity [19]. These data further indicated that *Tinospora cordifolia* was effective in infections due to its immunostimulant effects.

Table 2 - In vitro effect of incubation of Tinospora cordifolia (Tc) on PMN functions

a) Healthy volunteers (n = 15); test organism: *S. aureus*

Concentration of Tc, mg/ml	**% Phagocytosis**	**Phagocytic index**
0 (control)	35.7 ± 3.4	1.5 ± 0.1
0.2	39.3 ± 1.6	1.9 ± 0.3*
0.4	42.3 ± 3.8**	2.0 ± 10.3**
0.8	44.0 ± 16.9*	2.0 ± 0.3**

*Student's paired t-test; *, $p<0.05$ as compared to healthy volunteers; **, $p<0.05$; ***, $p<0.01$ as compared to control (MEM)*

b) Patients with obstructive jaundice (n = 13); test organism: *S. aureus*

Concentration of Tc, mg/ml	**% Phagocytosis**	**Phagocytic index**
0 (control)	28.9 ± 4.5*	1.4 ± 0.3
0.2	33.3 ± 9.7**	1.7 ± 0.5***
0.4	35.8 ± 17.6***	1.7 ± 0.4***
0.8	34.2 ± 5.8***	1.8 ± 0.4**

*Student's unpaired t-test; *, $p<0.05$ as compared to healthy volunteers; **, $p<0.05$; ***, $p<0.01$ as compared to control (MEM)*

c) Patients with tuberculosis (n=8); test organism *C. albicans*

Concentration of Tc, mg/ml	**% Phagocytosis**	**Phagocytic index**
0 (control)	26.7 ± 2.7	1.6 ± 0.2
0.2	27.9 ± 11.5*	1.4 ± 0.6
0.4	30.8 ± 12.7**	1.4 ± 0.6
0.8	29.0 ± 11.5**	1.7 ± 0.7

*Student's paired t-test; *, $p<0.05$; **, $p<0.01$ as compared to control (MEM)*

Pretreatment with *Tinospora cordifolia* was found to significantly reduce the mortality of *Escherichia coli*-induced peritonitis in a mouse model (16.7% in *Tinospora cordifolia* treated mice as compared to 100% in control mice) [20]. Bacterial clearance studies (up to 4 h after injection of *Escherichia coli*) revealed that in the *Tinospora cordifolia* treated mice, although the bacterial count increased initially, it dropped after the second hour. The phagocytic and intracellular bactericidal capacity of polymorphs of *Tinospora cordifolia*-treated mice were significantly increased (phagocytosis 56.7 ± 5.7%, intracellular killing capacity (ICK) 52.4 ± 5.5%) as compared to control (phagocytosis 34.3 ± 3.4%, ICK 30.5 ± 6.1%, $p<0.001$) [21].

Tinospora cordifolia has been evaluated in several animal models for immunosuppression. In a model of irreversible cholestasis, *Escherichia coli* sepsis was created [22]. Rats from the *Tinospora cordifolia*-treated groups resisted *Escherichia coli* infection and mortality was only 16.7%. Blood cultures of the surviving animals were sterile. In comparison, the control rats showed a mortality of 77.8 % and the blood culture of surviving animals from these groups showed the presence of *Escherichia coli.*

In mice, immunosuppression was created by injecting a single dose of cyclophosphamide. Infections were induced in such neutropenic mice with *Staphylococcus aureus*. As compared to a 75% mortality in the control animals, *Tinospora cordifolia* reduced mortality to 50%. The treated animals developed a significant leucocytosis and neutrophilia, and demonstrated significant inhibition of leucopenia and neutropenia as compared to control animals. PMN functions were also significantly increased in the treated animals [17, 18].

In a separate set of neutropenic mice (n = 10/group), *Klebsiella pneumoniae* sepsis was induced. All control mice died, whereas 70% of mice given *Tinospora cordifolia* alone survived. There was a significant leucocytosis in the *Tinospora cordifolia*-treated groups and a concomitant ablation in the cyclophosphamide-induced leucopenia that explained the protection [17].

In a third set of experiments, infection was induced with *Candida albicans*. Mice pre-treated with *Tinospora cordifolia* showed significant ($p < 0.01$) protection in mortality (42%) as compared to the control group (86%). This was comparable to the fluconazole-treated group (40%). When fluconazole was given in addition to pretreatment with *Tinospora cordifolia*, the mortality was further reduced to 30%. The *Tinospora cordifolia*-treated mice showed a remarkably lower number of colonies of *Candida albicans* in the kidneys, as compared to control mice [17].

Similar results have been seen with immunosuppression following hemisplenectomy in mice (n = 10/group). As compared to 100% mortality after *Escherichia coli* injection in the control group, *Tinospora cordifolia* treatment completely prevented mortality. In a *Staphylococcus aureus* model only 19.7% of the mice died in the *Tinospora cordifolia*-treated group as compared to 100% mortality in the control group.

When infection with *Candida albicans* was induced in laparotomised mice, only 42.1% of the untreated mice survived. On the other hand, in the group of laparotomised mice which were pretreated with *Tinospora cordifolia* prior to inducing infection the survival percentage was 86% [17].

White blood cells (WBC)

Normal mice

The effect of *Tinospora cordifolia* on peripheral leucocyte counts has been studied in some detail [23–25] and a dose and time dependent leucocytosis was found. At doses of 25 or 50 mg/kg no effect was observed whereas leucocytosis occurred at all other doses tested. Maximum was obtained on day 15 at 100 mg/kg and on day seven at 200 mg/kg. The onset was delayed until day two of therapy. When therapy with 200 mg/kg was continued for a further period of seven days a plateau effect was observed. In animals treated with 400 or 800 mg/kg, there was no significant difference in leukocytosis occuring at day 7 of therapy as compared to that observed with a dose of 200 mg/kg. However, this increase in the WBC count with higher doses was not maintained when therapy was continued beyond seven days [25].

Neutropenic mice

An aqueous extract of *Tinospora cordifolia* has been found to induce leucocytosis with predominant neutrophilia and blunt the leucopenic effects of cyclophosphamide (a cytotoxic drug used in cancer chemotherapy). These effects were comparable to those of lithium carbonate and glucan [23, 24].

In another study, the crude powdered stem of *Tinospora cordifolia* as well as the aqueous, ethanol, acetone and petroleum ether extracts were shown to ablate the cyclophosphamide-induced reduction in haemoglobin, leucocyte count and platelets. In this study, the petroleum ether extract was the most effective [26].

Effect on macrophages

Peritoneal macrophages

The aqueous extract of *Tinospora cordifolia* has been shown to stimulate peritoneal macrophages (% phagocytosis, % intracellular killing capacity of *Candida pseudotropicalis*) in a dose-dependent manner (25–100 mg/kg). This effect peaked at 200 mg/kg, a higher dose being inhibitory (300 mg/kg). The stimulatory effect was comparable to that of muramyl dipeptide [27].

Alveolar macrophages

Alveolar macrophages are very important components of the immunological response to tuberculosis (TB). Anti-TB therapy can alter their functions in a deleterious way and thus alter the clinical course in patients with TB. This experimental study evaluated the effects of *Tinospora cordifolia* when given in combination with anti-tubercular drugs.

Rats were divided into four groups depending on the drug therapy: group one was the control group and received distilled water (n = 16), group two received *Tinospora cordifolia*, orally 100 mg/kg (n = 12), group three received standard anti-tubercular therapy (consisting of intramuscular streptomycin, oral rifampicin, isoniazid and pyrazinamide in doses equivalent to the human dose for 15 days, n = 14), and group four was given standard anti-tubercular therapy along with *Tinospora cordifolia* (n = 14). After 15 days of therapy, alveolar macrophages were collected by broncho-alveolar lavage. Macrophage function was assayed in terms of

Table 3 - Effects of Tinospora cordifolia *on alveolar macrophages*

Grp No.	Treatment	% Phagocytosis	% Intracellular killing capacity
1	Distilled water (control)	33.4 ± 5.6	46.4 ± 5.1
2	*Tinospora cordifolia* (Tc)	44.3 ± 7.1*	48.8 ± 5.7
3	Antitubercular therapy	21.6 ± 5.659*	36.7 ± 8.1*
4	Antitubercular therapy + Tc	38.1 ± 8.5**	35.3 ± 6.5

**$p < 0.01$ (when compared to group 1), **$p < 0.01$ (when compared to group 3)*

% phagocytosis and % intracellular killing capacity of *Candida pseudotropicalis*. Results are depicted in Table 3.

Reticuloendothelial system

Tinospora cordifolia has been shown to increase the colloidal carbon clearance in rats [17] suggesting global activation of the macrophage system.

Macrophages play a key role in the action of Tinospora cordifolia

An experiment was performed in order to determine whether macrophages played a key role in the immunostimulatory effects of *Tinospora cordifolia.* To demonstrate this, a rise in white blood cell (WBC) count and neutrophilia were used as parameters to reflect non-specific immunostimulatory activity.

Lipofundin S (20%), a stable soyabean preparation, was chosen as a macrophage blocker. The effect of *Tinospora cordifolia* on WBC count and % neutrophils was studied in the presence and absence of Lipofundin S. Rats were given *Tinospora cordifolia*, 100 mg, twice a day for seven days. Lipofundin S was injected intravenously from day four to day seven (1 ml/day for four days). The leucocyte count was performed basally (day 0) and repeated at day four and day seven. The macrophage activity was assessed on day seven using *Staphylococcus aureus* as test organism.

Lipofundin S *per se* did not alter the WBC count but a decrease in the phagocytic activity of macrophages was seen (25.8 ± 10.8% as compared to 31.3 ± 1.2% in control rats, $p<0.05$). The total WBC counts on day four of treatment with *Tinospora cordifolia* were comparable to those obtained basally (0 day WBC count: 8066.66 ± 659.96/mm^3 with 46.5 ± 4.23% neutrophils) but the counts on day seven were significantly higher (WBC: 13250 ± 2491.48/mm^3, neutrophils 59.0 ± 1.7%; $p<0.001$ vs normal)

When Lipofundin S was given concurrently during this period, the rise in WBC count and neutrophils was inhibited (7066.6 ± 1556.34/mm^3, 41.0 ± 1.6% respectively; $p < 0.01$) and an associated decrease in phagocytic activity of macrophages (37.2 ± 6.1%), as compared to *Tinospora cordifolia* alone, was seen. This experiment indicates that activation of macrophages is essential for the non-specific effects of *Tinospora cordifolia* [30].

Effect on thymocytes

A study was conducted on 132 Swiss albino mice of either sex (age group 4–6 weeks, weight 18–25 gms) in order to study the effects of *Tinospora cordifolia* on thymocyte counts. After treatment with *Tinospora cordifolia*, thymocyte counts increased significantly ($8.96 \pm 0.13 \times 10^9$) as compared to animals receiving distilled water ($5.213 \pm 0.09 \times 10^9$, $p < 0.05$). In addition, the ability of petreatment with *Tinospora cordifolia* to reverse the lymphopenic effects of intraperitoneal hydrocortisone (125 mg/kg) was investigated in mice. When compared to control animals, the *Tinospora cordifolia*-treated mice showed a blunting of lymphopenia and restoration of a normal count on day eight after hydrocortisone injection. When *Tinospora cordifolia* was administered after hydrocortisone the effect on thymocytes was less pronounced.

Effects on bone marrow

The aqueous extracts of *Tinospora cordifolia* have been shown to increase the proliferative fraction of bone marrow which explains the leucocytosis [25]. The effect was associated with increased apoptosis in bone marrow cells at higher doses (400–800 mg/kg) of the extract [17]. Interestingly, at therapeutic doses, the extract did not per se increase apoptosis (as measured by acridine orange staining and counting by fluorescent microscopy), though it reduced apoptosis induced by cyclophosphamide. The extract also induced apoptosis in murine malignant S180 cells [28].

Miscellaneous studies

Tinopsora cordifolia has also been shown to increase the phagocytic functions of PMN though no significant effect was found on skin allograft reaction or antibody response [29].

Clinical studies

An exhaustive literature search reveals a remarkable paucity of published data on clinical studies documenting immunostimulant effects of most Indian medicinal plants. *Tinospora cordifolia* has been developed into a standardized formulation in our laboratory and evaluated for several clinical conditions. It has been found safe in Phase I human volunteer studies.

Use in obstructive jaundice

A study conducted in patients with obstructive jaundice [31] indicated that addition of *Tinospora cordifolia* to routine surgical procedures increased survival rates. Thus, when compared to a mortality of 61.5% (n = 13) in patients who underwent percutaneous transhepatic biliary drainage alone, addition of *Tinospora cordifolia* reduced this mortality to 25% (n = 16). Similarly, in another group where percutaneous transhepatic biliary drainage was not performed, *Tinospora cordifolia* reduced mortality from 57.1% (n = 14) in controls to 14.2% (n = 14). Treatment with *Tinospora cordifolia* led to an increase in PMN functions (30.4 ± 3.0% phagocytosis and 27.2 ± 6.2% IKC) as compared to 20.0 ± 8.5% phagocytosis and 11.2 ± 3.1% IKC in control patients.

Cirrhosis

Depression of Kupffer cell activity is a well recognized feature of cirrhosis. A significant depression of the phagocytic and intracellular killing capacity (ICK) of monocytes (20.6 ± 5.0% and 41.2 ± 12.9% respectively) was observed in 16 cirrhotics ($p < 0.05$ vs normal values: 23.9 ± 3.6% phagocytosis and 50.9 ± 6.3% ICK, n = 50).

Based on this finding, the effect of long term treatment (six months) with *Tinospora cordifolia* on the course of mild to moderate cirrhosis was evaluated in a placebo controlled, single blind, prospective study in 12 patients with cirrhosis. After six months, antipyrine clearance improved significantly (from 17.3 ± 3.8 h to 14.5 ± 3.9 h, $p < 0.05$) in patients given *Tinospora cordifolia* whereas no significant change was seen in the placebo group (from 17.0 ± 5.4 h to 19.3± 3.8 h). The monocyte function increased from 23.4 ± 5.7% phagocytosis to 40.3 ± 3.2% in the *Tinospora cordifolia*-treated patients but no change was seen in the placebo-treated group (18.5 ± 5.9 to 21.5 ± 5.0%). A similar result was seen in the ICK of monocytes. Thus, *Tinospora cordifolia* treatment increased the % ICK from 38.4 ± 4.8% to 45.8 ± 5.5% while in the placebo group the values were 35.3 ± 8.8% basally and 37.5 ± 3.5% after six months [30].

Asymptomatic carrier state of hepatitis B infection

The effect of *Tinospora cordifolia* was studied on viral elimination in asymptomatic carriers of Hepatitis B surface antigen, using seroconversion of HBsAg positivity as a criterion of success. Of the 24 carriers selected, 12 were randomly allocated to the *Tinospora cordifolia* group and the rest received placebo for a period of two months. A conversion rate of 37.5% was seen in the group receiving *Tinospora cordifolia* whereas in the placebo group the seroconversion was only 11.1%.

Tuberculosis

A clinical trial to evaluate the effect of *Tinospora cordifolia* on the chemotherapeutic course of patients with pulmonary tuberculosis was carried out whereby 50 patients with pulmonary tuberculosis between 13–60 years of age were included. This study was a double blind, placebo controlled, fixed dose, randomized trial. Patients received either Treatment A which consisted of standard anti-Koch's Therapy (AKT) along with *Tinospora cordifolia* or Treatment B which consisted of standard AKT along with placebo. The parameters assessed included clinical symptoms, radiological examination, complete hemogram, monocyte functions, sputum examination and a record of side effects. Patients were followed up after two and six months. Each symptom was graded as either '0' denoting absence of symptom or '1' indicating the presence of symptom. The scores for all the symptoms were added for each patient at each follow up to get composite scores.

Radiological assessment was performed as follows: the lesions were graded as mild, moderate or severe using a scale devised by the National Tuberculosis Association of USA (1961). The scores given were '0' for no lesion, '1' for mild involvement, '2' for moderate or '3' for severe involvement. For the purpose of comparison, the X-ray status (as per the above mentioned classification) was re-scored as '0' for basal status, '1' for improvement of one stage (e.g. from 3 to 2) at the second month follow up and '2' for improvement of two stages (e.g. from 3 to 1) and similarly at the sixth month follow up. Of the 50 patients recruited, 23 received treatment A and 27 received treatment B. None of the patients discontinued the treatment due to side-effects of AKT or *Tinospora cordifolia*. Minor side-effects reported were nausea, vomiting and joint pains. The number of patients complaining of joint pains in the placebo group was 37.5%. One patient in this group complained of joint pains even at the sixth month follow up. In the group given *Tinospora cordifolia* only 15% had similar complaints.

The clinical profile of the patients from the two groups was comparable at each follow up. The radiological assessment of the patients showed that 12/23 patients (52.2%) in the control group had the same X-ray status at the second month follow up, as compared to 4/18 patients (22.2%) in the *Tinospora cordifolia*-treated group, while the rest had a marked improvement. The difference was statistically significant ($p < 0.05$, Fisher's exact test). At the sixth month follow up, the extent of improvement was same in both of the groups.

Burns

Infection remains one of the most difficult problems in the therapy of burns. It is the commonest cause of death in burns patients who survive the resuscitative phase.

Since *Tinospora cordifolia* is an immunostimulant, a study was conducted to find out whether it modified the outcome in burns patients. This study was carried out in adult female burn patients with less than 50% thermal burns. Patients were randomly allocated to receive either *Tinospora cordifolia* or placebo so that the patient distribution was similar in both groups. Standard management of burns was given to both groups in the form of fluid replacement therapy, prophylactic antibiotics and daily dressings with silver sulfadiazine cream. Eusol dressings were given once the eschar started forming. The temperature, hydration, local wound status and nutrition were recorded daily while wound swabs were examined for culture sensitivity, serum immunoglobulin measured, and total and differential peripheral white blood cell (WBC) counts were performed on days 0, 7 and 14 after burns. All patients had a total WBC count higher than 10,000. The mean total WBC count in the *Tinospora cordifolia* group was lower than that of the control group. This was an interesting finding suggesting the capacity for *Tinospora cordifolia* to exert a modulatory (*rasayana*) effect. A progressive increase in the neutrophil count occurred on days 7 and 14 in the *Tinospora cordifolia*-treated group. This increase was statistically significant on day 14. The immunoglobulin levels fell in the first post-burn week and returned to normal on day 14 in the control group. In the *Tinospora cordifolia*-treated group, the mean IgG levels were higher on day 7, and increased further the second week. Moreover, the mean values of the drug treated group on day 7 and 14 were higher than those of the control group. This difference was statistically significant on day 14. Thus, *Tinospora cordifolia* seems to have a positive effect on serum IgG level in burns patient, and would thus enhance immunity in burns patients. The number of patients having 1–30% burns who survived were nine in the drug treated group and eight in the control group. Overall survival in both groups was equal. Thus, *Tinospora cordifolia* did not influence survival at this dose although it did exert a mild immunostimulatory effect. Further studies with higher doses seem warranted in this population of immunodepressed patients.

Breast cancer

A randomised, double blind, placebo controlled trial was conducted in collaboration with Tata Memorial Hospital, Mumbai, in order to evaluate the efficacy of *Tinospora cordifolia* in reducing the cytotoxic chemotherapy-induced leucopenia in patients with breast cancer [17]. For the study, 38 patients were recruited and randomised to receive either the active drug (*Tinospora cordifolia*, in syrup form) or matching placebo syrup for a period of 14 days prior to the first chemotherapy cycle. The drug administration was continued throughout the subsequent cycles (consisting of cyclophosphamide 750 mg/m^2, methotrexate 40 mg/m^2 and 5 flurouracil 750 mg/m^2 every three weeks) with a break of 4-5 days after each injection. A complete blood count was performed on days –10, 0, 4, 7, 10 and 14 in each cycle to detect the nadir. The absolute end point for each cycle of chemotherapy for every patient was the appearance of leucopenia (WBC count $< 3000/mm^3$) or the appearance of febrile neutropenia. In addition, an assessment of quality of life was performed at every visit and the incidence of delay in chemotherapy was recorded. Of the 38 patients studied, 19 received placebo and 17 received *Tinospora cordifolia*. There was no difference in the basal WBC counts of both groups, indicating that the groups were similar at the beginning. Treatment with *Tinospora cordifolia* did not increase the counts significantly. As expected, there was a significant leucopenia in both the groups. However, the number of patients with total WBC counts less than $3000/mm^3$ were significantly less ($p < 0.05$, chi square test) in the *Tinospora cordifolia* treated group (55%) than in the placebo treated group (70%). This effect was more evident in the first cycle than in subsequent cycles. Similarly, there were 24 cycles in the placebo group where the count fell below 2000, while there were only 14 in the *Tinospora cordifolia* treated group. In the group receiving placebo, counts fell below 500 in four patients while this happened in only one patient in the active drug-treated group.

Although these results suggest that *Tinospora cordifolia* is, at the given dose, not much more potent than placebo treatment, they point to the fact that there is merit in continuing this study, by further escalating the doses of *Tinospora cordifolia* and studying more patients so that the sample size is large enough to identify a difference between the two groups.

Withania somnifera Dunal (*Ashwagandha*)

Withania somnifera Dunal is called Indian ginseng because of its powerful anti-stress activities [32]. Apart from immunomodulatory effects, it also has a central nervous depressant action mediated via the γ-aminobutyric acid (GABA) receptors [33, 34].

Botany

A 1–2 m tall shrub, belonging to the family Solanaecae, *Withania somnifera* grows all over India. It flowers in autumn and the fruits are red and round (often called the Winter Cherry).

Chemistry

Alkaloids identified from the plant include nicotine, somniferine, somniferinine, withanine, withaferine, withananine and pseudo-withanine. Roots, which are the most commonly used part, have been shown to contain tropine, pseudotropine, 3-alpha tigloxytropane, choline, cuscohygrine, glycowithanolides (Sitoindosides IX and X) and other triterpenoids [35].

Ayurvedic uses

In Ayurvedic medicine, a topical preparation of the leaves or roots of *Withania somnifera* is applied on inflamed areas and abscesses to reduce inflammation. Taken internally, decoctions of the plant are prescribed as general tonics to patients with psychiatric diseases. It is also described as useful for the treastment of helminthic infections and blood disorders. It is well known for its aphrodisiac properties as well as for its utility in male and female infertility [36].

Pharmacological actions

Withania somnifera has been extensively investigated as an immunomodulatory agent. Thus, the aqueous extract of *Withania somnifera* has been shown to reduce cytotoxic drug-induced bone marrow suppression [23, 24, 37].

The root of *Withania somnifera* can exert both immunostimulant and immunodepressant activities. Two glycowithanolides (Sitoindosides IX and X) mobilise and activate macrophages and induce proliferation in murine splenocytes [38]. This effect has been suggested to be the basis of its use as a *rasayana* in Ayurveda.

However, withaferin-A, which was the first active principle isolated from *Withania somnifera* and also constituted the first member of a new class of phytosteroids (the withanolides), produced immunosuppression. Thus, it inhibited adjuvant arthritis in rats, graft vs host reaction in chicken, xenograft vs host reaction in mice, and depleted murine splenic cells *in vitro* [38–41]. This effect has been attributed to the glucocorticoid-like structure of withaferin-A [39]. *Withania somnifera* also reduces acute phase reactants [8] as well as α_2-macroglobulin during inflammation.

Apart from the immunomodulatory effects [42], cytotoxic, radiosensitising, antioxidative, and anti-stress effects of *Withania somnifera* have been described [8].

Clinical studies

Most clinical studies have focused on the anxiolytic potential of this plant. Only one report describes anti-ageing effects (as measured on the Alex Comfort Scale) of *Withania somnifera* in healthy, aged, male volunteers. This effect has, however, not been linked to immunomodulating effects [8].

Emblica officinalis Gaertn (*Amalki*)

The green fruit of *Emblica officinalis* is one of the richest sources of ascorbic acid which is embodied in its name "Emblica", derived from the Sanskrit "*Amlika*" meaning "sour". It is also called "*dhatri*" or "mother" because it is believed to exert beneficial effects similar to those of a mother.

Botany

The plant belongs to the family Euphorbiaceae and is also known as the Indian gooseberry. This deciduous tree grows to a medium height of 8–10 m. Its flowering season is autumn. Although fruits start appearing in winter, Ayurvedic texts [36] describe that they are optimally useful (in terms of active chemicals) in spring time. The cultivated variety growing in Varanasi (North India), having larger fruits than the one growing wild, is considered the best variety.

Chemistry

The pulp of the fruit (considered medicinally useful) contains 3.1% fibre, 14.1% carbohydrates, 0.5% proteins, 0.1% fats and 0.7% mineral matter.100 g of the fruit pulp yield about 600 mg of vitamin C. Sugars, tannins, and sitosterol are other compounds identified.

Ayurvedic uses

External application is advocated in alopecia or baldness, toothache, and ophthalmic conditions. It is prescribed internally for peptic ulcer, dyspepsia, piles, anaemia (along with iron preparations), tuberculosis and other chest infections (here, Ayurveda prescribes *Emblica officinalis* for its *rasayana* properties).

Pharmacological actions

There are few studies demonstrating immunomodulatory effects of *Emblica officinalis*. One report describes its ability to augment murine (BALB-c mice bearing Dalton's lymphoma ascites tumour) natural killer cells and antibody-dependent cellular cytotoxicity [43]. Further, the treated mice survived longer (35%) than non-treated animals.

In our laboratory we have demonstrated that the aqueous extract of *Emblica officinalis* stimulated the reticuloendothelial system as measured by the carbon clearance method [17]. Oral treatment with *Emblica officinalis* also increased the phagocytic and intracellular killing capacity of rat ($n = 10$) peritoneal macrophages (from a control of $32.1 \pm 0.9\%$ to $51.7 \pm 2.2\%$; $p < 0.01$).

Ocimum sanctum Linn

This small shrub is usually found in the front garden of most Indian homes. It has been imbued with religious powers. Its medicinal properties are also legendary.

Botany

Known as the Holy Basil or *Tulsi*, it is cultivated throughout India. This shrub grows to the height of 0.5 to 0.75 m. The leaves are very aromatic, about 3 cm long and slightly rounded. The flowers are in an inflorescence of about 12–14 cm length. The seed is small and black. It flowers in winter. There are two major varieties of *Tulsi*, viz. the white and the dark types. It is believed that the dark variety (*Krishna Tulsi*) is more medicinally active. There is also a wild variety of *Tulsi* which is larger.

Chemistry

The leaves yield an essential oil containing 71.3% eugenol, 3.2% carvacrol, 20.4% methyl eugenol, 1.7% caryophyllene [35], 6.4% nerol, 0.4% terpinen-4-ol, 0.2% decylaldehyde, 0.4% γ-selinene, 0.4% β-pinene, 2% camphene and 3.5% α-pinene [44].

Ayurvedic uses

Ayurveda has described *Ocimum sanctum* to have insecticide and pest repellent activities, and for this reason it is grown in most gardens. It is particularly said to act as a repellent against anopheles mosquitoes. The leaves are the most commonly used part and are applied locally on wounds. Topical application is believed to improve blood circulation. It has been prescribed for ear-ache. The juice of the leaves is also described as having digestive, laxative and antihelminthic properties. Apart from having a cardiotonic activity, its actions on the respiratory tract have made it a popular constituent of most therapies for respiratory infections. It also has antipyretic effects and has been prescribed for skin conditions such as leprosy [36].

Pharmacological actions

Ocimum sanctum [42] and *Ocimum gratissimum* [29] have been shown to stimulate phagocytic functions of PMN. This plant has also been been evaluated as an adaptogen [42]. In one study, rats were treated with the aqueous extract of *Ocimum sanctum* at a dose of 100 mg/kg/d for 15 days. This increased phagocytosis and intracellular killing (ICK) of alveolar macrophages from 21.7 ± 1.9% (phagocytosis) and 31.5 ± 3.4% (intracellular killing capacity, ICK) in controls to 44.7 ± 3.2% (phagocytosis) and 45.1 ± 2.7% (ICK), ($p < 0.001$). In a clinical study in children with recurrent respiratory tract infection, the effect of *Ocimum sanctum* on the course of infection was evaluated. Eighteen children with a history of more than eight episodes of respiratory tract infection per year were randomly divided into two groups (group one treated with placebo, n = 11 and group two with *Ocimum sanctum*, n = 7). The children were followed up at months 1, 3 and 6. Of children receiving placebo, ten out of eleven had a recurrence in this time period while only one child in group two developed infection. This was associated with improvement of polymorphonuclear cell functions [45].

The ability of methanolic and aqueous extracts of *Ocimum sanctum* to non-specifically stimulate immune cells has also been demonstrated in different studies [46, 47]. The primary antibody response in rats immunized with sheep red blood cells (SRBCs) as well as *Salmonella typhosa* was greater after treatment with *Ocimum sanctum*. In addition, *Ocimum sanctum* could reverse the immunosuppressant effect of stress. *Ocimum sanctum* has also been shown to inhibit cell-mediated immune responses [48, 49].

Other *rasayanas*

A number of other *rasayanas* from Ayurveda have been shown to stimulate the immune system in different models. As there are only isolated reports related to these plants they are presented in Table 4.

Non-*rasayanas*

Using random screening methods or taking hints from Ayurvedic uses (like in infections) several plants which are not *rasayanas* have also been identified as immunostimulants.

Table 4 - Other rasayanas *which have been investigated for immunomodulatory activity [8]*

Plant	Diseases for which primarily prescribed in Ayurveda
Acorus calamus	Epilepsy, psychosis
Aloe vera [50,51]	Liver diseases
Allium sativum [52,53]	Anti-aging, nervous disorders (spice)
Asparagus racemosus [17,18]	GI cytoprotective, galactogogue, progestational
Bacopa monnieri [54]	CNS diseases
Borrhevia diffusa	Renal diseases
Celestrus panniculatus	CNS diseases
Convolvulus pluricaulius	CNS diseases
Cuminum cyminum	no defined disease (spice)
Embelia ribes	Anthelminthic
Glycerrhiza glabra [55]	Respiratory infections, cough
Ipomea digitata	used as a tonic
Leptadenia reticulata	Renal diseases
Piper longum	Asthma
Semicarpus anacardium	Intestinal colic, piles
Sphaeranthus indicus	Arthritis
Terminalia chebula [17]	Eye diseases, obstipation
Terminalia bellerica	Eye diseases, respiratory disorders

Picrorrhiza kurroa Royle ex Benthe (*kutaki*)

More well known for its effects on the liver, *Picrorrhiza kurroa* has been shown by several groups to have immunomodulatory activity.

Botany

Picrorrhiza kurroa belongs to the family Scrophulariaceae (Fig Wort family). It has radish like tuberous stems, with dentate leaves. It flowers in summer and the root is the most used plant part.

Chemistry

The root contains an active bitter principle called picrorrhizin (15%) as well as cathartic acid, glucose and wax. Additionally, kutkin, apocynin, picroside I, II and III as well as kutkoside have been identified [44].

Ayurvedic uses

The root of *Picrorriza kurroa* has been described as having a mild laxative effect. It also stimulates digestion, and has a choleretic effect. It is particularly useful in jaundice, reducing some of the symptoms associated with this condition. It has been described as having anthelminthic and antipyretic effects and has been claimed to reduce edema, thus reducing the preload on the heart.

Pharmacological effects

Atal et al. [29] have reported immunostimulating properties of the ethanol extract of this plant. It has been found to enhance delayed type hypersensitivity by 80% as well as increase the antibody response to antigens and the phagocytic function of PMN. At the same time, oral treatment of animals led to hastening of allograft rejection. The leaves of *Picrorrhiza kurroa* have been found to enhance B cell-mediated immunity as well as PMN phagocytosis [8]. Administration of picroliv, a standardized extract of the root and rhizome of *Picrorrhiza kurroa* (containing mainly iridoid glycosides), led to a significant increase in hemagglutinating antibody titre, plaque forming cells, and response to sheep red blood cells (delayed type hypersensitivity).There was also an increase of the macrophage migration index, phagocytosis of *Escherichia coli*, and chemiluminescence of peritoneal macrophages as well as lymphocyte proliferation as measured by ^{3}H-thymidine uptake. At the same time, golden hamsters were protected form *Leishmania donovani* infections [56].

Surprisingly, aqueous extracts of roots of *Picrorrhiza kurroa* have been found to inhibit both pathways of complement activation. After fractionation the maximum effects were found in the methanol and ethylacetate fractions [57, 58]. The methanol-insoluble extracts were found to contain primarily carbohydrates and proteins [59].

Apocynin isolated from the root of *Picrorrhiza kurroa* inhibits the neutrophil oxidative burst and is perhaps responsible for the noted anti-inflammatory activity [60]. It also reduced IL-6 levels in animals [61].

Azadharichta indica A. juss

Colloquially known as "*neem*" this plant has attracted international attention. Apart from immunostimulatory activity, it has also been shown to have insecticidal, pesticidal and microbicidal activity.

Botany

Belonging to the Meliacea family, *Azadharichta indica* grows to a height of 8–10 m. It has a thick bark which yields a thick, creamy gum. The leaves are small and sickle shaped. The flowers are white and fragrant, while the fruits are small and green in colour. The seed of the ripe fruit yields neem oil. The flowering season is spring though fruits may be found throughout the year.

Chemistry

Several compounds have been isolated from different parts of the plant. Azadirachtin, found in the seed, is believed to be one of the active ingredients. Nimbidin, nimbin, sodium nimbidinate and nimbidol are other compounds isolated from the oil. The leaves yield meliacin, nimbolide, quercetin and β-sitosterol. The bark contains several bitter principles, peptidoglycans, nimbin, nimbidic acid, nimbiol and deacetylnimbin [62, 63].

Ayurvedic uses

The oil is widely used externally for wound healing purposes. Internally, it is recommended for its anthelminthic effects, for jaundice, irritable bowel syndrome, respiratory infections, gynaecological diseases and as a contraceptive [36].

Pharmacological actions

Azadharichta indica (*neem*) has been shown to have non-specific immunostimulatory activity [64]. *Neem* acts by activating macrophages (increased phagocytosis) and also increases the expression of MHC-II antigens indicating enhancement of their antigen-presenting ability. In vitro treatment of mice splenocytes with extracts of *Azadharichta indica* stimulates production of IL-2, IFNγ and TNFα, reflecting activation of T_{H1} (type of T) cell response [64, 65]. Since the T_{H1} type of response has been associated with cell-mediated immunity, the therapeutic effects of Azadharichta indica as reported in Ayurvedic literature [36] may be mediated via activation of cellular immune reactions. In fact, the contraceptive, anti-bacterial, anti-viral and anti-chlamydial effects of *Azadharichta indica* have been found to be mediated through the immune system [66].

An additional effect on cellular immunity of the aqueous extract of the bark is the stimulation of lymphocyte function. A dose-dependent increase in Migration Inhibitor Factor (MIF), a lymphokine which attracts macrophages to the site of action has been seen [67]. There are reports on the ability of polysaccharides found in aqueous extracts of neem bark to induce production of interferon [68].

One study has reported that aqueous extracts of the neem leaf produced anti-complement activity specifically in the classic pathway, but no stimulation of PMN phagocytosis or respiratory burst as measured by nitroblue tetrazoleum reduction [8]. Two polymers are believed to be responsible for the anti-complement activity of *Azadharichta indica* [69]. Further, the aqueous extract of the bark also reduced both classical and alternative complement pathway activity [70]. The effect was found to be dose and time dependent and most pronounced in the classical pathway.

The crude aqueous bark extract inhibits generation of chemiluminescence by activated PMN. Catechins have been found to be responsible for this activity [71].

Nimba arishtas (which are commercially available preparations of *Azadharichta indica*) and the crude water extract of *neem* have been shown to inhibit both complement pathways as well as activated PMN cells *in vitro* [58]. *Arishtas* contain self-generated alcohol which increases the shelf life of the preparation. The flowers of *Woodfordia fruticosa* are added to *arishtas* for fermentation. It has been reported that addition of these flowers to *Nimba arishtas* increases its immunomodulatory effects. Interestingly, this activity was not found to be due to microbial interference, but rather to immuno-active constituents released from the flowers [72]. The partially purified leaf extracts of *Melia azadharich* L. have been reported to reduce mortality induced by Tacaribe viral encephalitis to 15% [73]. This was associated with reduced viral titres and an improved humoral immune response with increased levels of neutralizing antibodies.

Clinical studies

A clinical study conducted in patients with psoriasis given 300 mg per day of neem leaf extract (supplemented with coal tar application topically) showed reduction in erythema, desquamation and infiltration of psoriatic lesions [8].

Miscellaneous

Several other Indian medicinal plants which are not described in Ayurveda as *rasayana*, *balya* or *jeevaniya* have been found to stimulate the immune system. A summary of these plants is presented in Table 5. *Shilajit* (asphalt) is not a medicinal plant but deserves to be mentioned for its immunomodulatory properties [8]. It is a complex mixture of organic and inorganic compounds found as an exudate on special rocks in the Himalayan regions. It has been found to activate mouse peritoneal macrophages and fibroblasts when injected intraperitoneally, although this

*Table 5 - Non-*rasayana *plants which have shown putative immunomodulatory effects*

Plant	Primary Ayurvedic use / pharmacological activities [36]
Aconitum heterophyllum	Respiratory infections in children
Andrographis paniculata [76, 77] (ethanol extract, antigen specific and non-specific immunity in mice)	Hepatoprotective
Boswellia serrata [78, 64] (inhibits PMN infiltration in mice)	Anti-inflammatory
Centella asiatica [54]	CNS diseases
Clitorea ternatea	Cathartic
Curcuma longa	Anti-inflammatory, anti-septic
Desmodium gangeticum	Arthritis
Dendrophthoe falcata [76] (leucocytosis, neutrophilia, increased ADDC)	CNS diseases
Holorrhena antidysenterica	Diarrhea
Mangifera indica [64, 74, 79]	Laxative
(Increased phagocytosis of macrophages)	Malaria, anthelmintic
Nyctanthes arbor tristis [80]	
(Increased DTH and macrophage	Carminative
migration index)	Arthritis
Piper betel	Emetic
Pluchea lanceolata	CNS diseases, arthritis
Randia dumatorum	Respiratory infections, asthma,diarrhoea
Sphaeranthus indicus	Digestive
Tylophora indica [29]	
Zingiber aromaticum [55]	

Note: The Ayurvedic use mentioned is the main one. The plants may be used as adjuvants for treatment of several other disorders.
Other plants without reference are listed in [8].

effect was significantly less when shilajit was injected subcutaneously and in *in vitro* studies [74]. Further, Ghosal et al. [75] have shown that the fulvic acid present in *shilajit* is responsible for the immunomodulatory activity (mast cell stabilisation).

Specific problems related to research on Ayurvedic drugs

Herbal research is either based on random screening followed by bioassay-directed fractionation or a reliance on ethnomedicine. The last approach has provided leads for research (including immunomodulatory activities [81]) and many effective plant-based prescriptions have been developed from traditional systems of medicine from countries like China, Japan, Korea and Germany.

Ayurveda, the Indian traditional system of medicine also offers a vast source for research. However, one finds, especially in the area of immunostimulant agents, a number of lacunae. There are anecdotal reports on different plants and only few have been followed up and developed into clinical formulations. This is because research on Ayurvedic medicines is fraught with a number of difficulties which need to be addressed [82].

Firstly, all standard and ancient textbooks of Ayurveda are written in Sanskrit, the classical Indian language. Although a number of translations in vernacular as well as English are available [3, 4], the interpretation of Sanskrit stanzas in terms of contemporary science is difficult and subject to wide individual variations. Further, many diseases were unknown in ancient times and are therefore not described in old texts. Thus, for example, iatrogenic diseases like those caused by cytotoxic or immunosuppressive drugs never existed. Hence the question remains – how to find a lead? For example, there are two more concepts in Ayurveda that deserve indepth investigation since it is likely that they may reveal an immunostimulant potential of the plants just as *rasayana* or *balya* concepts have done so far.

Drugs that act on "*ama*" represent one such concept. *Ama* are immunologically active, but nutritionally insignificant, complexes generated in the intestine due to improper digestion of food [83]. *Ama* has been implicated by Ayurveda to be part of the pathogenesis of several diseases like rheumatoid arthritis, ulcerative colitis and liver disease, all of which we know today have an immunological background. Table 6 lists plants which act on *ama*. Although these plants cannot be included as classical immunostimulants (as per the definition) [54], they can be called immunoactive agents, since they are described as modifying immune-related diseases.

Several plants are prescribed in Ayurveda as antiallergic agents. It is likely that this activity can be attributed to stimulation of T suppressor cells. Thus, these drugs would qualify as immunomodulatory agents. *Picrorrhiza kurroa* has been extensively investigated for antiallergic activity [84, 85]. In these studies the root of *Picrorrhiza kurroa* was shown to blunt the sensitivity of guinea pigs to histamine and sympathomimetic amines as well as to prevent allergen and PAF-induced bronchial obstruction. However, the effects of *Picrorrhiza kurroa* on T cell subsets needs to be explored in order to confirm its immunomodulatory properties.

Piper longum is another plant often used for the therapy of bronchial asthma and other allergic disorders [36]. It has been found to reduce passive cutaneous ana-

Table 6 - Plants prescribed in Charaka Samhita as having actions on Ama

***Deepak* drugs**	***Pachak* drugs**
Ferula narthex	*Aconitum heterophyllum*
Garcinia pedunculata	*Berberis aristata*
Piper longum	*Cissampelos pareira*
Piper nigrum	*Curcuma longa*
Piper retrofractum	*Cyperus rotundas*
Plumbago zeylanica	*Aleatory cardomonium*
Semicarpus anacardium	*Emblica officinalis*
Trachyspermum ammi	*Picrorrhiza kurroa*
Zingiber officinalis	*Plumbago zeylenica*
	Saussurea lappa
	Semicarpus anacardum
	Terminalia bellerica
	Terminalia chebula

Note: These drugs are of two types
*(1) those which increase digestion capacity to prevent formation of ama (*deepak*) and*
*(2) those which digest ama (*pachak*).*

phylaxis in rats and protect guinea pigs against antigen induced bronchospasm [86]. In a clinical study conducted on 20 children having bronchial asthma the effect of increasing dosages of *Piper longum* (150–450 mg/day) was investigated. After five weeks of therapy, eleven of these children had no recurrence while three improved with a moderate response. In three patients the response was poor [87]. These data indicate the potential of *Piper longum* in modulating allergic processes.

Hence, attention should be given to the conceptual framework of Ayurveda (or any other traditional or folk medicine) while looking for leads for research [82, 88].

Another major aspect of research on Ayurvedic drugs is that Ayurveda (as it is an ancient science) prescribes the whole extract of the plant. This was, until recently, not acceptable to modern science. Chemical fractionation and isolation of single active components was the trend. Now, however, there is an increasing awareness that although, for academic purposes and for standardization of the compound, it is necessary to know what the active ingredient is, for clinical use a formulation that is a "whole standardized extract" is accepted [89]. In our laboratory we have found that the highest pharmacological activity was obtained with an aqueous extract of the stem of *Tinospora cordifolia* as compared to extracts prepared with methanol, hydroalcohol or petroleum ether. A similar observation has also been made with *Withania somnifera*, as mentioned earlier [42].

Table 7 - The effects (as measured by carbon clearance (min)) of rasayanas *at different times of the year**

Drug	Winter (Nov–Dec)	Spring (March)
Asparagus racemosus	17.8 ± 11.5	49.2 ± 20.1
Emblica officinalis	11.2 ± 7.0	57.3 ± 25.5
Withania somnifera	20.8 ± 9.0	58.0 ± 16.1
Tinospora cordifolia	25.3 ± 5.6	70.4 ± 24.2

**Note the high standard deviation in the hotter months. There was also higher mortality at this time.*

An important facet of Ayurvedic medicine is that polyherbal therapy is often prescribed. Thus, a number of plants are combined for their synergistic, additive or adjuvant effects (either to increase efficacy or reduce side-effects). Research on individual plant formulations therefore may be frustrating. We have therefore concentrated our work on plants which are prescribed as "single" entities (e.g. *Tinospora cordifolia*, *Emblica officinalis*, *Asparagus racemosus*, *Terminalia chebula*). Dosage may also serve as a point of argument. Given as a single plant, the dose recommendations will be different from those given for the polyherbal formulation.

Rasayana therapy is always prescribed as a pretreatment. This is because *rasayanas* are expected to be "pro-host". We have found in most of our studies with *rasayanas* that pretreatment is essential for maximum benefits. For example, pretherapy of at least four days is required for the effects of *Tinospora cordifolia* (leucocytosis and bone marrow proliferation) [25] or *Emblica officinalis* (protection of pancreas in pancreatitis) [90].

Chronopharmacology plays an important role in Ayurveda. *Rasayanas* are described as potent drugs and have been advised to be used only in the winter months. India, it is worth noting, has a mild winter and spring is often a fairly warm season. In order to investigate the validity of this recommendation we measured the reticulo-endothelial system (RES) activity by estimating clearance of colloidal carbon following therapy with *Rasayanas* in winter and spring months. Table 7 summarizes the results and shows that the *rasayanas* were not effective in the warmer season. There was also somewhat higher mortality in rats treated with rasayanas in summer.

In spite of these problems, research on Ayurveda has flourished recently. It has been, and will continue, to be a rich source for immunostimulants [91]. Thus, accurate scientific translations and correct interpretations of stanzas in Ayurvedic texts will provide excellent leads which can form the basis of further research.

Acknowledgements
We acknowledge the encouragement from Dr. P. M. Pai, Dean of Seth GS Medical College and KEM Hospital. We also thank Mr. Anthony Fernandes for assistance during the word processing.

References

1 Dahanukar SA, Thatte UM (1989) Therapeutic Approaches. In: *Ayurveda Revisited.* Popular Prakashan, Mumbai, 74–130
2 Golub ES (1987) The clonal nature of the immune response. In: *Immunology: A synthesis.* Sinauer Associates, Inc., Massachusetts, USA, 1–13
3 P. Sharma (ed) (1983) Chikitsasthana. In: *Charaka Samhita*, Chapter 6; Stanzas 7, 8, Chaukhambha Orientalia, Varanasi
4 Shastri AK (ed) (1993) Sutrasthana. In: *Sushrut Samhita*, Chapter 1; Stanza 15, Chaukhambha Orientalia, Varanasi
5 Dahanukar SA, Thatte UM (1996) In: *Ayurveda unravelled.* National Book Trust, New Delhi
6 Dahanukar SA (1987) *Study of influence of plant products on adaptive processes.* Ph.D. Thesis, University of Bombay
7 Thatte UM, Dahanukar SA (1997) The 'Rasayana' Concept: Clues from immunomodulatory therapy. In: Upadhyay S (ed): *Immunomodulation.* Narosa Publishing House, New Delhi, 141–148
8 Katiyar CK, Brindavanam NB, Tiwari P, Narayana DBA (1997) Immunomodulator products from Ayurveda: Current status and future perspectives. In: Upadhyay S (ed): *Immunomodulation.* Narosa Publishing House, New Delhi, 163–187
9 Sarma DNK and Khosa RL (1993) Chemistry and pharmacology of *T. Cordifolia* Miers. *Indian Drugs* 30(11): 549–554
10 Gangan VD, Pradhan P, Sipahimalani AT, Banerji A (1994) Cordifolisides A, B, C: norditerpene furan glycosides from *Tinospora cordifolia. Phytochemistry* 37(3): 781–786
11 Swaminathan K, Sinha UC, Ramakumar S, Bhatt RK, Sabata BK (1989) Structure of columbin, a diterpenoid furanolactone from *Tinospora cordifolia* Miers. *Acta Crystallogr* C, 45(Pt 2): 300–303
12 Swaminathan K, Sinha UC, Bhatt RK, Sabata BK Tavale SS (1989) Structure of tinosporide, a diterpenoid furanolactone from *Tinospora cordifolia* Miers. *Acta Crystallogr* C, 45(Pt 1): 134–136
13 Kidwai AR, Salooja KC, Sharma V, Siddiqui S (1949) Chemical examination of *Tinospora cordifolia* Miers. *Journal of Scientific & Industrial Research* VIIIB(7): 115–118
14 Rao EV, Rao MV (1980) Studies on the polysaccharide preparation (Guduchi satwa) derived from *Tinospora cordifolia. Indian J Pharm Sci* 43(3): 103–106

15 Sainis KB, Sumariwalla PF, Goel A, Chintalwar GJ, Sipahimalani AT, Banerji A (1997) Immunomodulatory properties of stem extracts of *Tinospora cordifolia*: Cell targets and active principles. In: Upadhyay S (ed) *Immunomodulation.* Narosa Publishing House, New Delhi, 155–162
16 Mathew S, Kuttan G (1996) Antioxidant activity of *Tinospora cordifolia* and its usefulness in the amelioration of cyclophosphamide induced toxicity. *Amala Research Bulletin* 16: 113–121
17 Dahanukar SA, Thatte UM (1997) Current status of Ayurveda in phytomedicine. *Phytomedicine* 4(3): 297–306
18 Thatte UM, Dahanukar SA (1989) Immunotherapeutic modification of experimental infections by Indian medicinal plants. *Phytotherapy Res* 3(2): 43–49
19 Dahanukar SA, Thatte UM, Pai N, More PB, Karandikar SM (1988) Immunotherapeutic modification by *Tinospora cordifolia* of abdominal sepsis induced by caecal ligation in rats. *Ind J Gastroenterol* 7(1): 21–23.
20 Thatte UM, Chhabria S, Karandikar SM, Dahanukar SA (1987) Immunotherapeutic modification of E.coli induced abdominal sepsis and mortality in mice by Indian medicinal plants. *Indian Drugs* 25(3): 95–97
21. Thatte UM, Kulkarni MR, Dahanukar SA (1992). Immunotherapeutic modification of E.coli peritonitis and bacteremia by *Tinospora cordifolia. J Postgrad Med* 38(1): 13–15
22 Rege NN, Nazareth HM, Bapat RD, Dahanukar SA (1989) Modulation of immunosuppression in obstructive jaundice by *Tinospora cordifolia. Ind J Med Res* 90: 178–183
23 Thatte UM, Chhabria S, Karandikar SM, Dahanukar SA (1987) Protective effects of Indian medicinal plants against cyclophosphamide neutropenia. *J Postgrad Med* 33: 185–188
24 Thatte UM, Dahanukar SA (1988) Comparative study of immunomodulating activity of Indian medicinal plants, lithium carbonate and glucan. *Meth & Find Exptl Clin. Pharmacol* 10: 639–644
25 Usha D (1995) Immunomodulatory actions of *Tinospora cordifolia.* A dissertation for the M.D. examination; University of Bombay
26 Patil M, Patki P, Kamath HV, Patwardhan B (1997) Antistress activity of *Tinospora cordifolia* (wild) Miers. *Indian Drugs* 34(4): 211–215
27 Rege NN, Dahanukar SA (1993) Quantitation of microbicidal activity of mononuclear phagocytes: An *in vitro* technique. *J Postgrad Med* 39(1): 22–25
28 Thatte UM, Dahanukar SA (1997) Apoptosis: Clinical relevance and pharmacological manipulation. *Drugs* 10: 1–21
29 Atal CK, Sharma ML, Kaul A, Khazuria A (1986) Immunomodulating agents of plant origin. I: Preliminary screening. *J Ethnopharmac* 18: 133–141
30 Rege NN (1996) Evaluation of hepatoprotective effects of *Tinospora cordifolia.* Ph.D. Dissertation in Pharmacology, University of Bombay
31 Bapat RD, Rege NN, Koti R, Desai NK, Dahanukar SA (1995) Can we do away with PTBD? *HPB Surgery* 9: 5–11

32 Bhattacharya SK, Goel RK, Kaur R, Ghosal S (1987) Antistress activity of Sitoindosides VII and VIII, new acylsteryglucosides from *Withania somnifera*. *Phytother Res* 1: 32–37
33 Kulkarni SK, Sharma A, Verma A, Ticku MK (1993) GABA receptor mediated anticonvulsant action of *Withania somnifera* root extract. *Indian Drugs* 30: 305–12
34 Mehta AK, Binkley P, Gandhi SS, Ticku MK (1991) Pharmacological effects of *Withania somnifera* root extract on GABA, receptor complex. *Indian J Med Res* 94: 312–315
35 Chopra RN, Chopra IC, Varma BS (1969) In: *Supplement to Glossary of Indian Medicinal Plants*. Publications and Information Directorate, New Delhi, 102
36 Gogtay VK (1982) In: *Dravyagunavigyan*, Continental Prakashan, Pune
37 Davis L, Kuttan G (1996) Amelioration of cyclophosphamide induced toxicity using *Withania somnifera*. *Amala Research Bulletin* 16: 109–112
38 Ghosal S, Lal J, Srivastava R, Bhattacharya S, Upadhyay S, Jaiswal A, Chattopadhyay U (1989) Immunomodulatory and CNS effects of sitoindosides IX and X, two new glycowithanolides from *Withania somnifera*. *Phytother Res* 3: 201–206
39 Bahr V, Hansel R (1982) Immunomodulating properties of 5,20α(R)-dihydroxy-6α,7α-epoxy-l-oxo(5α)-witha-2,24-dienolide and solasodine. *Planta Medica* 44: 32–33
40 Cassady JM, Chang CJ, McLaughlin JL (1981) Recent advances in the isolation and structural elucidation of antineoplastic agents from higher plants. In: Beal JL, Reinhard E (eds): *Natural Products as Medicinal Agents*. Hippokrates Verlag, Stuttgart, 93– 124
41 Blasko G, Cordell CA (1988) Chemistry of plant derived anti-cancer agents. In: Wagner H, Hiroshi H, Farnsworth NR (eds): *Economic and Medicinal Plant Research*, Vol 1. Academic Press, London, 119–191
42 Wagner H, Nörr H, Winterhoff H (1994) Plant Adaptogens. *Phytomedicine* 1: 63–76
43 Suresh K, Vasudevan DM (1994) Augmentation of murine natural killer cell and antibody dependent cellular cytotoxicity activated by *Phyllanthus emblica*, a new immunomodulator. *J Ethnopharmacology* 44 (1): 55–60
44 Rastogi RP, Mehrotra BN (1991) In: Rastogi RP (ed): *Compendium of Indian medicinal plants*. CDRI and PID, New Delhi, Vol 2: 536
45 Rege NN, Mahajan J, Sheth S, Shah MD, Dahanukar S (1990) Protective role of Ocimum sanctum in recurrent respiratory tract infection. *Abstract, Tenth National Congress on Respiratory Diseases*, 12–15 Dec., Bombay
46 Bhattacharya SK, Gupta VS, Maiti PC, Sen P (1988) Effect of Ocimum sanctum Linn on humoral immune responses. *Indian J Med Res* 87: 384–86
47 Godhwani S, Godhwani JL, Vyas DS (1988) *Ocimum sanctum* – A preliminary study evaluating its immunoregulatory profile in albino rats. *J Ethnopharmacol* 24: 193– 198
48 Sen P (1993) Therapeutic potentials of *Tulsi*: From experiences to facts. *Drugs: News and Views* 1(2): 15–20
49 Mediratta PK, Dewan V, Bhattacharya SK, Gupta VS, Maiti PC, Sen P (1988) Effect of *Ocimum sanctum* Linn on humoral immune responses. *Indian J Med Res* 87: 384–386
50 't Hart LT, van Enckevort PH, van Dijk H, Zaat R, de Silva KTD, Labadie RP (1988) Two functionally and chemically distinct immunomodulatory compounds in the gel of *Aloe vera*. *J Ethnopharmacol* 23: 61–71

51 't Hart LT, van den Berg AJ, Kuis L, van Dijk H, Labadie RP (1989) An anti-complementary polysaccharide with immunological adjuvant from the leaf parenchyma gel of *Aloe vera. Planta Med* 55(6): 509–512

52 Hirao Y, Sumioka I, Nakagami S, Yamamoto M, Hatono S, Yoshida S, Fuwa T, Nakagawa S (1987) Activation of immunoresponder cells by the protein fraction from aged garlic extract. *Phytother Res* 1(4): 161–164

53 Lau B, Woolley J, Marsh C, Barker G, Koobs D, Torrey R (1986) Superiority of intralesional immunotherapy with *Corynebacterium parvum* and *Allium sativum* in control of murine transitional cell carcinoma. *J Urology* 136: 701–705

54 Wagner H, Proksch A (1985) Immunostimulatory drugs of fungi and higher plants. In: Wagner H, Hiroshi H, Farnsworth NR (eds): *Economic and Medicinal Plant Research*, Vol 1. Academic Press, London, 113– 153

55 Hikino H (1985) Recent research on oriental medicinal plants. In: Wagner H, Hiroshi H, Farnsworth NR (eds): *Economic and Medicinal Plant Research*, Vol 1. Academic Press, London, 53–85

56 Puri A, Saxena RP, Sumati, Guru PY, Kulshreshtha DK, Saxena K, Dhawan B (1992) Immunostimulant activity of Picroliv, the iridoid glycoside fraction of *Picrorrhiza kurroa*, and its protective action against *Leishmania donovani* infection in hamsters. *Planta Med* 58(6): 528–532

57 Simons JM, 't Hart, Labadie RP, van Dijk H, De Silva K (1990) Modulation of human complement activation and the human neutrophil oxidative burst by different root extracts of *Picrorrhiza kurroa. Phyother Res* 4: 207–211

58 Labadie RP (1990) Immunomodulatory activity studies on single plant constituents and compound extracts. *Actes du 1er Colloque European d'Ethnopharmacologie; Metz 22–25 mars*, 291–297

59 Simons JM, 't Hart, van Dijk H, Fischer FC, De Silva K, Labadie RP (1989) Immunomodulatory compounds from *Picrorrhiza kurroa*: isolation and characterization of two anti-complementary polymeric fractions from an aqueous root extract. *J Ethnopharmacol* 26: 169–182

60 't Hart BA, Bakker NP, Labadie RP, Simons JM (1991) The newly developed neutrophil oxidative burst antagonist apocynin inhibits joint-swelling in rat collagen arthritis. *Agents Actions* 32(Suppl): 179–184

61 't Hart BA, Simons JM, Knaan Shanzer S, Bakker NP, Labadie RP (1990) Antiarthritic activity of the newly developed neutrophil oxidative burst antagonist apocynin. *Free Radic Biol Med* 9(2): 127–131

62 Asolkar LV, Kakkar KK, Chakre OJ (1992) In: *Second supplement to glossary of Indian medicinal plants with active principles*, Part I. Publications and Information Directorate, New Delhi, 108–111

63 Van der Nat JM, Van der Sluis WG, de Silva KT, Labadie RP (1991) Ethnopharmacognostical survey of *Azadirachta indica* A. Juss (Meliaceae). *J Ethnopharmacol* 35(1): 1–24

64 Upadhyay SN (1997) Therapeutic potential of immunomodulatory agents from plant

products. In: Upadhyay S (ed): *Immunomodulation*. Narosa Publishing House, New Delhi, 149–154

65 Upadhyay SN, Dhawan S, Garg S, Talwar GP (1992) Immunomodulatory effects of neem (*Azadharichta indica*) oil. *Int J Immunopharmacol* 14(7): 1187–1193

66 Garg S, Talwar GP, Upadhya SN (1994) Comparison of extraction procedures on the immunocontraceptive activity of neem seed extracts. *J Ethnopharmacol* 44(2): 87– 92

67 Van Der Nat JM, Klerx JPAM, Van DK, de Silva KTD, Labadie RP (1987) Immunomodulatory activity of an aqueous extract of *Azadirachta indica* stem bark. *J Ethnopharmacology* 19: 125–131

68 Fujuwara T, Takeda T, Ogihara Y, Shimizu M, Nomura T, Tomita Y (1982) Studies on the structure of polysaccharides from the bark of *Melia azadirachta. Chem Pharm Bull* 30: 4025–4030

69 Van der Nat JM, 't Hart LA, Van der Sluis WG, van den Berg AJ, de Silva KT, Labadie RP (1991), Characterization of anti-complement compounds from *Azadirachta indica. J Ethnopharmacol* 27(1–2): 15–24

70 Bamunuarachchi A, Abeysekera A, de Silva KTD, Labadie RP (1984) Evaluation of effects of Sri Lankan plants on human complement *in vitro*. *Pharmaceutisch Weekblad* 119: 901–902

71 Van der Nat JM, Van der Sluis WG, 't Hart LA, Van Dijk H, de Silva KT, Labadie RP (1991) Activity-guided isolation and identification of *Azadirachta indica* bark extract constituents which specifically inhibit chemiluminescence production by activated human polymorphonuclear leukocytes. *Planta Med* 57(1): 65–68

72 Kroes BH, Van den Berg AJ, Abeyesekera AM, de Silva KT, Labadie RP (1993) Fermentation in traditional medicine: the impact of *Woodfordia fruticosa* flowers on the immunomodulatory activity, and the alcohol and sugar contents of *Nimba arishta. J Ethnopharmacol* 40(2): 117–125

73 Columbie FC, Andrei GM, Laguens RP, de Torres RA, Coto CE (1992) Partially purified extracts of *Melia azadarach* L. inhibit tacaribe virus growth in neonatal mice. *Phytother Res* 6: 15

74 Bhaumik S, Chattopadhyay S, Ghosal S (1993) Effect of *Shilajit* on mouse peritoneal macrophages. *Phytother Res* 7: 425–427

75 Ghosal S, Lal J, Singh SK, Dasgupta G, Bhaduri J, Mukhopadhyay M, Bhattacharya SK (1989) Mast cell protecting effects of shilajit and its constituents. *Phytother Res* 3(6): 249–252

76 Handa SS, Sharma A (1997) Pharmacological studies on Indian medicinal plants. In: Chauhan CK (ed): *Reviews of Research in Pharmacology in India (1988–1993)*. CK Chauhan, Mumbai-22, 176–215

77 Puri A, Saxena R, Saxena RP, Saxena KC, Srivastava V, Tandon JS (1993) Immunostimulant agents from Andrographis paniculata. *J Nat Proceedings* 56: 995– 999

78 Sharma ML, Khajuria A, Kaul A, Singh S, Singh GB, Atal CK (1988) Effect of salai guggal ex-*Boswellia serrata* on cellular and humoral responses and leucocyte migration. *Agents Action* 24: 161–164

79 Guha S, Chattopadhyay U, Ghosal S (1993) Activation of peritoneal macrophages by mangiferin, a naturally occuring C-glucosyl xanthone. *Phytother Res* 7: 107–110
80 Puri A, Saxena R, Saxena RP, Saxena KC, Srivastava V, Tandon J. (1994) Immunostimulant activity of *Nyctanthes arbor tristis* L. *J Ethnopharmacol* 42(1): 31–37
81 Labadie RP, Van der Nat J, Simons JM, Kroes BH, Kosasi S, Van den Berg A, 't Hart L, Van der Sluis W, Abeysekera A, Bamunuarachchi A, De Silva K (1989) An ethnopharmacognostic approach to the search for immunomodulators of plant origin. *Planta Med* 55: 339–348
82 Dahanukar SA, Karandikar SM (1983) Rethinking on Research in Ayurvedic Medicines. *Indian Drugs* 20(5): 177–182
83 Thatte UM, Dahanukar SA (1986) Ayurveda and contemporary scientific thought. *Trends in Pharmacological Sciences* 7; 247–251
84 Mahajani SS, Kulkarni RD (1977) Effect of disodium cromoglycate and picrorrhiza kurroa root powder on sensitivity of guinea pigs to histamine and sympathomimetic amines. *Int Archs Allergy Appl Immun* 53: 137–144
85 Dorsch W, Stuppner H, Wagner H, Gropp M, Demoulin S, Ring J (1991) Antiasthmatic effects of *Picrorrhiza kurroa*: Androsin prevents allergen- and PAF-induced bronchial obstruction in guinea pigs. *Int Archs Allergy Appl Immun* 95: 128–133
86 Dahanukar SA, Karandikar SM (1984) Evaluation of antiallergic activity of *Piper longum*. *Indian Drugs* 21(9): 377–383
87 Dahanukar SA, Karandikar SM, Desai M (1984) Efficacy of *Piper longum* in childhood asthma. *Indian Drugs* 21(9): 384–388
88 Labadie RP. (1986) Problems and possibilities in the use of traditional drugs. *J Ethnopharmacol* 15(3): 221–230
89 Rawls R (1996) Europe's strong herbal view. *C&EN*, Sept.23, 53–60
90 Hazra A (1997) Protective effect of *Emblica officinalis* in experimental pancreatitis in rats. M.D. Dissertation in Pharmacology, University of Bombay
91 Smit HF, Woerdenbag HJ, Singh RH, Meulenbeld GJ, Labadie RP, Zwaving JH (1995) Ayurvedic herbal drugs with possible cytostatic activity. *J Ethnopharmacol* 47: 75–84

Immunostimulants in traditional Chinese medicine

Pei-Gen Xiao[1] *and Chang-Xiao Liu*[2]

[1]Institute of Medicinal Plant Development, Chinese Academy of Medical Sciences, Beijing, 100094, P.R. China; [2]Tianjin Institute of Pharmaceutical Research, State Pharmaceutical Administration of China, 308 An-Shan West Road, Tianjin, 300193, P.R. China.

Introduction

Chinese materia medica (Chinese traditional drugs or Chinese drugs), *Zhongya* in Chinese, is an integral part of traditional Chinese medicine and Chinese civilization. Historically, Chinese traditional medicine rose from mythical medicine to a system of Chinese drugs and herbal medicine. The first book on materia medica, *Shen-nong Bencao Jing*, known as "the canon of materia medica", was compiled in the second century BC by the folklore under the pseudonym of Shennong, the Holy Farmer. It is well-known that China was and is one of the leading nations when the use of medicinal plants is considered. This has further developed so that medicinal plants are today playing an outstanding role within the framework of official health services in China. China is endowed with an abundant resource of medicinal plants, more than five thousand plants have been identified as medicinal. The latest edition of *The Chinese Pharmacopoeia* (the 1995 edition) records more than 700 items of Chinese drugs origining from medicinal plants.

Chinese drugs are classified into many categories, usually into 15–20 classes, according to their clinical effects such as diaphoretics, antitussives, diuretics, digestives, etc. These are comparable to those in western medicine, there is, however, an important group of drugs which are indispensable in Chinese medicine but not familiar nor accepted in western medicine. These have been translated as tonics, restoratives or strengthening agents. Considering their mode of pharmacological actions, it has been proposed to classify them as biomodulators. Biomodulators modulate the physiological and biochemical activities of the body's systems at many levels. Among these drugs, Chinese drugs which stimulate immune activity occupy an important place in Chinese medicine.

Medicinal plants with immunostimulating activity

There is a large number of medicinal plants and relevant prescriptions recorded in the Chinese medical literature aimed at improving the well-being of aged people, as

Immunomodulatory Agents from Plants, edited by H. Wagner

well as the prevention of diseases and the prolongation of life-span. In the well-known *Compendium of Materia Medica* (*Bencao Gangmu*) compiled by the famous Chinese traditional doctor Li Shi-Zhen during the years 1552–1578, more promising antiageing drugs are presented. Some drugs and herbs possessing immunostimulating, immunoregulating or antiageing activities have been selected from the medical literature and experimental studies for research and development by modern scientific methods concerning chemical, pharmacological and clinical aspects.

According to the mode of action, Chinese traditional drugs and herbs with immunostimulating activity may be divided into three types: (1) drugs and herbs enhancing the phagocytic activity; (2) drugs with a stimulating effect on cell functions and (3) drugs with a stimulating effect on humoral immune functions [1–4]. Some drugs representative of the three types of Chinese traditional drugs and herbs having immunostimulating activity are listed in Tables 1–3.

The main chemical constituents isolated from Chinese traditional drugs and herbs with immunoregulation or immunostimulating activity are listed in Table 4. Among them the polysaccharides and saponins are predominant.

In this chapter an introduction is given to the pharmacological and clinical studies on the immunostimulating or immunoregulating activities of *Acanthopanax senticosus*, *Angelica sinensis*, *Astragalus membranaceus*, *Bupleurum chinense*, *Glycyrrhiza uralensis*, *Panax ginseng*, *Cordyceps sinensis*, *Cynanchum auriculatum*, *Epimedium brevicornum*, *Ganoderma lucidum*, *Lycium barbarum*, *Polygonatum sibiricum*, *Polygonum multiflorum* and *Polyporus umbellatus*.

Angelica sinensis

Radix Angelicae sinensis, *Danggui* in Chinese, is the root of *Angelica sinensis* (Oliver) Diels (*Umbelliferae*). Ethnopharmacologically, the Chinese *Angelica* root is reputed as a most valuable drug for women. It is a 'sweet, pungent and warm drug', which 'enters the liver, heart and spleen meridians'. The functions are to replenish blood, to invigorate blood, to stop pain, and to moisten the intestines. It is used to nourish the blood, improve the rhythmicity and tonicity of uterine muscles, in the treatment of menstrual disorder and as an emollient and laxative for chronic constipation in aged and debilitated humans [5].

Pharmacologically and clinically, Chinese *Angelica* possesses broad activities (Table 5). *Angelica* polysaccharide and ferulic acid are the major constituents of Radix Angelicae Sinensis. The isolated polysaccharide as well as the extract of Radix Angelicae sinensis can significantly increase the phagocytic activity of rat peritoneal macrophages. Administration of the cytostatic drug endoxan along with *Angelica* polysaccharide is capable of maintaining the non-specific immunities of the body at normal levels. Radix Angelicae extract in combination with ferulate sodium can significantly improve the engulfing rate of Congo red by rat monocytes and they

Table 1 - Chinese traditional drugs and herbs with phagocytosis enhancing activity

Chinese drug	Plant origin
Radix Codonopsis Piloculae	*Codonopsis pilosula* (Franch.) Nannf
Rhizoma Atractylodis Macrocephalae	*Atractylodes macrocephala* Koidz.
Radix Ginseng	*Panax ginseng* C. A. Mey.
Radix Scutellariae	*Scutellaria baicalensis* Georgi
Rhizoma Coptis	*Coptis chinensis* Franch.
Radix Astragali	*Astragalus membranaceus* (Fisch.) Bge.
Rhizoma Smilacis Glabrae	*Smilax glabra* Roxb.
Rhizoma Glycyrrhizi	*Glycyrrhiza uralensis* Fisch.
Rhizoma Dioscoreae	*Dioscorea opposita* Thunb.
Cortex Acanthopanacis	*Acanthopanax senticosus* (Rupr. et Maxim). Maxim.
Fructus Psoraleae	*Psoralea corylifolia* L.
Herba Epimedii	*Epimedium brevicornum* Maxim.
Radix Morindae Officinalis	*Morinda officinalis* How
Radix Stephaniae Tetrandrae	*Stephania tetrandra* S. Moore
Flos Lonicerae	*Lonicera japonica* Thunb.
Flos Chrysanthemi	*Chrysanthemum morifolium* Ramat.
Folium Isatidis	*Isatis tinctoria* L.
Radix Isatidis	*Isatis indigotica* Fort.
Herba Houttuyniae	*Houttuynia cordata* Thunb.
Herba Andrographitis	*Andrographis paniculata* Thunb.
Herba Oldenlandiae	*Oldenlandia diffusa* Nees (Willd.) Roxb.
Cortex Phellodendri	*Phellodendron chinense* Schneid.
Radix Bupleuri	*Bupleurum chinensis* DC.
Radix et Rhizoma Rhei	*Rheum palmatum* L.
Herba Artemisiae Chinghao	*Artemisia annua* L.
Radix Ophiopogon	*Ophiopogon japonicus* (Thunb.) Ker-Gawl.
Radix Platycodi	*Platycodon grandiflorum* (Jacq.) A. DC.
Radix Rhapontici	*Rhaponticum uniflorum* (Linn.) DC.
Herba Taraxaci	*Taraxacum mongolicum* Hand.-Mazz.
Radix Asteris	*Aster tataricus* L.f.
Herba Lysimachiae	*Lysimachia christinae* Hance
Fructus Aristolochiae	*Aristolochia contorta* Bge.
Caulis Aristolochiae manshuriensis	*Aristolochia manshuriensis* Kom.
Rhizoma Ligustici Chuanxiong	*Ligusticum chuanxiong* Hort.
Radix Salviae Miltiorrhizae	*Salvia miltiorrhiza* Bge.
Radix Paeoniae Rubra	*Paeonia lactiflora* Pall.

Table 2 - Chinese traditional drugs and herbs with stimulating cell-immune activity

Chinese drug	**Plant origin**
Radix Codonopsis Pilosulae	*Codonopsia pilosula* (Franch.) Nannf
Radix Ginseng	*Panax ginseng* C. A. Mey.
Rhizoma Atractylodis macrocephalae	*Atractylodes macrocephala* Koidz.
Ganoderma Lucidum	*Ganoderma lucidum* (Leyss. ex Fr.) Karst.
Semen Coicis	*Coix lacryma-jobi* L. var. mayuem (Roman) Stapf
Radix Polygoni Multiflori	*Polygonum multiflorum* Thunb.
Rhizoma Polygonati	*Polygonatum sibiricum* Red.
Caulis Spatholobi	*Spatholobus suberectus* Dunn
Rhizoma Ligustici Chuanxiong	*Ligusticum chuanxiong* Hort.
Radix Rehmanniae	*Rehmannia glutinosa* (Gaertn.) Libosch.
Radix Paeoniae Rubra	*Paeonia obavata* Maxim.
Flos Carthami Tinctori	*Carthanmus tinctorius* Linn.
Herba Rhapontici	*Rhaponticus uniflorum* (Linn.) DC.
Semen Vaccariae	*Vaccaria segetalis* (Neck.) Garcke
Radix Salviae Miltorrhizae	*Salvia miltiorrhiza* Bge.
Herba Epimedii	*Epimedium brevicornum* Max.
Fructus Lycii	*Lycium barbarum* Linn.
Fructus Mori	*Morus alba* L.
Cortex Eucommiae	*Eucommia ulmoidea* Oliv.
Fructus Schisandrae	*Schisandra chinensis* Baill
Remulus Loranthi	*Loranthus parasiticus* (L.) Merr.
Radix Rehmanniae parapariti	*Rehmannia glutinosa* Libosch.
Rhizoma Imperatae	*Imperata cylindnica* Beauv.
Herba Violae	*Viola yedoensis* Makino
Herba Taraxaci	*Taraxacum mongolicum* Hand.-Mazz.
Caulis Lonicerae	*Lonicera japonica* Thunb.
Fructus Ligusitri Lucidi	*Ligustrum lucidum* Ait.
Radix Scrophulariae	*Scrophularia ningpoensis* Hemsl.
Flos Lonicerae	*Lonicera japonica* Thunb.
Flos Chrysanthemi	*Chrysanthemum morifolium* Ramat.
Rhizoma Coptidis	*Coptis chinensis* Franch.
Radix Scutellariae	*Scutellaria baicalensis* Georgi
Semen Cuscutae	*Cuscuta chinensis* Lam.

also increase the phagocytic activity of rat peritoneal phagocytes [4]. Oral administration of *Angelica* decoction has no significant effect on the E-rosette forming cells, but improves the effectiveness of plasma antibodies.

Table 3 - Chinese traditional drugs and herbs with stimulating humoral immune activity

Chinese drug	Plant origin
Radix Angelici Sininensis	*Angelica sinensis* (Oliv.) Diels
Cortex Cinnamomi	*Cinnamomum cassia* Presl.
Rhizoma Curculiginis	*Curculigo orchioides* Gaertn.
Semen Cuscutae	*Cuscuta chinensis* Lam.
Rhizoma Polygonati	*Polygonatum sibircum* Red.
Herba Cynomorii	*Cynomirium songaricum* Rupr.
Radix Scrophulariae	*Scrophularia ningpoensis* Hemsl.
Raidix Asparigi	*Asparagus cochinchinensis* (Lour.) Merr.
Radix Ophiopogonis	*Ophiopogon japonoca* (Thunb.)Kerr.-Ga.
Radix Ginseng	*Panax ginseng* C. A. Mey.
Radix Polygalae	*Polygala tenuifolia* Willd.
Fructus Ligustri Lucidi	*Ligustrum lucidum* Ait.
Rhizoma Zingiberis Receno	*Zingiber officinale* (Willd.) Rosc.
Radix Astragali	*Astragalus membranaceus* (Fisch.) Bge.
Radix Salviae Miltiorrhizae	*Salvia miltiorrhiza* Bge.

Angelica sinensis and its component ferulic acid increase the DNA synthesis and IL-2 production of mice spleen lymphocytes after concanvalin A (ConA) costimulation. At doses of 15–20 g/kg of Radix Angelicae and at doses of 12.5–25 mg/kg of ferulic acid by ip administration for seven days, the thymus and spleen weight was increased; phagocytosis of macrophage, carbon clearance rate, the production of hemolysines and response of lymphoid cells immune against sheep red cells (SRBC) was seen. The spleen index, thymus index and clearance rate were also increased. Radix Angelicae and ferulic acid also showed a remarkable effect on the proliferation of spleen lymphocytes in ConA-stimulated mice [6].

Acanthopanax senticosus

Cortex Acanthopanacis, *Ciwujia* in Chinese, is the root bark of *Acanthopanax senticosus* (Rupr. et Maxim.) Maxim. (*Araliaceae*). According to Chinese Medicine, the properties and taste of this drug are pungent, bitter and warm. The drug 'enters the liver and kidney meridians', dispels wind and dampness, strengthens the tendons and bone, and improves urination [7].

Cortex Acanthopanacis can increase the phagocytic activity of guinea pig peritoneal macrophages as well as the phagocytic functions of the rat reticuloendothe-

Table 4 - The chemical substituents form Chinese traditional drugs and herbs with immuno-stimulating activity

Compounds	Plant origin
Lentinan	*Lentinus edodes* (Berk) Sing.
Artemisinine	*Artemisia annua* L.
Angelica polysaccharides	*Angelica sinensis* (Oliv.) Diels
Ferulate sodium	
Polyporus polysaccharides	*Polyporus umbellatus* (Pers.) Fr.
Ophipogon saponins	*Ophiopogon japonicus* (Thunb.) Ker-Gawl
Bupleurum polysaccharide	*Bupleurum chinensis* DC.
Lycium polysaccharides	*Lycium barbamum* Linn.
Isatis polysaccharides	*Isatis indigotica* Fort.
Safflower yellow	*Carthamus tinctorus* Linn.
Ecdysterone	*Rhaponticum uniflorum* (Linn.) DC.
Curcumin	*Curcuma longa* Linn.
Paeonol	*Paeonia suffruticosa* Andr.
b-3,4-Dihydroxyphenyl lactate sodium	*Salvia miltiorrhiza Bge.*
Salvianolic acid A	
Salvianolic acid B	
Rosmarinic acid	
Nifedipine	*Scutellaria baicalensis* Georgi
Glycyrrhizin	*Glycyrrhiza uralensis* Fisch.
Astragalus polysaccharides	*Astragalus membranaceus* (Fisch.) Bge.
Astragalus saponins	
Schisanrenol	*Schisandra chinensis* Baill.
Schisandrone	
Schisandiol	
Schisandrin	
Ginsenosides	*Panax ginseng* C. A. Mey.
Ginseng polysaccaride	
Panaxatriol ginsenoside	
Acanthopanax saponin B	*Acanthopanax senticosus* (Rupr. et Maxim) Maxim.
Acanthopanax saponin D	
Acanthopanax saponin E	

lial system. It increases the gross weight of spleen and the number of splenic macrophages. It is also noted to enhance the production of specific immunoglobulins. Intraperitoneal injection of the root bark extract can increase the splenic plaque

Table 5 - Pharmacological and clinical effects of Radix Angelicae sinensis

1. Modulation of the tonicity and rhythmicity of the uterus
2. Modulation of cardiovascular activities, relieving local circulatory stasis
3. Anti-thrombotic effect, decrease of platelet aggregation
4. Anti-inflammatory effect
5. Central sedative and analgesic effects
6. Hematopoietic effect
7. Modulation of immune activities

forming cell (SPFC) numbers in rats. Cortex Acanthopancis can increase T-cell population and the rate of E-rosette cell formation in patients with cor pulmonale. It also leads to a significant increase in the number of high-efficiency IgMs and the total amount of complement factors. This drug also enhances the morphological transformation of rat lymphocytes and the production of antibodies, boosting the immunity of the body against pathogens. The drug exhibits activities against infection and tumors. The polysaccharide containing extract from the bark leads to a significant interferon induction. The mechanism of action is probably due to the inhibiting effect on the degradation of RNA responsible for the interferon production. The immunological regulatory activity manifested by the bark extract can probably be attributed to the ability of its polysaccharides to induce the non-specific immune system [8]. It has also been shown to significantly increase the serum cAMP level, but it has no significant effect on cGMP levels.

Intraperitoneal administration of an extract containing eleutherosides B and D of *Acanthopanax senticosus* to mice at a daily dose of 18 mg/animal for one week increased the cytostatic activity of natural killer cells by about 200%. The eleutherosides stimulated macrophage T cell and possibly B cell-mediated immunity [9].

In a study on the immunomodulatory activity of the ethanol extract of *Acanthopanax senticosus*, the extract, administrered orally to healthy volunters for four weeks, showed a drastic increase in the absolute number of immune competent cells, especially T-lymphcytes [10].

The polysaccharides PES-A and B from *Acanthopanax senticosus* significantly increased the weight of spleen and thymus in mice and promoted the production of specific antibodies together with the phagocytosis of peritoneal macrophages [11].

The polyssacharide PES-A and B were found to decrease toxic effects of thioacetamide and phytothemagglutinine in mice and to enhance resistance to X-ray irradiation [12]. PES can markedly increase the serum levels of anti-bovine serum albumin (BSA) IgG and total IgG can stimulate the immune activity of mouse against invasion of foreign substances [13].

Astragalus membranaceus

Radix Astragali is the dried root of *Astragalus membranaceus* (Fisch.) Bge. or *A. membrabaceus* var. *mongholicus* (Bge.) Hsiao (*Leguminosae*), belonging to the traditional non-toxic medicine. Ethnopharmacologically it can strenghthen one's general health and it is used as a common tonic for vital energy (*Qi*) and *Yin*. The 'sweet' and 'warm' drug enters the lung and spleen meridians. Its functions are to replenish vital energy and cause *Yang* to ascend, to benefit vital energy and stabilize the exterior, to remove toxins, to promote healing, to promote water metabolism and to reduce edema. It is used to replenish the vital energy and to stop perspiration in the treatment of spontaneous perspiration, night sweating, prolapse of the uterus and anus, to dispel pus and accelerate the healing of wounds for the treatment of chronic ulcers, and as a diuretic for chronic nephritis with edema and proteinuria [14].

Radix Astragali can impove both specific and non-specific immunological functions of the body and has been shown to protect hepatic cells from injuries, and to possess infection- and tumor-suppressive effects. It can cause an increase in the size of the spleen, a diminution of the thymus gland, and a decrease in T cell value. It inhibits T cell functions, while those of the B cells are enhanced [15]. The drug can inhibit the complement-induced immunohemolysis and lead to a recovery in the decreased rat E-rosette formation rate caused by hydroxycorticosteroids, and to an elevation in the E-rosette rate in normal animals. To a certain degree, Radix Astragali can enhance the function of macrophage Fc fragment receptors. Though this drug possesses certain positive effects on the peritoneal macrophage Fc fragment receptors of normal rats, the effect is most pronounced in immunologically compromised animals. Increasing attention has been paid to the effect of this drug in both directional regulation of immunological functions and to its role in induction of interferon [4].

Recent pharmacological studies have shown that Radix Astragali can inhibit the biosynthesis of glycogen and dilate coronary as well as renal vessels. It also serves as a cardiac tonic, diuretic and antibacterial agent. More interestingly, it possesses an antiinfluenza action and may prevent respiratory infections. Both effects are believed to be related to the enhancement of immunological functions.

Studies on the effects of Radix Astragali on the regulation of the immune system are presented below:

(1) The drug and its refined extracts increase the plasma level of cAMP, liver cGMP and spleen cAMP and cGMP in mice all after administration of the crude extracts of this drug [16] (Tab. 6).
(2) The drug can also increase the levels of plasma cAMP, IgM and IgE in healthy volunteers after oral administration (Tab. 7).

These changes in the cyclic nucleotide level might be related to some extent to the important regulators of the immune response. It is suggested that there exists a link between an increased level of cAMP and inhibition of lymphocyte proliferation, generation of lymphokines, T lymphocyte mediated cyctoxicity and several other lymphocyte functions [17]. Three polysaccharides from *Astragalus mongholicus*, astragalan I, II and III, showed wide variety of immunological effects on mice. They increased the weight of spleen as well as the number of spleen cells, augmented the response of the mouse spleen against sheep red blood cells and stimulated the phagocytic activity of peritoneal macrophages. Astragalan I, however, inhibited the response of spleen cells to sheep red blood cells. Astragalan II showed similar but weaker effects, while astragalan III showed no significant effects [16].

In conclusion, Astragali polysaccharides (APS) show remarkable immuno-modulatory effects on cell-mediated and humoral immunity as well as monocyte-macrophage activity. APS has a stimulating effect on all types of immunocytes, T cells, B cells, and NK cells. It increases the size and weight of the spleen as well as the levels of DNA, RNA and protein of the spleenocytes. It increases the plasma, and spleen levels of both cAMP and cGMP. Other organs, such as the liver, may have an uneven response with a rise of cAMP and a fall of cGMP which is congruent with the finding that the level of the intracellular cAMP is closely related to the immuno-activity of the lymphocytes [18].

Beside these immunological effects Radix Astragali can also increase the muscular contractility of rats and, by reinforcing the adrenal cortical function, it can improve the stress performance of guinea pigs and regulate serum cAMP and cGMP levels in rats as well as those of rat hepatic and spleenic tissues. Since an Astragalus saponin fraction causes an elevation of rabbit serum cAMP level, promotes DNA synthesis in regenerating hepatic cells, accelerates the replication of hepatic cells, significantly enhances the incorporation of ^{3}H-lysine in rat plasma and accelerates protein synthesis in the liver, a general enhancing effect on the protein metabolism is demonstrated [18].

Saponin astramembrainin I at a dose of 10 mg/kg i.v. injected into rabbits induced accumulation of cAMP in plasma, affected deoxyribonucleic acid (DNA) biosynthesis in hepatectomized mice and increased incorporation of ^{3}H-thymidine into regenerating mouse liver [19]. These effects meet many of the requirements of an adaptogen.

In clinical application, Radix Astragli was used for the treatment of chronic hepatitis. It elevated serum glutamic-pyruvic transaminase (SGPT), stimulated phagocytosis of the reticuloendothelial cells of patients with chronic hepatitis and enhanced the cellular immunity in particular [20].

Bupleurum chinense

The dried root of *Bupleurum chinense* DC. (Apiaceae), radix Bupleuri, is listed officially in the Chinese Pharmacopoeia and used commonly in traditional Chinese

Table 6 - Effect of Radix Astragali on plasma and tissue cAMP and cGMP in mice

	Group	No of animals	cAMP Mean± SD (pmol/ml of plasma,	cGMP Mean± SD pmol/g of tissue)
Plasma	Control	12	96.8 ± 9.3	48.6 ± 14.0
	Radix Astragali	12	144.3 ± 11.0**	37.0 ± 11.0*
Liver	Control	12	1060 ± 14 0	41.30 ± 7.50
	Radix Astragali	12	800 ± 280**	54.89 ± 14.31**
Spleen	Control	12	1040 ± 340	55.00 ± 11.31
	Radix Astragali	12	1440 ± 300**	82.40 ± 18.10***

$^{*}p<0.05$, $^{**}p<0.01$ and $^{***}p<0.001$, compared with control group.

Table 7 - The effect of Radix Astragali on plasma cAMP, IgM and IgE in healthy subjects

	Unit	Before	After
cAMP	pmol/ml	26.67	42.33
IgM	μg/ml	133.33	147.5
IgE	μg/ml	577.08	751.67

medicine. As well as the official *Bupleurum* species, *B. falcatum* L. and *B. marginatum* Wall ex DC. have also been used [21]. Ethnopharmacologically, Radix Bupleuri is classified as a bitter and cold drug. It enters 'the meridians of pericardium, liver, gallblader and triple *Jiao*'. The functions are to release enterior symptoms, 'to clear heat, to pacify the liver, to relieve stagnation, and to elevate *Yang-Qi*'. It is used as an antipyretic for intermittent fever, to relieve stagnancy of vital energy of the liver for pains in sides and chest, and for visceroptosis. It is used in the treatment of influenza, fever, malaria and menstrual disorders [22].

Chemically, some triterpene saponin and sapogenin compounds, Saikosaponin A. B1, B2, B3, B4, C, D, E and F, and saikogenin A, B, C, D, E and F, were isolated from the root of Bupleurum species. In addition to the saponins, a pharmacologically active essential oil was obtained from *B. chinense* [21, 23].

The polysaccharide isolated from *B. kummingense* showed an immunomodulatory action on the proliferative response of mouse splenocytes to mitogens as measured by ^{3}H-thymidine incoporation [24].

The pectic polysaccharide, bupleuran 2IIb, administered i.p. to mice with a dose of 50 mg/kg enhanced the clearance of immune complexes from circulation *in vivo*. This result suggests that the use of the Bupleurum polysaccharide may provide a beneficial effect on the treatment of immune complex-mediated autoimune disease [25]. A saponin fraction from *B. fruticosum* stimulated phagocytosis whereas saikosaponin decreased the spleen cell proliferative response to T cell mitogen but increased the response to B cell mitogen. Macrophages, which were treated with this compound showed a significant increase of phorbol myristate acetate (PMA)-induced chemiluminescence [26].

The essential oil of *Bupleurum* species markedly suppressed the hind paw swelling induced by carrageenin in mice and rats. The mechanism of anti-inflammatory action however might be related with the inhibitory effect of the synthesis or release of prostaglandin E (PGE) and bradykinin [27].

Cordyceps sinensis

Cordyceps, *Dongchongxiacao* in Chinese, is the fruiting body of *Cordyceps sinensis* (Berk.) Sacc. (*Clavicipitaceae*) growing on the larval of *Heplalus armoricanus* Oborthur. According to Chinese medicine, the properties of this traditional drug are 'sweet and warm', it enters 'the lung and kidney meridians'. The functions of this drug are to stimulate lung and kidney, to stop bleeding, and resolve phlegm. It is used for the treatment of impotence, nocturnal emission, night sweat, chronic renal insufficiencies, leukopenia, bronchitis and chronic cough with hemoptysis, hyperlipidaemia and climactic syndromes [28, 29].

In China, many institutions have initialized studies on the chemical composition and pharmacological significance of this drug. *Cordyceps sinensis* possesses broad bioactivities, such as increasing the coronary blood flow, promoting the immune system, inhibiting human nasopharyngeal carcinoma cells, inhibiting saliva secretion, exhibiting sedative and anti-inflammatory action, prolonging sleep induced by pentobarbital and raising endurance in the swimming test. A comparative investigation has been undertaken between a cultured fungal colony of Cordyceps and the wild specimen in order to search for substitutes of the natural specimen. Both the cultured and wild specimens of Cordyceps exalted significant effects on the immunological organs of rats. This drug can increase the size of the spleen, decrease the size of the thymus, increase phagocytic activity of the hepatic Kupffer's cells, and enhance the production of splenic macrophages [30]. Both specimens, *Dongchongxiacao* and *Chongcao*, can enhance the levels of macrophages and at the same time activate the functions of the phagocytic system. They enhance not only the phagocytic activity of macrophages, but also increase the alkaline phosphatase activity of macrophages suggesting a direct relationship between these two effects [31]. This drug has also been noted to counteract the inhibitory effect of corticosteroids on the phagocytic activity of macrophages and to inhibit the graft-versus-host-reaction (GVHR) [32]. Cordyceps and its culture broth had no significant effect on normal rat T cells, but exhibits a significant protective effect on defective T cells resulting from azathioprine administration.

Cordyceps polysaccharides can enhance lymphocyte transformation, leading to an elevation of serum IgG concentration [33]. Cordyceps and the fungus itself can increase the gross weight of spleen and accelerate the metabolism of splenic nucleic acid and proteins. They can also cause an increase in RNA concentration and a decrease in protein concentration of the spleen. They increase the splenic DNA synthesis, which might be the reason for the altered RNA and protein metabolism. The polysaccharides cause an acceleration of splenic regeneration and growth, leading to an increase of immunological function as well as of body resistance to pathogenic factors.

In the clinic, a Cordyceps preparation was shown to be of therapeutic value in the treatment of chronic hepatic diseases, hyperchlolesterolemia and other diseases commonly associated with the process of ageing. It has also been noted to improve sexual potency in aged people [34].

Two preparations of Cordyceps, called *Jinshuibao* and *Jinshukang* are produced by Jiangxi Pharmaceutical Co. Ltd. The Jinshuibao capsule Cordyceps have equal effects as the *Cordyceps sinensis* drug. It is used for the treatment of chronic bronchitis, sexual dysfunction, hyperlipemia, menstrual disorder, pains in the loins and abdomen, leucorrhea, senile weakness, cardiovascular diseases, liver cirrhosis, and in supplementary tumor treatment. In 56 cases with cancer, Jinshuikang capsule significantly improved the immune functions and raised the quality of life of the patients [35]. As shown in Table 8, the immune and humoral cell functions are markedly increased after treatment [36].

Jinshuikang Cordyceps paste is a refined decoction paste used only in traditional Chinese medicine It consists of Cordyceps extract obtained from a submersed fermentation strain of Cordyceps, combined with *Bulbus Fritillariae* cirrhosae and loquat leaves. Pharmacologically the actions can be described as relieving cough, making expectoration easy, relieving asthma, resisting oxygen-deficiency, resisting fatigue, resisting cold and as an anti-inflammatory. It is enhancing phagocytosis of red culo-endothetial cells, enhancing resistance to disease, improving the adaptability of an organism to external environment and enhancing immunocompetence as well as modulating functions [37].

Cynanchum auriculatum

Radix Cynanchi auriculati, *Baishouwu* in Chinese is the dried root of *Cynanchum auriculatum* Royle (*Asclepiadaceae*), Ethnopharmacologically this drug is regarded as the white species of *Hoshouwu*, and used as a tonic for *yin*-insufficiency with

Table 8 - Improving effect on immune functions of Jinshuibao capsule in cancer patients

Immune function	Change before and after treatment Control group Mean ± SD	 Drug group Mean ± SD
WuT3	−8.7 ± 8.3	9.19 ± 9.65**
WuT4	−6.3 ± 8.68	4.19 ± 8.7**
WuT8	−1.35 ± 8.62	1.50 ± 7.09*
T4/T8	−0.21 ± 0.38	0.11 ± 0.98
LBT	−18.1 ± 18.3	12.1 ± 13.8**
IgG	2.14 ± 5.29	−0.35 ± 5.36
IgA	0.25 ± 0.85	−0.37 ± 5.36
IgM	0.14 ± 0.42	0.036 ± 0.55

$^{*}p < 0.05$ and $^{**}p < 0.01$ compared with control group

symptoms of dizziness, insomnia, dyspesia and debility. Chemically, this drug contains phospholipids, amino acids and steroid glycosides, cynanuricuricuoside A, B and C, as well as the trace elements Zn, Cu, Se [38]. Clinically, this drug has been tested for the treatment of impotency, seminal emission and development of sperm.

The total phospholipid fraction of the drug increases significantly the ratio of the acid naphthyl aceterase (ANAE)(+) lymphocytes, and prevents the inversed ratio of ANAE(+) to ANAE(−) lymphocytes caused by peritoneal injection of cyclophosphamide [39]. The steroid glycosides showed various inhibitory effects against Sarcoma 180, Lewis lung cancer and Ehrlich carcinoma, and prolonged the survival time of the cancer-transplanted animals [40]. Both the steroid glycosides and the powdered drug form decreased significantly the serum total cholesterol level [41].

Epimedium brevicornum

Herba Epimedii, *Yingyanghuo*, also known as *Xianlingpi* in China, from the leaves and stems of *Epimedium brevicornum* Maxim., or *E. sagittatum* (Sieb. et Zucc.) Maxim., *E. pubescens* Maxim. and *E. koreanum* Nakai., has been used in ethnopharmacology as a tonic to replenish the vital function, especially sexual neurasthenia. It is also used for the treatment of climacteric hypertension and as an antirheumatic agent against rheumatic pain [42]. The drug contains polysaccharides (EPS), a series of flavonoids among them 8-isoprenyl flavanone (EPF), and icariin(ICA) as the major flavones [43].

Pharmacological investigations have demonstrated its endocrine functions, its immunomodulating functions, its antiviral activity, and its cardiovascular effects.

Preparations of *Herba Epimedii* have already been used in clinics [44]. EPS enhance the immune response to sheep red blood cell (SRBC) immunization, increase T lymphocyte proliferation and the phagocytic activity of peritoneal macrophages. EPS and ICA exerted a mutual synergistic effect [45, 46].

Studies on the immunopharmcological effects of EPS, EPFI and ICA indicate that all compounds contribute to the stimulating effect on the immune functions, with EPS as the most potent ones. When these constituents are administered simultaneously they exhibit synergistic effects. Investigations on the antiageing effects of EPS, EPF, and D-galactose injected into mice showed significant changes in most of the measured parameters, including a decrease in splenic T and B lymphocyte proliferation, a decrease of SOD activity in the liver, a significant increase of MDA in the liver as well as of lipofusion in brain and liver. EPS and EPF were able to antagonize significantly the D-galactose-induced decrease of splenic lymphocyte proliferation (SPL) from the very early stage of injection (Tab. 9).

It is notable that EPS stimulates both suppressor T cells and helper T cells while ICA enhances only the helper T cell and depresses the suppressor T cells. This suggests that the two active substances of the plant, act as complements as well as counterparts in modulating the immune system [46]. *Herba Epimedii* has found wide clinical and pharmacological application (Tab. 10), mainly for the treatment of cardiovascular diseases, hypertension and neurasthenia.

Several Epimedium-containing preparations for senile patients have been produced from a thorough study of this drug [47] i.e an oral formulation called "*kangbao*" prepared from of *Herba Epimedii* and another six Chinese drugs. Experimental findings indicated that the preparation raises serum gonadal hormone levels in aged rats, and replenishes "kidney-yang" in rats with hydroxy- corticosteroid-induced "kidney-yang deficiency". It can promote human lymphocyte DNA synthesis, as well as accelerate the rate of lymphocyte transformation. It also enhances immunological lymphocyte activities and significantly improves humoral and cellular immunities. Clinical observations revealed that the administration of this preparation to middle-age and aged patients with signs of asthenia can result in an increase of appetites and improvements of body vigor. There are also significant improvements of the objective physical evaluation indices. It can facilitate recovery from post-stroke complications, leading to a generalized state of well-being with satisfactory performance on motor functions, skeletomuscular function, fine movement, visual acuity and balance, and favorable findings concerning blood viscosity and electrocardiograms [4].

Ganoderma lucidum

Fructificatio Ganodermae, named *Lingzhi* in Chinese, consists of the dried fruit body of *Ganoderma lucidum* (Leyss. ex Fr.) Karst. and other related species (*Polyporaceae*).

Table 9 - The postive effect of Epimedium extracts EPS and EPF on D-galactose-induced changes in immune functions and lipid peroxidation in mice

Group	SPL. T cell (%)	SPL. B cell (%)	MDA (%)	Lipofusion %
Control	100	100	100	100
D-G	27	24	131	249
D-G+EPS	78	54	112	104
D-G+EPF	40	46	118	111
D-G+EPS+EPF	84**	61**	103**	94**

*****p < 0.01 compared with D-G group.*

Table 10 - The clinical and pharmacological effects of Herba Epimedii

1. Stimulation of sex behavior and sex hormonal activity
2. Modulation of neuro-endocrine activities (ACTH and adreno-corticosterone)
3. Modulation of cardiovascular activity, relief of hypertension
4. Central sedative effect
5. Modulation of the activities of immune system, antiallergic effect
6. Antihyperglycemic and antilipemic effects
7. Antiulcer activity

Ethnopharmacologically, *Ganoderma* has a tradition as long as ginseng in China and the drug is usually administered in the form of a liquid extract or in tablets as a sedative and as a tranquilizer in the treatment of dizziness and insomnia due to neurasthenia and hypertension, and as a tonic for symptoms of weakness or debility in various chronic diseases. It is also used for the treatment of bronchitis and asthmatic conditions [48].

Chemically, *Ganoderma* contains polysaccharides, nucleosides, lanostane-type triterpenes, steroids, amino acids and polypeptides. Pharmacologically, *Ganoderma* decreases spontaneous motor activity, prolongs pentobarbital sleep, inhibits pilocarpine-induced salivation, protects mice from nicotine-induced convulsions and death, and lowers rectal temperature in animal experiments. *Ganoderma* preparations were found to increase the tolerance of mice to hypoxia and promote the heart and brain uptake of ^{86}Rb, to rapidly increase the coronary blood flow in anaesthetized dogs, and to prevent the elevation of total serum cholesterol levels in normal and Triton WR 1339-induced hyperlipemic mice. In addition, *Ganoderma* had a significant cardiotonic action on isolated frog hearts and on pentobarbital sodium-induced hearts [3]. Significant antitussive and expectorant actions were shown on coughing induced by concentrated ammonia aerosol and in phenol red tests by intraperitoneal injection of *Ganoderma* preparations. Ascorbic acid content of rat adrenals was diminished significantly one hour after subcutaneous injection of the *Ganoderma* spore preparations [5]. The polysaccharide fraction of *Ganoderma* markedly increased the phagocytic abilita of abdominal macrophages of mice against chicken erythrocytes, as seen by an increase in the percentage and index of phagocytosis relative to controls.

As far as the immunoregulatory effects of *Ganoderma* are concerned, phagocytic function of the murine mononuclear phagocyte system was markedly enhanced by i.p. administration of a *Ganoderma* spore extract, 100 mg/kg a day for seven days, while the delayed-type hypersensitivity (DTH) in normal mice induced by sheep blood cells (SRBC), 2,4-dinitrochlorobenzene, or allotropic splenocytes, was significantly inhibited by the injection of *Ganoderma* spore extract. Moreover, the primary antibody response to SRBC and the hemolysin production of murine splenocytes were inhibited by the same dose of *Ganoderma* spore extract after s.c. or i.p. injection [43].

Ganoderma spore extract clearly suppressed the graft versus host reaction *in vivo* and the mixed lymphocyte reaction of murine splenocytes *in vitro* which might infer that it is appropriate for use in tissue transplantation. Further studies illustrate that *Ganoderma* spore extract inhibits *in vitro* murine spleen cell proliferation induced by ConA or LPS as well as IL-2 production of murine splenocytes stimulated by ConA. The immunoregulatory activation of *Ganoderma* might be at least in part responsible for the benificial effects in treating hypersensitivity or autoimmune diseases [49].

The polysaccharides of *Ganoderma* can increase the phagocytic activity of rat peritoneal macrophages against chicken RBC. Both the phagocytic rate and phagocytic index were significantly increased, indicating that *Ganoderma* indeed can enhance the non-specific immunity [37]. *Ganoderma* and its preparations have attracted much more attention in the field of immunodeficiency diseases and cancer prevention (especially for the well-being of the aged people). Administration of *Ganoderma* can increase the immunoglobulin (IgA) concentration in the sputum of chronic bronchitis patients.

Ganoderma enhances the formation of RBC 2,3-DPG *in vivo*. It also regulates nucleic acid and protein metabolism. The polysaccharides of *Ganoderma* can hasten the incorporation of ^{3}H-leucine in plasma proteins, resulting in an accelerated plasma protein synthesis in the liver. These findings clearly indicate that *Ganoderma* can affect the metabolism of nucleic acid and proteins, and thus accelerate protein synthesis. *Ganoderma* has certain protective effects on rats exposed to radiation. The results of experiments on the effect of *Ganoderma* in eliminating plasma free hydroxyl radicals show that it is active both *in vitro* and *in vivo*. Thus it is also evident that *Ganoderma* has a commendable antioxidant effect [4].

Studies of *Ganoderma lucidum* spore extract on DTH induced by SRBC, 2,4-dinitrochlorobenzene, and allotropic splenocytes showed a significant inhibiting effect on the DTH reaction. It was concluded that the extract may be effective by inhibiting cell-mediated immunity in mice [51].

Some diseases, including dermatosclerosis, dermatomyositis, systemic lupus erythematosis, psoriasis, and myasthenia gravis, etc. may be the result of a disorder of immune responses. The *Ganoderma lucidum* spore extract showed inhibiting effects on DHT, decreased the primary antibody response in mice and also, in a dose related manner, suppression of murine splenocytes or human tonsil mononuclear cell proliferation *in vitro*. It inhibited a mixed lymphocyte reaction and decreased the IL-2 level. These results indicate that the inhibitory actions on both the cellular and humoral immunity might explain the use of this drug for the treatment of autoimmune disorders [52].

Ganoderma can improve the general tolerance of rats to hypoxia, particularly that of the myocardium. It can lower the total body oxygen consumption and has been shown in rats to increase the arterial blood flow in isolated rat hearts. *Ganoderma* can compensate pituitin-induced ECG changes (T-wave changes) in rabbits and is noted to be inhibitory to isolated frog hearts. It has an insidious hypotensive effect on anesthesized rabbits, but no effect on their respiration. Administration of *Ganoderma* can maintain the myocardial ATP and glucose levels at a relatively higher level. These findings indicate that *Ganoderma* possesses properties beneficial to the myocardial metabolism of hypotic animals [4].

Clinically, *Ganoderma* is used for the treatment of coronary disease, hyper-lipidaemia, hypertension, chronic bronchitis, neurasthenia and insomnia, progressive muscular destrophy and atrophic myotonus, leukopenia, cancer, neurosis, treatment of collagen diseases such as dermatomyositis, dermatosclerosis and lupus erythematosus, and other diseases associated with ageing. In general, it has been used as a non-toxic tonic beneficial to all viscera. How to quantify the different *Ganoderma* preparations for treatment of the various diseases is a problem that has still to be solved.

Glycyrrhiza uralensis

Licorice root (Radix Glycyrrhizae), *Gancao* in Chinese, is well-known in both East and West, and has been used since ancient times as a useful drug in traditional and folklore medicine. It consists of the dried root and rhizome of *Glycyrrhiza uralensis* Fisch., *G. inflata* Bat. or *G. glabra* L (*Leguminosae*). It is a 'sweet and mild drug' and enters 'the heart, lung, spleen and stomach meridians'. Its functions are to tonify the spleen and replenish vital energy, to moderate the lungs and stop coughs, to relax spasms and stop pain, to moderate the action of herbs, to reduce 'fire' and release toxins. It is used to invigorate the functions of the heart and spleen for the treatment of sympotoms due to the deficiency of vital energy of these viscera, as a spasmolytic and antitussive for peptic ulcers and cough, as an antiphlogistic for sore throat, boils and carbuncles, and as an antitoxicant for drug poisoning[40]. Licorice is also employed as a sweetening and flavouring agent in pharmaceutical preparations and tobacco.

The pharmacological activities of licorice are mainly, if not all, due to the main saponin, glycyrrhizin and its aglycone, glycyrrhetinic acid. About 30 non-glycosidic flavonoid compounds have been isolated from licorice including flavones, flavanones chalcones, isoflavones, isoflavanones, isoflavones, pterocarpans, coumestans and 3-arylcoumarins. Anti-stress ulcerogenic, anti-allergic and anti-inflammatory activities in mice and rats have been demonstrated for the licorice constituents and their derivatives. Immunological activity, antiviral action, estrogen and testosterone effects, histamine effects, insulin-like effects, effects on the central nervous system, mineralocortid and glucocorticoid effects, as well as interferon inducing activity and antitumor promoting effects have also been observed with some licorice compounds. Glycyrrhizin to some extent inhibits prostaglandin E_2 (PGE_2) biosynthesis in activated rat peritoneal macrophages, whereas in cell-free experiments glycyrrhizin and glycyrrhetinic acid showed little inhibitory effect on cyclooxygenase [54, 55].

The *in vitro* immunomodulatory activities of a number of saponins and glycyrrhicic acids have been described. Addition of these saponin preparations to mouse spleen cell cultures resulted in significantly increased cell proliferation. Isolated B-cells were also induced to proliferate in the presence of this saponin. On the other hand, glycyrrhicic acid stimulated both T and B lymphocytes in an equal manner. The selective proliferation of subtypes of lymphocytes correlated with restimulation responses by polyclonal mitogens. In comparison, similar exposure of lymphocytes to glycyrrhizic acid produced markedly increased responses to phytohaemagglutinin (PHA), ConA, pokeweed mitogen (PWM) and lipopolysaccharide (LPS). Incubation of lymphocytes in the presence of saponins (?) caused effector cell generation as determined in a one-way mixed lymphocyte reaction. In the case of lymphocyte cultures in the presence of sappiness (saponins?) or glycyrrhizic acid, the supernatants contained active soluble factors. This was demonstrated by the observation that glycyrrhizic acid exhibited the most profound immunomodulatory activity *in vitro* [56].

The influences of glycyrrhizic amide, a derivative of glycyrrhizin, on immunoregulation and PGE_2 and cAMP levels of mice spleen has been investigated. This compound significantly increased the spleen weight, tissue mg/g body weight was increased from 4.3 to 5.50, the phagocytotic index of carbon particle clearance rose from 1.23 to 4.41, and the number of leucocytes in the peripheral circulation rose from 5.87 to 10.1. It also significantly increased the PGE_2 and cAMP levels of mouse spleen. The PGE_2 levels of spleen were enhanced from 17.7 to 31.8 pg/mg tissue, and the cAMP level from 0.56 to 1.12 pmol/mg tissue. There were no significant differences in PGE_2 levels in the peripheral circulation. The compound stimulated PGE_2 secretion and increased the number of spleen lymphocytes, while indomethacin inhibited it. These studies suggest that glycyrrhizic amide has immunoregulatory functions by influencing the PGE_2 and cAMP levels [57].

Lycium barbarum

Fructus Lycii, *Gongqizi* in Chinese, the dried fruit of *Lycium barbarum* L. (*Solanaceae*), is one of the most commonly prescribed *Yin*-modulators. Ethnopharmacologically, this drug is widely used as a tonic for the treatment of general debility with a deficiency of vital essence. It replenishes the *Yin* component and blood elements, improves eyesight, vertigo, lumbago, impotence and other symptoms of *Yin* deficiency of the kidney-orbit and liver-orbit. In traditional Chinese medicine, it has been documented extensively as a favourite ingredient in recipies for elderly people. The drug contains simple sugars, polysaccharides, betaine, zeaxanthin and physalein [43].

The results of pharmacological studies have demonstrated that Lycium poly-saccharides (LYPS), the major active ingredients, enabled the old animals to restore atrophy of the thymus, increase the percentage of T lymphocytes, and promote proliferation of lymphocytes, phagocytosis of macrophages, antibody content and PEC number [43]. LYPS have been shown to increase the DANN-biosynthesis in thymus and to induce a high degree of lymphocyte transformation in both thymus and spleen cells. Other effects include an increase in macrophages and reticula endothelial system (RES) phagocytosis, a hematopoietic effect and the anti-lymphocytoxic effect of cyclophosphamide [18].

This drug possesses a number of regulatory effects on metabolic processes. It is reported to be a biostimulator or growth-promoting drug in demented animals. It increases the egg production after addition to the diet of chickens. It promotes hematopoesis and reduces or regulates the high blood sugar level. This drug also protects from liver damage due to carbon tetrachloride. Traditional medicinal preparations for sick persons and the elderly usually contain it as one of the ingredients. Experiments on mice indicate that it has anti-ageing effects (13). LYPS also demonstrated an ability to improve sexual disorders in elderly animals [59].

An *in vivo* stimulating effect of *Lycium barbarum* on tumor weight, number of splenocytes, proliferation of splenocytes, and NK activity in S180 tumor-bearing mice was registered. The cellular immunity of the organism was restored by LYPS and tumor-inhibition was the final result [58]. An experiment showed that the *Lycium barbarum* extracts can enhance T lymphocyte functions and the levels of cytokine IL-2, r-IFN and TNF, which are of importance for the immune surveillance. It has been suggested that the extract has a beneficial effect in keeping people younger as well as preventing neoplastic and other diseases caused by the decrease in immune surveillance function [60].

A study on its immune-modulation mechanism showed that *Lycium barbarum* acts through an enhancement of the IL-2 level in tonsillar mononuclear cell (TMNC) supernatants, a promotion of the IL-2R expression, and an increase in the TNF and IL-6 activity in the blood serum. These cytokines together with other ones (IL-1, IL-3, IL-4 etc.) are part of a network, modulating each other and resulting in an immunostimulation effect [60].

In the treatment of neoplastic diseases, this drug is accepted as an adjuvant to radiotherapy or chemotherapy to stimulate the host defense system against cancer cells as well as to render the patient in a better state to tolerate the toxic effects of irradiation or chemotherapy [18]. Clinical trials of this drug with 294 aged patients have shown that LYPS (100 mg p.o. per day administered for 60 days) distinctly increased the amount and activity of peripheral T lymphocytes, and stengthen the phagocytic potential of macrophages. The total curative rate was 88.1% in the treatment of various symptoms of senility (Tab. 11). Furthermore, it is not only an optimal remedy for the improvement of immunological functions in senile patients but also a stimulating agent for the treatment of immunodeficiency caused by malignant and various other diseases [61].

In a clinical trial, 43 subjects aged around 60 years and older were included into this study. Dry fruit of *Lycium barbarum* was orally administered daily at a dosage of 50 g for ten days. Five indices of immune function were tested before and after the 10 day treatment. The results indicated that this drug was able to reverse or promote most of the immune responses from the levels naturally occurring in the elderly adults in comparison to that of the younger. The values of lysozyme, IgG, IgA, and lymphocyte blastogenesis were 24.59 μg/ml, 1457 mg/dl, 189.99 mg/dl and 23.79 SI, respectively, before treatment and rose to 76.92 μg/ml, 1729.22 mg/dl, 261.93 mg/dl and 184.18 SI after administration, respectively. The differences between each value were significant ($p<0.05$). These data suggest that *Lycium barbarum* can restore age-related immune deficiency [62].

Panax ginseng

Ginseng, Radix Ginseng (*Renshen* in Chinese), one of the tonics in traditional Chinese medicine, consists of the dried roots of Asiatic ginseng, *Panax ginseng* C. A. Mey. (*Araliaceae*). According to the literature, ginseng has been known in Chinese ethnopharmacology for more than 3000 years. Its medicinal use has been adequately explored not only in China and Korea but also in Japan, Russia and the United States of America. A large number of the articles based on original research on ginseng have been published by Chinese scholars [63–67]. Radix Ginseng is a 'sweet, slightly bitter and mild drug' and enters 'spleen and lung meridians'.

Table 11 - Clinical efficacy of Lycium polysaccharides for symptoms of senility

Symptoms	Cases	Efficacy rate (%)
Dizziness	71	91.5
Fauguing easily	78	84.6
Opprresion in chest	43	83.7
Sleeplessness	70	85.7
Poor appetite	32	100
Total	294	88.1

Ethnopharmacologically, the functions of this drug are to replenish vital energy (*Qi*), prevent collapse and strengthen *Yang*, to tonify the spleen and lungs, to promote body fluids, to relieve thirst and to calm the heart and to soothe the mind. The various pharmacological and clinical activities reported, are listed in Table 12 [67].

28 ginsenosides and polysaccharides are the main active constituents of ginseng and have been isolated from the root, root-stock, stems, leaves, flowers and flower-buds of the ginseng plant. Ginsenosides are triterpenoid glycosides, which can be divided into three types: the oleanolic acid-, panaxadiol- and panaxatriol types, the latter belonging to the dammaran type. Ginsenoside Ro is an oleanolic acid saponin, while the other ginsenosides are derived from panaxadiol or panaxatriol. In addition to ginsenosides and polysaccharides, flavonoids, daucosterin, mucilaginous substances, amino acids, bitter substances, vitamins, choline, pectin, fatty oils and essential oils have been found in different parts of the ginseng plant [67]. In order to secure the source and guarantee the quality of ginseng, tissues culture of ginseng was carried out. The chemical components of ginsenosides in the cultured cells of ginseng were almost the same as those in the root of cultivated ginseng. As shown in Table 13, a difference was found in the ratio among the three types of saponins [68].

Early studies revealed that ginseng possesses biomodulatory effects on the higher centers of the central nervous system, facilitating both physical and mental activities. It has a noteworthy effect on the endocrine system, regulating the blood sugar level as demonstrated in alloxan diabetics. Recent experimental and clinical studies concluded that it has a wide range of effects, such as a remarkable anti-shock effect in circulatory failure, modulatory effects on the immune functions, modulation of cellular metabolic processes, modulation of neuroendocrine system activities, improvement of learning and memory processes, and others (see Tab. 12).

Ginseng root polysaccharides have been found to markedly stimulate phagocytosis of the reticuloendothelial system and the production of antibodies. They caused an increase of serum complement in guinea pigs, raised serum IgG levels in

Table 12 - The clinical and pharmacological activities of ginseng

1.	Anti-stress activity
2.	Anti-circulatory shock effects and modulation of cardiovascular activities
3.	Improvement or facilitation of learing and memory processes
4.	Modulation of neuro-endocrine system activities, hypothalamic adrenal-gonadal system
5.	Modulation of cellular metabolic processes on carbohydrate, fat and protein metabolism
6.	Promotion of hematopoesis
7.	Modulation of immune functions
8.	Protection against radiation and liver toxicities

mice and increased the B to T cell ratio. The numbers of plaque forming cells (PFC) and specific rosette forming cells (SRFC) in tumor-bearing mice immunized with SRBC were markedly increased after oral administration of ginseng polysaccharides (400–800 mg/kg for ten days). The polysaccharides also increaed both serum hemolysin and SRBC hemolysis mediated by spleen cells *in vitro*. The polysaccharides had however, no significant effect on these immunological parameters in normal mice. Most of the studies confirm the host-mediated antitumor activity of the polysaccharides [67].

Two polysaccharides isolated from the tissue cultures of ginseng and cultivated ginseng root caused, at a concentration of 20 and 40 mg/kg i.v. injection, a marked increase in spleen weight, enhanced the carbon clearance rate in mice and significantly promoted the production of serum specific antibody hemolysins as well as the IgG level in mice. They also enhanced DTH of footpad induced by SRBC in mice, but had no effect on graft-versus-host-reaction (GVHR) in mice [69].

Ginsenosides induce a significant increase of serum corticosterone and decrease of liver glycogen, and stimulate the synthesis of kidney DNA and RNA in mice. It could be suggested that ginsenosides have an analogous effect in humans [70]. In one investigation it has also been found that ginsenosides influence the circadian variation of plasma corticosterone and liver glycogen in rats [71], which, after long term administration, could result in the well documented anti-fatigue property of ginseng [72].

Since only recently a mediate influential linkage between the immune and the cardiovascular system has been found it might be of interest to draw light on the effects of ginseng on platelet aggregation and vascular and hemodynamic parameters. Ginsenosides inhibit the rabbit platelet aggregation induced by arachidonic acid (AA), adenosin diphosphate (ADP), collagen and thrombin *in vitro* and *in vivo*. For the inhibitory effect three mechanisms of action can be suggested: (1) The rise of the cAMP level in platelets may be one cause of the inhibitory effect on platelet aggregation since the cAMP level in platelets treated with ginsenosides is markedly

Table 13 - Comparison of ginsenosides of tissue culture with cultivated ginseng

	Sidegenin content (%)			
	Oleanolic acid	Panaxadiol	Panaxztriol	Total amount
Liquid culture	0.0699	0.0614	0.0359	0.167
Soild culture	0.0600	0.138	0.114	0.277
Cultivated ginseng	0.205	0.276	0.169	0.650

elevated. Ginsenosides stimulate adenylate cyclase in platelet membranes and inhibit the activity of platelet phosphodiestase (PDE). (2) Ginsenosides inhibit the production and release of thromboxane B_2 (TXB_2), ADP, AA and collagen, and induce the production of a considerable amount of TXB_2 and by this increase the cAMP level in platelets. (3) Ginsenosides interfere with the AA metabolism of rabbit platelets, they block the biosynthesis of platelet PGI_2 (see Tab. 14), and inhibit also cyclo-oxygenase and thromboxane synthesis [73–76].

Earlier pharmacological studies have demonstrated that ginseng possesses a wide range of cardioavascular activities including effects on the heart, heart rate, blood pressure and vasculature. Recent studies on the cardiovascular system focused on the following aspects: (1) effect on cardiac performance and hemodynamics. Ginsenosides (i.v. injection, 25 mg/kg) caused a significant decrease of artery pressure (AP), dp/dtmax of left ventricular pressure (LVP), and decreasing of heart rate (HR) in dogs. The renal blood flow was also remarkably reduced by i.v. injection of ginsenosides. (2) Ginsenosides possess protective properties against myocardial infarct, and it can be suggested that the effect on PGI2/thromboxan A_2 (TXA_2) seems to contribute to the myocardial protective properties. (3) Ginsenosides show a prejunctional excitatory effect on sodium release and a postjunctional inhibitory effect on histamine release and Na^+-response, both involving interference with the calcium influx processes [77, 78].

Ginsenosides markedly prolong the time of survival in normobaric hypoxia stress mice, and regenerate locomotory activity in mice. They possess anti-stress activities and show effects on neurotransmitters. The observed anti-heat stress effects of ginsenosides may be mediated by brain monoamines and the hypothalamus (HPA) system. Ginsenosides selectively modulate the circadian variations of brain 5-hydroxytryptamine (5-HT), 5-hydroxy-indole-3-acetic acid (5-HIAA), norepinedrine (NE) and dopamine (DA) levels, but as a function of the time of the light-dark cycle [79, 80].

Ginsenoside Rg_1 and Rb_1 have been found to have nootropic properties. They improve memory and learning processes in normal animals as well as in animals with impaired cognitive functions. The mechanism of action is due to a multiplicity of biological effects: (1) they influence the brain's cholinergic mechanism and

Table 14 - The effects of ginsenosides on the production of TXB_2, PGI_2 and the utilization of ^{14}C-arachidonic acid

Ginsenosides (mg/kg)	TXB_2 production ratio (%)	PGI_2 Production ratio (%)	AA utilization ratio (%)
0.25	6.83 ± 2.99	1.00 ± 0.25	91.58 ± 1.64
0.5	2.18 ± 0.33	1.01 ± 0.13	89.00 ± 3.08
1.0	1.05 ± 0.18	1.26 ± 0.39	63.80 ± 6.21
2.0	0.64 ± 0.19	1.20 ± 0.45	44.30 ± 6.12
Control	24.80 ± 3.49	2.81 ± 1.10	97.10 ± 4.54

increase the synthesis and release of Ach; (2) they decrease 5-HT levels in the brain; (3) they promote nucleotide and protein metabolism in the brain; and (4) they have a free radical scavenging effect. Therefore one may conclude that ginseng can be useful as a nontropic agent in antiageing therapy [79, 80].

The most outstanding clinical results are: improved resistance to the adverse effects of antitumor medicines and protection of the blood formation system. In clinical trials, the administration of ginseng tablets for 30 days raised the WBC by 64.5% [81]. In an other trial, a ginseng decoction improved the brain and immune functions in old patients with cancer [82].

Polygonum multiflorum

Radix Polygoni multiflori, *Heshouwu* in Chinese, the dried tuberous roots of *Polygonum multiflorum* Thunb. (*Polygonaceae*), is ethnopharmacologically used mainly as a decoction. It is a 'bitter, sour and warm drug' and enters 'the liver and kidney meridians'. Its functions are to nourish the blood, to replenish the vital essence, to moisten the intestine, to move the stool and to release toxins. It is used to replenish the vital essence of the liver and kidney and to nourish the blood for the treatment of anemia, early graying of hair, aching back and knees, neurasthenia and hyper-cholesteremia [83].

The drug contains lecithin, several anthraquinones (chrysophanol, emodin, rhein, physicon and chrysophanolanthrone), 2,3,4,5-tetrahydroxy-stilbene-2-O-β-D-glucoside, and is rich in trace elements for example Ca, Fe, Zn, Mn, Cu, Sr [84].

Pharmacological studies have shown that this drug can prolong the life cycle of somatic cells. A study using a scanning electron microscope revealed that treated cells remained in a state of active growth until maturation, while cells of the control group showed signs of senility and degeneration. Studies also revealed that Radix Polygoni multiflori increased the cellular antioxidant activity, lowered the lipofusion content of myocardial cells, increased the superoxide dismutase (SOD) activity, and showed a significant inhibitory effect on the formation of oxidized lipids. It protected old mice against atrophy of the thymus [72]. This drug could lengthen the life-span, raise plasma high density lipoprotein cholesterol level (HDL-C) and HDL-C total cholesterol (TC) ratio, and reduce plasma LPO level in senile Japanese quails.

Polygonatum sibiricum

Rhizoma Polygonati, the dried rhizome of *Polygonatum sibiricum* Red, with 'sweet and neutral' properties, enters 'the spleen, lung and kidney meridians'. The functions are to nourish the *Yin* and moisten the lungs, to tonify the spleen and promote vital energy [86].

Rhizoma Polygonati is effective in increasing the phagocytic activity of monocytes and macrophages, thus reinforcing cellular immunity.The effect of this drug on hepatic oxidation of lipids was tested in rats poisened by tetrachlorocarbon. It significantly decreases the level of malondialdehyde (MDA) in the liver, implying its effectiveness in antagonizing the oxidative process of lipids. Rhizoma Polygonati effectively protects rats from hypoxic assaults and it is a cardiotonic in cardiac failure. This drug has a significant effect on increasing the coronary blood flow and on counteracting piuitrin-induced acute myocardial ischemia [4].

Polyporus umbellatus

Umbellate pore-fungus, *Zhuling* in Chinese, is the pore-fungus of *Polyporus umbellatus* (Pers.) Fr. (*Polyporaceae*). This drug is widly used in traditional Chinese medicine. The properties and taste are sweet or without taste and neutral. It enters the kidney and urinary meridians. The functions are to transform dampness and promote water metabolism. The indications for use of Umbellate pore fungus are dysuria, turbid urine, edema, diarrhoea and profuse leukorrhea [87].

An extract of *Polyporus umbellatus* which contains polysaccharides (β-glucans) as the major components was found to inhibit tumor S180 in mice, resulting in a complete tumor regression in 6–7% of treated mice. The treated mice were reimplanted with sarcoma cells 1–6 months after tumor regression, but again no sign of tumor growth was observed. The i.v. and i.p. injections were the most effective routes for administering medication. The isolated polysaccharides were shown to increase the formation of B cells in the spleen. It significantly increased the phagocytosis of macrophages in the peritonium of tumor-bearing mice, the plasma corticosterone levels and liver glyconeogenesis in mice bearing hepatoma was restored, and the activity of liver glucose 6-phosphatase and of liver fructose 1,6-diphosphatase were elevated. The consumption and waste of large amounts of energy are the special biochemical characteristics of tumor tissue. Polysaccharides of *Polyporus umbellatus* polysaccharides augmented the glycogen storage in tumor-bearing mice and demonstrated elevated enzyme activities in glyconeogenesis. These polysaccharides, used in combination with cyclophosphamide, mitomycin and methotrexate, can increase the therapeutic effect on mice bearing U14 tumors and reduce the spontaneous metastatic foci of Lewis lung cancer. The number of hepatoma H22 cells in mice was reduced to 39% on day ten after daily i.p. injection of 200–400 mg/kg of these polysacharides for five days [88].

No marked acute and subchronic toxicity, irritation of mucous membrane or hemolytic or pyrogenic reactions were observed.

More than 300 patients with malignant tumors including lung, uterus, stomach, intestine, liver tumors and leukemia tumor, took part in clinical trials with the polysaccharides of *Polyporus umbellatus*. Some advanced stage lymphosarcocoma patients showed no side-effects or harmful reactions after two years of treatment and observation.

Discussion and conclusion

The immunological system is very closely linked to several diseases and the process of ageing. Immunological dysfunctions in the aged are usually manifested as a decline in cellular immunity, deregulation of humoral immunity, or an increase in the positive rate of autoimmunity. Many Chinese research reports indicate that anti-ageing herbs and their active compounds or active components possess potential in increasing the immunological functions in animals and the human body.

Immunomodulators directly modify a specific immune function or have a net positive or negative effect on the activity of the immune system. Chinese traditional and herbal drugs and their active compunds have been shown to be an important source of immunomodulators [4, 89]. There are two categories of activity, adjuvants and immunostimulation activity in immunomodulators [26, 89].

Chinese drugs with immunostimulating activities can be divided into two types: those that increase the non-specific immunity, and those that modulate the specific immunity and the regulation of humoral immunity. With regard to the increase in non-specific immunity, Chinese drugs are found to have the ability to increase the phagocytic activity of monocytes or macrophages: examples are Radix Polygoni Multiflori (*heshouwu*), Fructicatic Ganodermae (*lingzhi*), Cortex Acanthopanacis (*ciwujia*), Radix Astragali (*huangqi*), Radix Angelicae sinensis (*danggui*) and Herba Epimedii (*yingyanghuo*). With regard to the increase of specific immunity, Radix Astragali (*huangqi*), Radix Polygonati (*huangjing*), Radix Ginseng (*renshen*) and Cortex Acanthopanacis (*ciwujia*) as well as their polysaccharides can increase the cellular immunity; ginseng saponins, Radix Astragali (*huangqi*) and Radix Angelicae sinensis (*danggui*) can increase humoral immunity. Radix Ginseng (*renshen*), Radix Astragali (*huangqi*) and Cordyceps (*dongcong-xiacao*) are effective enhancers of almost all immunological functions.

The immunological mechanism of the body is subject to multiple regulatory factors. In a number of studies on the relation between cAMP, cGMP levels and immunological functions, it has been indicated that Chinese drugs with immunostimulating activity improve the immunological status, and also change the cAMP and cGMP levels. The increase in cAMP levels leads to a stimulation of a series of immunological reactions. In aged people, the humoral immunity is very deranged; IgE tends to be on the low side, and both IgA and IgG levels are elevated. In terms of traditional Chinese medicine, these drugs regulate the Yin, Yang energy, and cause an appropriate adjustment towards the normal level.

It is worth mentioning that several polysaccharides have been shown to be immunostimulators in experimental research and clinical application.

Through these studies, we may not only find some promising immunostimulator, but also clarify the mechanism of action of some medicinal plants. We conclude that it is very useful to study the immunostimulatory action of Chinese traditional and herbal medicines, and to develop new drugs with high efficacy and low toxicity under the coorperation of phytochemists, pharmacologists, immunologists and clinical doctors.

References

1 Yang CY (1993) Antiageing constituents from Chinese herbal medicine. *Northwest Pharmaceut J* 8(1): 36–39

2 Qian YK (1994) *Applied Immuno Technique*. Beijing Medical University & Peking Union Medical University Press, Beijing, 108–111

3 Qian YK (1994) *Clinical Immunology*. Beijing Medical University & Peking Union Medical University Press, Beijing, 58–61

4 Clien KJ, Zhaiig WP (1987) Advances on Antiageing herbal medicine in China. *Abstracts of Chinese Medicines* l (2): 309–330

5 Liu CX, Xiao PG (1993) *Danggui (Angelica sinensis). An Introduction To Chinese Materia medica*. Beijing Medical University & Peking Union Medical University Press, Beijing, 168

6 Gao XD, Wu WT (1994) Effect of Danggui (Angelica sinensis) and ferulic acid on immune system. *Third International Congress on Ethnopharmacology and its Contemporary Utilization*. China Pharmaceutical Association, Beijing, B-58

7 Geng JY, Huang WQ, Ren TC, Ma XF (1991) *Wujiapi (Acanthopanax senticosus). Medicinal Herbs*. New World Press, Beijing, 82

8 Yaiig JC (1984) Studies on immunepharmacological activity of Cortex Acanthopanax. *Chin Trad Herb Drugs* 15(6): 278–280

9 Barenboim GM, Sterlina AG, Bebyakova NV, Ribokas AA, Fuks BB (1986) Investigation of the pharmacokinetics and mechanism of action of *Eleutherococus glycosides*. VIII. Investigation of natural killer activation by the *Eleutherococcus* extract. *Khim Farm Zh* 20: 914–917

10 Bohn B, Nebe CT, Berr C (1987) Durchflußzytometrische Untersuchungen auf immunmodulatorische Wirkungen von *Eleutherococcus senticosus* Extrakt. *Arzneim-Forsch* 37: 1193–1196

11 Liu CX, Xiao PG (1993). *Polysaccharides of Acanthopanax. An Introduction To Chinese Materia Medica.* Beijing Medical University & Peking Union Medical University Press, Beijing, 276–277

12 Xu RS, Feng SC, Fan ZY, Ye CQ, Zhai SK, Slien ML (1982) Immuno-potentiating polysaccharides of *Acanthopanax senticosus* (Rupr. et Maxim.) Hams. In: Wang Y (ed): *Chem Natl Prod, Proc Sino-Am Symp 1980.* Sci Press, Beijing, 271–274

13 Zhu CA,Tu GR, Shen ML (1982) Effect of polysaccharide from *Acanthopanax senticosus* on mouse serum type-specific antibodies. *Chin Pharm Bull* 17: 178

14 Liu CX, Xiao PG (1993) *Huangqi (Astragalus membranaceus). An Introduction to Chinese Materia Medica.* Beijing Medical University and Peking Union Medical University Press, Beijing, 165

15 Sheng ML (1984) Immunopharmacological study of Radix Astragali. *Chinese Journal of Integrated Traditional Medicine and Western Medicine* 4(10): 615–617

16 WangZG (1987) Chinese traditional tonic remedies. *Proceedings of the International Symposium on Traditional Medicines and Modern Pharmacology.* Chinese Pharmacological Association, Beijing, 37–44

17 Wang YL (1986) Studies on immunopharmacology of Radix Astragali. *Acta Acad Med Nanjing* 6 (1): l5–16

18 Zhou JH (1987) Bio-modulation: A modern interpretation of traditional Chinese medicine. *Proccedings on International Symposuim on Traditional Medicine and Modern Pharmacology.* Chinese Pharmacological Association, Beijing, 3–20

19 Zhang YD, Shen JP, Song J, Wang YL, Shao YN, Li CF, Zhou SH, Li YF, Li DX (1984) Effects of Astragalus saponin I on cAMP and cGMP level in plasma and DNA synthesis in regenerating liver. *Acta Pharm Sin* 19: 619–621

20 Zhou QJ (1985) Chinese medicinal herbs in treatment of viral hepatitis. In: Chang HM, Yeung HW, Tso WW, Koo A (eds): *Advances in Chinese Medicinal Materials Research.* World Scientific Press, Singapore, 215–219

21 Tang WC, Eisenbrand G (1992) *Bupleurum Chinese drugs of plant origin.* Springer-Verlag, Berlin, Heidelberg, New York, 23–232

22 Liu CX, Xiao PG (1993) *Bupleurum chinense. An Introduction To Chinese Materia Medica.* Beijing Medical University & Peking Union Medical University Press, Beijing, 98

23 Pu QL, Ji XR, Li P, Huang L, Guo QX, Chen XX (1981) Studies on three constituents of the essential oil of *Bupleurum chinense* DC. *Acta Chim Sin* 41: 559–561

24 Zhang LX, Pan SL, Huang K-X, Sun KX (1986) Immunomodulatory action of *Bupleu-*

rum kummingense polysaccharide on lymphocyte proliferation. *Acta Acad Med Shanghai* 13: 20–23
25 Matesumoto T, Yamada H (1996) The pectic polysaccharide from *Bupleurum falcatum* L. enhance clearance of immune complexes in mice. *Phytotherapy Res* 10: 585–588
26 Lacaille-Dubois MA, Wagner H (1996) A review of the biological and pharmacological actions of saponins. *Phytomedicine* 2: 363–386
27 Zhang CC, Stin XB, Liu JY, Lu SQ, Lu CY (1985) Antiinflammatory effect of spinasterol. *Acta Pharm Sin* 20: 257–261
28 Liu CX, Xiao PG (1993) *Dongchongxiacao* (*Cordyceps sinensis*). *An Introduction to Chinese Materia Medica*. Beijing Medical University and Peking UnionMedical University Press, Beijing, 175
29 Liang YL, Liu Y, Yang JW, Liu CX (1997) Studies on Pharmacological Activities of Cultivated *Cordyceps sinensis*. *Phytotherapy Research* 11(3): 237–239
30 Chen DM (1985) Study on immune function of Cordyceps. *Chinese Journal of Integrated Traditional and Western Medicine* 5(1): 42–44, 50
31 Zhang SL (1985) Pharmacological activity of *Cordyceps sinensis*. *Chinese Journal of Integrated Traditional and Western Medicine* 5(1): 45–47
32 Chen YP (1983) Immune pharmacology of *Cordyceps sinensis*. *Bulletin of Chinese Materia Medica* 8(5): 33–35
33 Zang QZ (1983) Studies on pharmacological actions of *Cordyceps sinensis*. *Chinese Traditional Herba and Drugs* 14(5): 221–223
34 Shao G (1985) Clinical study of *Cordyceps sinensis*. *Chinese Journal of Integrated Traditional and Western Medicine* 5(II): 652–654
35 Jiangxi Jinshuibao Pharmaceutical Co. Ltd (1995) *Jinshuibao Cordyceps capsule*
36 Zhou DY, Lin LZ (1995) Effect on immune functions of *Jinshuibao* capsule in cancer patients. *J Chinese Trad Med Administ* 15 (suppl): 36–38
37 Jangxi Jinshuikang Pharmaceutical Co. Ltd (1996) *Introduction to the Jinshuikang Cordyceps paste*
38 Chen JJ, Zhang ZX, Zhou J (1990) Cynauricusides A, B and C, steroid glycosides from the root of *Cynanchum auriculatum*. *Acta Botanica Yunnanica* 12: 197–210
39 Gong SS,Yan RN, Dang Y, Fu CY, Wu BQ (1983) Effects of total phospholipids and ecdysterone isolated from Chinese herba on cell immunity in mice. *Chinese Journal of Geriatrics* 2: 193–197
40 Gu LG, Gong SS (1991) Antineoplastic effect of steroid glycoside from the root of *Cynanchum auriculatum*. *Acta Beijing College of Traditional Chinese Medicine* 14: 323–33
41 Niu JZ, Ye BK, Wang DF, Zhang Y, Ben ZE, Yang CZ, Wang ZG, Yang MJ, Glio SG, Li GM (1988) The protective effect on hyperlipidemic rat liver by *Cynanchum auriculatum*. *Acta Medica Sinica* 3: 26–43
42 Liu CX, Xiao PG (1993) Tonics. *An Introduction To Chinese Materia Medica*. Beijing Medical University and Peking Union Medical University Press, Beijing, 165–177

43 Xiao PG, Xing ST, Wang LW (1993) Immunological aspects of Chinese medicinal plants as antiageing drugs. *J Ethnopharmacol* 38: 167–175

44 Guo BL, Xiao PG (1994) Ethnopharmacological investigation of traditional Chinese drug-Yinyanghuo. *3rd International Congress on Ethnopharmacology and its Contemporary Utilization.* China Pharmaceutical Association, Beijing, C-24

45 Wang LW, Wang JH, Shi TR, Liti HQ, Zhao DZ, Wang Z (1988) Effect of *Polygonum muliltiflorum* on the life-span and lipid metabolism in senile Japanese quails. *Chinese Integrat Trad West Med* 8: 223–224

46 Xing ST (1988) Immunopharmacological research and usage of active ingredients of tonics in Chinese traditional medicine. *Bull Acad Milit Med Sci* 2: 219

47 Zhou JH (1986) Biomodulation: A modern interpretation of traditional Chinese medicine. *Proceedings International Symposium on Traditional Medicines and Modern Pharmacology.* Chinese Pharmacology Society, Beijing, 3–20

48 Liu HB (1990) Studies on antiageing effects of Chinese traditional medicine: Effects of *Epimedium koreanum* flavonoids and polysaccharides on immune functions and lipid prexidation in D-galatose injected mice. *Medical Science Thesis.* Academy of Military Medical Sciences,Beijing

49 Xie ZP, HuangXK (1980) *Terms of Chinese Traditional Medicine in English.* Beijing Medical University Press, Beijing, 159

50 Zhang LH, Xiao PG (1993) Studies of antihyperlipidemic and antihyperglycemic effects from *Ganoderma lucidum. Phytotherapy Research* 7: 200–202

51 Zhang LH, Xiao PG (1993) Inhibitory actions of *Ganoderma lucidum* spore extract on delayed-type hypersensitivity in mice. *Phytotherapy Research* 7: 203–204

52 Zhang LH, Huang Y, Wang LW, Qian YK, Xiao PG (1994) Immunological effect of *Ganoderma* lucidum spore extract *in vivo* and *in vitro. 3rd International Congress on Ethnopharmacology and its Contemporary Utilization.* China Pharmaceutical Association, Beijing, C-12

53 Liu CX, Xiao PG (1993) *Gancao* (*Glycyrrhiza uralensis*). *An Introduction to Chinese Materia Medica.* Beijing Medical University and Peking Union Medical University Press, Beijing, 166

54 Shoji S (1987) Chemistry and pharmacology of licorice. *Proceedings of the International Symposium on Traditional Medicine and Modern Pharmacology.* Chinese Pharmacological Association, Beijing, 45–61

55 Tsai TH, Chen CF (1990) *Glycyrhiza Radix.* Sanlian Press, Taipei, 1–129

56 Cliavati SR, Francis T, Campbell JB (1987) An *in vitro* study of immunomodulatory effects of some saponins. *Int J Immunopharmacol* 9(6): 675–783

57 Xing ST (1988) The effects of *Lycium barbarum* on the immunological function in the elderly over 60 years old. *Pharmacology and Clinics of Chinese Materia Medica* 4: 43

58 Liu JL, Zhang LH, Qlan YK (1994) Immune tumor-inhibition of *Lycium barbarum* on S 180-bearing mice. *3rd International Congress on Ethno-pharmacology and Its Contemporary Utilization.* China Pharmaceutical Association, Beijing, D-34

59 Long Z, Zhang X, Qian YK (1 994) *Lycium barbarum* agent (LBA) in improving

immune function and antiageing and antitumor. *3rd International Congress on Ethnopharmacology and Its Contemporary Utilization.* China Phamaceutical Association, Beijing, B-60
60 Du SY, Zliang X, Qian YK (1994) The immunomodulatory effects of Lycium barbarum extractions and its mechanism. *3rd International Congress on Ethnopharmacology and Its Contemporary Utilization.* China Pharmaceutical Association, Beijing, C-35
61 Gu SN (1990) Elevated effect of Lycium barbarum polysaccharides combined with the complex therapy on 20 cases of primary hepatocarcinoma. *Pharmacology and Clinics of Chinese Materia Medica* 6: 35
62 Xu SY, Lin ZB, Zhu XY (1987) Summary of group discussion on antiinflamma-tory and immunopharmacological drugs in traditional medicine and modern pharmacology. *Proceedings of the International Symposium on Traditional Medicine and Modern Pharmacology.* Chinese Pharmacological Association, Beijing, 237–248
63 Liu CX (1975) Introduction on research of ginseng. *Information on Traditional Chinese Medicines* (2): 9–11
64 Wang BX (1980) Progress of pharmacological studies on ginseng. *Acta Pharmaceut Sin* 15: 312–320
65 Wang BX (1985) *Ginseng Research.* Tianjin Scl & Tech Press, Tianjin
66 Liu CX, Xiao PG (1993) Radix Ginseng (Renshen). *An Introduction to Chinese Materia Medica.* Beijing Medical University & Peking Union Medical University Press, Beijing, 165–166
67 Liu CX , Xiao PG (1992) Recent advances on ginseng research in China. *J Ethnopharmacology* 36: 27–38
68 Huang BQ, Duing JY (1989) Comparison of immune function between polysaccharides from tissue culture of *Panax ginseng* and from Ginseng root. *J China Pharm Univ* 20: 216–218
69 JC, Li YP, Xue LS (1988) Influence of ginseng saponins on the circadial rhythm in brain monoamine neurotransmitters. *Proceedings of 5th Southeast Asian and Western Pacific regional Meeting of Pharmacologists.* Chinese Pharmacological Association, Beijing, s30.02
70 Li JC, Tao R, Ma KC, Zhang QJ, Bi JW (1987) Circadial variation of ginseng total saponins on plasma corticosterone and hepatic glycogen in rats. *J Shenyang College of Pharmacy* 4(4): 249–253
71 Zhang BF, Pan WJ, Shu Q, Dai YR (1986) Effects of saponins of GLS and GKS on DNA, RNA and protein synthesis in liver and kidney of mice. *J Shenyang College of Pharmacy* 3(4): 255–258
72 Mo ZX, Huang YH , Li XH (1988) Effects of ginsenosides on the function, morphology and CAMP level of rabbit platelets. *Proceedings of 5th Southeast Asian and Western Pacific Regional Meeting of Pharmacologists.* Chinese Pharmacological, Beijing, s31.01
73 Yang Y, Chen Z, Luo G, Zliang Y (1988) The mechanism of inhibitory effects of panaxdiol saponin on rabbit platelet aggregation. *Proceedings of 5th Southeast and West*

Pacific Regional Meeting of Pharmacologists. Chinese Pharmacological Association, Beijing, 033.06

74 Shen JJ, Jin YY, Wu YS and Zhou X (1987) Effects of ginseng saponins on Arachidonic acid metabolism in rabbit platelets. *Acta Pharmaceut Sin* 22: 166–169

75 Chen X, Zhu QY, Li LY and Tang XL (1982) Effect of ginsenosides on cardiac performance and hemodynamics of dogs. *Acta Pharmacolog Sin* 3: 235–239

76 Li Y, Deng HW and Chen X (1987) The protective effect of ginsenosides and its components on myocytes anox/reoxygenation and myocardial reperfusion injury. *Acta Pharmaceut Sin* 22: 1–5

77 Zhang FL, Meehan AG and Rand MJ (1988) Effects of ginsenosides on noradrenergic transmission, histamine response and calcium influx in rabbit ear isolated artery. *Proceedings of 5th Southeast Asian and Western Pacific Regional Meeting of Pharmacologists*. Chinese Pharmacological Association, Beijing, 041.07

78 Cheng XJ, Shi X, and Lin B (1988) Effects of ginseng root saponins on brain and serum corticosterone in normobaric hyposis stress mice. *Proceedings of 5th Southeast Asian and Western Pacific Regional Meeting of Pharmacologists*. Chinese Pharmacological Association, Beijing, 31.05

79 Zhang JT (1989) Progress of research on three kinds of anti-ageing drugs. *Information of the Chinese Pharmacological Association* 6(3–4): 4

80 Lu G, Cheng XJ, Yuan WX (1988) Effect of ginseng root saponins on serum corticosterone and brain neurotransmitters of hypobaric hypoxic mice. *Proceedings of 5th Southeast Asian and Western Pacific Regional Meeting of Pharmacologists*. Chinese Pharmacological Association, Beijing, s31.03

81 Xue XM (1986) Protective effect of ginseng preparation on blood system in tumor patients. *Chin Trad Patent Drugs* 11: 20–21

82 Mo JY (1988) Clinical application of ginseng solution. *Chinese Trad Patent Med* 3: 18–20

83 Xie Z, Huang XK (1980) *Heshouwu. Common Terms of Traditional Chinese Medicine in English*. Beijing Medical College Press, Beijing, 272–273

84 Deng WL, Gong SR (1987) Recent advances on the research of *Heshouwu*. *Chin Trad Herb Drugs* 18: 42–46

85 Chen XG, Cui ZY, Cliang YD, Wang BX (1991) Effects of the extract of *Polygorum multiflorum* on some biochemical indicators related to ageing in old mice. *Chin Trad Herb Drugs* 22: 357–359

86 Geng JY, Huang WQ, Ren TC , Ma XF (1991) *Zhuling. Medicinal Herbs*. New World Press, Beijing, 95

87 Geng JY, Huang WQ, Ren TC, Ma XF (1991) *Huangjing. Medicinal Herbs*. New World Press, Beijing, 244–245

88 Xiao PG, Chen KJ (1987) Clinical trails of Chinese herbs in a number of chronic conditions. *Phytotherapy Res* 1(2): 53–57

89 Zhang LH, Huang Y, Wang LW, Xiao PG (1995) Several compounds from Chinese traditional and herbal medicines as immunomodulators. *Phytotherapy Res* 9: 315–322

Index

PIR
Progress in Inflammation Research

T Cells in Arthritis

Miossec, P.,
Hôpital Edouard Herriot, Lyon, France /
van den Berg, W.B.,
University Hospital Nijmegen, Netherlands /
Firestein, G.S.,
UCSD, La Jolla, USA (Ed.)

Rheumatoid arthritis (RA) is the most common and most severe form of inflammatory arthritis. The pathogenesis of RA has been the subject of intense research for several decades. The prevailing hypotheses have changed over the years, and have attempted to incorporate the most recent data. Although T cells represent an important component of the cells which infiltrate the joint synovium, their contribution at a late stage of the disease remains a matter of debate.

The goal of this book is to outline the major arguments and data suggesting that T cells may, or may not, be central players in the pathogenesis of chronic RA. While each of the editors and authors has his/her own bias (as will be clear by reading the respective chapters), our hope is that the readers will enjoy a complete and balanced view of the critical questions and experiments. This is not just an intellectual exercise since the direction of future therapeutic interventions depends heavily on how one interprets the pathogenesis of RA and the contribution of T cells.

Contents

PIR – Progress in Inflammation Research
Miossec, P., et al. (Ed.)
T Cells in Arthritis
1998. 238 pages. Hardcover
ISBN 3-7643-5853-X

PIR
Progress in Inflammation Research

Fatty Acids and Inflammatory Diseases

Schröder, J.-M.,
Department of Dermatology, University of Kiel, Germany (Ed.)

Fatty acids play an important role in the barrier function of skin and represent a major source of proinflammatory mediators such as prostaglandins, leukotrienes and other lipids in inflammatory skin disorders. This book combines the two major functions of fatty acids in skin biology.
In the first part the biosynthesis of fatty acids in skin with its role in barrier function as well as the role of dietary fatty acids on skin cell function and in the treatment of inflammatory skin diseases is presented. The second part deals with skin as a source of proinflammatory eicosanoids, especially with the keratinocyte as a major cellular source. Metabolism of eicosanoids in skin, its role in psoriasis and atopic dermatitis as well as pharmacological inhibition of eicosanoid biosynthesis is reviewed.
The book finishes with a chapter describing the methods used for quantification of fatty acids and derivatives in skin inflammation.
Anyone interested in skin physiology would benefit from the overviews about the two sites of fatty acids' function in skin integrity and in skin inflammation.

Contents

PIR – Progress in Inflammation Research
Schröder, J.-M., (Ed.)
Fatty Acids and Inflammatory Diseases
1998. Approx. 250 pages. Hardcover
ISBN 3-7643-5847-5
Due in December 1998

FSC
www.fsc.org
MIX
Papier | Fördert
gute Waldnutzung
FSC® C083411

Kolibri 360 GmbH
Ferdinand-Jühlke-Straße 7
99095 Erfurt, Deutschland
produktsicherheit@kolibri360.de